## DATE DUE

# MANUAL OF
# *BEDSIDE*
# *MONITORING*

# MANUAL OF
# BEDSIDE
# MONITORING

Springhouse Corporation
Springhouse, Pennsylvania

# STAFF

**Executive Director, Editorial**
Stanley Loeb

**Senior Publisher**
Matthew Cahill

**Clinical Manager**
Cindy Tryniszewski, RN, MSN

**Art Director**
John Hubbard

**Senior Editor**
Stephen Daly

**Clinical Project Editor**
Betsy Saulter, RN, MSN

**Drug Information Editor**
George J. Blake, RPh, MS

**Editors**
Judith A. Lewis, Neal Fandek, Gale Sloan

**Copy Editors**
Cynthia C. Breuninger (supervisor), Jennifer George Mintzer, Doris Weinstock

**Designers**
Stephanie Peters (associate art director), Elaine Ezrow, Kris Gabage, Susan Hopkins Rodzewich, Amy Smith

**Illustrators**
Michael Adams, Jackie Facciolo, Jean Gardner, John Gallagher, Linda Gist, Frank Grobelny, Bob Jackson, Robert Neumann, Judy Newhouse, Gary Phillips, George Retseck, Larry Ward

**Typography**
Diane E. Paluba (manager), Elizabeth Bergman, Joyce Rossi Biletz, Phyllis Marron, Robin Mayer, Valerie Rosenberger

**Manufacturing**
Deborah Meiris (director), T. A. Landis (manager), Anna Brindisi, Kate Davis,

**Production Coordination**
Patricia W. McCloskey

**Editorial Assistants**
Maree DeRosa, Beverly Lane, Mary Madden

**Indexer**
Barbara Hodgson

BDM-011293

Library of Congress Cataloging-in-Publication Data
Manual of bedside monitoring.
    p.   cm.
    Includes bibliographical references and index.
    1. Patient monitoring. 2. Nursing. I. Springhouse Corporation.
    [DNLM: 1. Monitoring, Physiologic – nursing. WB 142 M294    1994]
RT48.55.M36 1994
610.73 – dc20
DNLM/DLC                                                                    93-38015
ISBN 0-87434-658-4                                                          CIP

# CONTENTS

# CONTRIBUTORS AND CONSULTANTS

**Linda S. Baas,** RN, PhD, CCRN
Assistant Professor
University of Cincinnati
College of Nursing and Health

**Carol A. Basile,** RN,C, BSN, CCRN
Research Study Coordinator
Department of Pulmonary Medicine
Hospital of the University of Pennsylvania
Philadelphia

**Ruth E. Blauer,** RN, MS, CNA
Director, Education Department
Rutland (Vt.) Regional Medical Center

**Vicki L. Buchda,** RN, MS
Director, Special Care Unit
Maryvale Samaritan Medical Center
Phoenix, Ariz.

**Sherry Buffington,** RN, CCRN, CLA (ASCP)
Staff Nurse, ICCU
Doylestown (Pa.) Hospital

**Robin Donohoe Dennison,** RN, MSN, CCRN, CS
Cardiopulmonary Nursing Consultant
Continuing Education for Health Professionals, Inc.
Winchester, Ky.

**Marcy L. Diethorn,** RN, MSN
Director, Professional Education Services
Baxter Healthcare Corp.
Edwards Critical-Care Division
Irvine, Calif.

**Tina R. Dietrich,** RN, BSN, CCRN
Nurse Consultant
Bethlehem, Pa.

**Julie LaPiana Evarts,** RN, MSN, CRNP
Neonatal Nurse Practitioner
Pennsylvania Hospital
Philadelphia

**Harriett Wagner Ferguson,** RN,C, MSN, EdD
Associate Professor
Temple University
Philadelphia

**Margaret A. Fitzgerald,** RN,C, MS, FNP
Assistant Professor, Graduate Nursing
Simmons College
Boston
Family Nurse Practitioner
Lawrence, Mass.

**Ellie Z. Franges,** RN, MSN, CCRN
Patient Care Manager
Lehigh Valley Hospital
Allentown, Pa.

**Diane Broadbent Friedman,** RN, MSN, CS
Research Nurse Coordinator
Milton S. Hershey Medical Center
Hershey, Pa.

**Paula Harrison Gillman,** RN, MSN, CCRN
Clinical Affairs Specialist
Baxter Healthcare Corp.
Edwards Critical-Care Division
Irvine, Calif.

**Susan J. Hart,** RN,C, MSN, CCRN
Critical Care Independent Nurse Consultant
Florham Park, N.J.
Adjunct Professor, College of Nursing
Seton Hall University
South Orange, N.J.
Staff Nurse, ICU
Morristown (N.J.) Memorial Hospital

**Jan M. Headley,** RN, BS
Senior Education Consultant
Baxter Healthcare Corp.
Edwards Critical-Care Division
Irvine, Calif.

**Patricia E. Heslop,** BSN, RN, CCRN
Critical Care Nurse Clinician
Newcomb Medical Center
Vineland, N.J.

**JoAnn Hungelmann,** RN, DNSc
Associate Professor
Loyola University of Chicago

**Pamela Kasold,** RN, BSN, CCRN
Clinical Education Manager
St. Jude Medical, Inc.
Cardiac Assist Division
Chelmsford, Mass.

**Charles Krozek,** RN, MN
Nursing Education Coordinator
Saint John's Hospital and Health Center
Santa Monica, Calif.

**Dianne M. Lameier,** RN, MSN
Electrophysiology Clinical Nurse Specialist
University of Cincinnati Medical Center

**Barbara Leeper,** RN, MN, CCRN
Cardiovascular Clinical Nurse Specialist
Baylor University Medical Center
Dallas

**Margaret Massoni,** RN, MSN, CS
Assistant Professor
College of Staten Island
City University of New York

**Patricia A. McGaffigan,** RN,C, MS
Clinical Education Manager
Nellcor, Inc.
Hayward, Calif.

**Judith E. Meissner,** RN, MSN
Senior Associate Professor
Bucks County Community College
Newtown, Pa.

**Cheryl Milford,** RN, MS, CCRN
Nursing Staff Development Specialist
Ohio State University
Columbus, Ohio

**Doris A. Millam,** RN, MS, BSN, CRNI
I.V. Therapy Clinical Nurse Specialist
Holy Family Hospital
Des Plaines, Ill.

**Susan Russell Neary,** RN,C, MS, ANP, GNP
Assistant Professor, Graduate Nursing
Simmons College
Nurse Practitioner, Home Care
Beth Israel Hospital
Boston

**Frances W. Quinless,** RN, PhD
Chair, Department of Nursing Education
and Services
University of Medicine and Dentistry of
New Jersey
Newark, N.J.

**Suzanne D. Skinner,** RN, MS
Nursing Education Consultant
Severna Park, Md.

**Johanna K. Stiesmeyer,** RN, MS, CCRN
Critical Care Clinical Educator
El Camino Hospital
Mountain View, Calif.

**Sarah E. Whitaker,** RN,C, MSN
Lecturer
University of Texas at El Paso

# *F*OREWORD

Because of the rapid pace of technological developments in health care, nurses must continually adapt to new challenges. And nowhere is this more evident than at the front line of nursing care — at the patient's bedside.

Constant advances in bedside monitoring techniques and equipment have virtually redefined the nurses' role in patient care. Today you're likely to encounter telemetry units (once limited to critical care settings) at a cardiac patient's bedside, and you'll be routinely called on to use external fetal monitoring techniques once reserved for high-risk pregnancies.

To perform your duties effectively in such situations, you need to combine clinical observation skills with a clear understanding of often-complex monitoring techniques and bedside equipment. The question is: How do you stay current without drowning in a sea of manufacturer's manuals and technical journals? *Manual of Bedside Monitoring* is your answer.

In this concise, well-organized book, you'll find start-to-finish instructions on every type of monitoring used today. Chapter 1 covers conventional and newer methods for monitoring the patient's vital signs. You'll also find instructions for performing pulse amplitude and arterial pressure monitoring. Chapter 2 explores monitoring cardiovascular status, beginning with a cardiac physiology review and continuing with ECG, continuous cardiac, ST-segment, CVP, pulmonary artery and capillary wedge pressure monitoring.

Chapter 3 shows you how to monitor respiratory status by such methods as spirometry, arterial blood gas, pulse oximetry, and transcutaneous monitoring. Chapter 4 simplifies the often bewildering field of neurology by explaining how to monitor neurologic vital signs and intra-cranial pressure. Chapter 5 describes monitoring fluid and electrolyte status; you'll review how to measure patient intake and output, how to manage I.V. fluid administration, and how to interpret urine specific gravity measurements.

Chapter 6 guides you through G.I. and nutritional status monitoring techniques, from bowel sounds monitoring to patient monitoring during total parenteral nutrition. Chapter 7 assists you in mastering the intricacies of fetal and neonatal monitoring — fetal heart rate monitoring, internal and external fetal monitoring, and apnea monitoring. Finally, you'll find helpful appendices to help you recognize common arrhythmias and manage your patient's pain.

More than 120 helpful illustrations, photographs, tables, and charts enhance the text, giving you further insight into pathophysiology, assessment, and the latest advances in monitoring techniques and equipment.

To help you use this book, each procedure appears in the same easy-to-follow format. Each starts with an introduction that defines and briefly describes the monitoring procedure and its purpose.

Next, *Equipment* lists all the items you'll need to perform the procedure and, where appropriate, identifies the items available as kits. *Preparation of equipment* explains all the steps you must take before beginning the procedure.

*Implementation* takes you step-by-step through the procedure in clear, concise style. Where necessary, you'll also find suggestions for patient teaching and discharge planning. Next, *Special considerations* lists additional important concerns related to the procedure, such as ways to avoid common problems, variations in performing the procedure, nursing alerts, and insights from the latest research.

Where appropriate, the *Complications* section alerts you to possible patient problems resulting from the procedure, and explains how to manage or prevent them. Finally, *Documentation* tells you which procedure-specific items you should include in your notes or on the patient's medical record.

*Manual of Bedside Monitoring* covers every monitoring technique you're likely to perform in today's ever-changing clinical setting. As you monitor your patients, you'll turn to this comprehensive, easy-to-use manual to help you master new equipment or refresh your nursing intervention skills.

Whether you're caring for a critically ill patient in a cardiac care unit or assuring a pregnant patient that her labor is progressing smoothly, using this book will boost your confidence. Designed to save you time and improve your skills, it will help you provide quality patient care at the patient's bedside.

**Jan M. Headley, RN, BS**
Senior Education Consultant
Baxter Healthcare Corp.
Edwards Critical-Care Division
Irvine, Calif.

# MANUAL OF
# BEDSIDE
# MONITORING

# MONITORING VITAL SIGNS

## Introduction

Taking vital signs may be considered a routine nursing function, but remember that it provides extremely important information. During your initial examination, you'll record baseline values. Then you'll take vital signs at regular intervals. For a hospitalized patient, you'll usually take vital signs every 4 to 6 hours. For a patient in a critical care area, you'll take them every 15 minutes to every 2 hours. When a patient first returns from surgery or any invasive procedure, or whenever an unstable patient is undergoing drug titration, you may take vital signs as often as every 5 to 15 minutes.

Your initial measurements can alert you to a problem that needs immediate attention. But, usually, a series of readings will provide much more valuable information than any single set of vital signs. Always analyze vital signs together, not separately, because two or more abnormal vital signs can provide important clues to a patient's problem. A rapid, thready pulse and low blood pressure, for instance, can suggest shock.

Before you take a patient's vital signs, try to help him relax by providing a quiet, calm environment. Physical or emotional stress can alter your measurements. If you obtain an abnormal value, take the vital sign again.

When taking a patient's vital signs, you'll typically measure temperature, pulse, respiration, and blood pressure.

## Temperature monitoring

Temperature can be measured with a mercury, digital electronic, tympanic membrane, or chemical-dot thermometer. Oral temperature in adults normally ranges from 97° to 99.5° F (36.1° to 37.5° C); rectal temperature is usually 1° F higher; axillary temperature, the least accurate, reads 1° to 2° F (0.6° to 1.1° C) lower. Temperatures obtained with a tympanic membrane thermometer closely correlate with core body temperatures (98.6° F plus or minus 1° F).

Temperature normally fluctuates with rest and activity. Lowest readings typically occur between 4 and 5 a.m.; the highest readings occur between 4 and 8 p.m. Other factors also influence temperature, including sex, age, emotional condition, and environment. Keep the following principles in mind. Women normally have higher temperatures than men, especially during ovulation. Normal temperature is highest in neonates and lowest in elderly persons. Heightened emotions raise temperature; depressed emotions lower it. A hot external environment can raise temperature; a cold environment can lower it.

## Equipment

Mercury or electronic thermometer for oral or rectal use, tympanic membrane thermometer, or chemical-dot thermometer ▪ water-soluble lubricant or petroleum jelly (for rectal temperature) ▪ facial tissue ▪ disposable thermometer sheath or probe cover (except for chemical-dot thermometer) ▪ alcohol sponge.

## Preparation of equipment

A thermometer may be included as part of the admission pack. If it is, keep it at the patient's bedside and, on discharge, allow him to take it home. If you use an electronic thermometer, make sure it has been recharged.

### For a mercury thermometer

• Hold the thermometer between your thumb and index finger at the end opposite the bulb.
• If the thermometer has been soaking in a disinfectant, rinse it in cold water. *Rinsing removes chemicals that may irritate oral or rectal mucous membranes or axillary skin.* Avoid using hot water *because it expands the mercury, which could break the thermometer.* Using a twisting motion, wipe the thermometer from the bulb upward.
• Then quickly snap your wrist several times while holding the thermometer to shake it down. *Shaking causes the mercury to descend into the bulb.* The mercury will then expand in response to the patient's body temperature and be forced upward.

• To use a disposable sheath over the mercury thermometer, first disinfect the thermometer with an alcohol sponge. Next, insert it into the disposable sheath opening; then twist to tear the seal at the dotted line. Pull it apart. *Using a sheath decreases contamination and reduces cleaning time.*

### For an electronic thermometer
• Insert the probe into a disposable probe cover. If taking a rectal temperature, lubricate the probe cover *to reduce friction and ease insertion.* Leave the probe in place until the maximum temperature appears on the digital display.

### For a chemical-dot thermometer
• Remove the thermometer from its protective dispenser case by grasping the handle end with your thumb and forefinger, moving the handle up and down to break the seal, and pulling the handle straight out. Be sure to keep the thermometer sealed until use *because opening it activates the dye dots.*

### For a tympanic membrane thermometer
• Lift the probe from the base unit.
• Cap the probe with a disposable cover.

## Implementation
• Explain the procedure to the patient, and wash your hands.

### Taking an oral temperature
• Position the tip of the thermometer under the patient's tongue, as far back as possible, on either side of the frenulum linguae. *Placing the tip in this area promotes contact with abundant superficial blood vessels and contributes to an accurate reading.*
• Instruct the patient to close his lips but to avoid biting down with his teeth. *Biting can break a mercury thermometer, cutting the mouth or lips or causing ingestion of broken glass or mercury.*
• *To register temperature,* leave a mercury thermometer in place for at least 2 minutes, a chemical-dot thermometer for 45 seconds, or an

electronic thermometer until the maximum temperature is displayed. (With some electronic units, a buzzer sounds when the maximum temperature is reached; with others, a light appears.)
• For a mercury thermometer, remove and discard the disposable sheath, and then read the temperature at eye level, noting it before shaking down the thermometer. For an electronic thermometer, note the temperature; then remove and discard the probe cover. For the chemical-dot thermometer, read the temperature as the last dye dot that has changed color, or fired, and then discard the thermometer and its dispenser case.

### Taking a rectal temperature
• Don gloves.
• Position the patient on his side with his top leg flexed, and drape him to provide privacy. Then fold back the bed linens to expose the anus.
• Squeeze the lubricant onto a facial tissue *to prevent contamination of the lubricant supply.*
• Lubricate about ½″ (1.3 cm) of the thermometer tip for an infant or about 1½″ (3.8 cm) for an adult. *Lubrication reduces friction and thus eases insertion.* This step may be unnecessary when using disposable rectal sheaths *because they're prelubricated.*
• Lift the patient's upper buttock, and insert the thermometer about ½″ for an infant or 1½″ for an adult. Gently direct the thermometer along the rectal wall toward the umbilicus. *This will avoid perforating the anus or rectum or breaking the thermometer.* It also will help ensure an accurate reading because the thermometer will register hemorrhoidal artery temperature instead of fecal temperature. Feces may increase the patient's apparent temperature *because of the heat given off during decomposition.*
• Hold the mercury thermometer steadily in place for 2 to 3 minutes or the electronic thermometer until the maximum temperature is displayed. *Holding it prevents damage to rectal tissues caused by displacement or loss of the thermometer into the rectum. Note:* Electronic thermometers usually

provide a separate rectal probe that may be color coded to distinguish it more easily from the oral probe.
• Carefully remove the thermometer, wiping it as necessary.
• Wipe the patient's anal area *to remove any lubricant or feces.*
• Remove and discard your gloves, and wash your hands.

### Taking an axillary temperature
• Position the patient comfortably with the axilla exposed.
• Gently pat the axilla dry with a facial tissue *because moisture conducts heat.* Avoid harsh rubbing, *which generates heat.*
• Ask the patient to place his hand over his chest and to grasp his opposite shoulder, lifting his elbow.
• Position the thermometer in the axilla with the tip pointing toward the patient's head.
• Tell the patient to continue grasping his shoulder and to lower his elbow and hold it against his chest. *This promotes skin contact with the thermometer.*
• Leave a mercury thermometer in place for 10 minutes; leave an electronic thermometer in place until it displays the maximum temperature. Axillary temperature takes longer to register than oral or rectal temperature *because the thermometer isn't enclosed in a body cavity.*
• Grasp the end of the thermometer and remove it from the axilla.

### Taking a temperature with a tympanic membrane thermometer
• Insert the probe deeply enough in the ear canal to seal the opening.
• Press the trigger to activate the temperature scan.
• Listen for the beep that signals a completed temperature reading (in a few seconds).
• Remove and discard the probe cover, and return the probe to the base unit.

### Special considerations
Oral temperature measurement is contraindicated in patients who are unconscious, disoriented, or seizure-prone; in young children and infants; and in patients with oral or nasal impairment that necessitates mouth breathing. In these instances, a tympanic membrane thermometer may be more appropriate. With this method, the reading is unaffected by mouth breathing or other patient activity, and the thermometer responds quickly to subtle thermal changes.

Rectal temperature measurement is contraindicated in patients with diarrhea or recent rectal or prostatic surgery or injury *(because it may injure inflamed tissue)* or recent myocardial infarction *(because anal manipulation may stimulate the vagus nerve, causing bradycardia or another rhythm disturbance).*

Drinking hot or cold liquids, chewing gum, or smoking may alter oral temperature readings. Wait 15 minutes after these activities before taking a temperature. Bathing may alter axillary temperature.

Use the same thermometer and route for repeated temperature taking *to avoid spurious variations caused by equipment or route differences.* Store chemical-dot thermometers in a cool area *because exposure to heat activates the dye dots.*

You can take an oral temperature even when the patient is receiving nasal oxygen *because oxygen administration raises oral temperature by only about 0.3° F (0.17° C).*

### Documentation
Record the time, route, and temperature on the patient's chart.

## Pulse monitoring

Blood pumped by the heart into an already full aorta during ventricular contraction creates a fluid wave that travels from the heart to the peripheral arteries. This recurring wave — called a pulse — can be palpated at locations on the

## Pulse points

Shown below are anatomic locations where an artery crosses bone or firm tissue and can be palpated for a pulse.

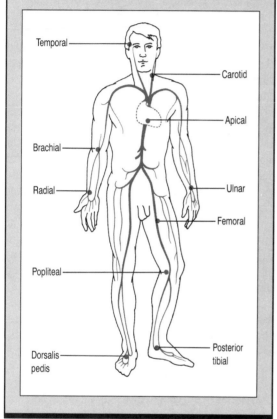

Temporal
Carotid
Apical
Brachial
Radial
Ulnar
Femoral
Popliteal
Dorsalis pedis
Posterior tibial

first by auscultation at the apex of the heart, the second by palpation at the radial artery. Some heart beats detected at the apex aren't strong enough to be detected at peripheral sites. When this occurs, the apical pulse rate is higher than the radial; the difference between the two rates is the pulse deficit.

Pulse taking involves determining the rate (number of beats per minute), rhythm (pattern or regularity of the beats), and amplitude (force of each beat). If the pulse is faint or weak, use a Doppler ultrasound stethoscope if available.

### Equipment
Watch with second hand ▪ stethoscope (for auscultating apical pulse) ▪ Doppler ultrasound stethoscope if necessary.

### Preparation of equipment
If you're not using your own stethoscope, disinfect the earpieces with an alcohol sponge before and after use *to prevent cross-contamination.*

### Implementation
• Wash your hands, and tell the patient that you intend to take his pulse.
• Make sure the patient is comfortable and relaxed *because an awkward, uncomfortable position may affect the heart rate.*

#### Taking a radial pulse
• Place the patient in a sitting or supine position with his arm at his side or across his chest.
• Gently press your index, middle, and ring fingers on the radial artery inside the patient's wrist. You should feel a pulse with only moderate pressure; *excessive pressure may obstruct blood flow distal to the pulse site.* Don't use your thumb to take the patient's pulse *because its own strong pulse may be confused with the patient's.*
• After locating the pulse, count the beats for 60 seconds, or, if it's more convenient, count for 30 seconds and multiply by 2. *Counting for a full minute provides a more accurate picture of irregularities.* While counting the rate, assess pulse

body where an artery crosses over bone or firm tissue. (See *Pulse points.*) In adults and children over age 3, the radial artery in the wrist is the most common palpation site because it's easily accessible and the artery can be compressed readily against the radius. In infants and children under age 3, use a stethoscope to listen to the heart itself instead of palpating a pulse. Because auscultation is done at the heart's apex, this pulse is called the apical pulse.

An apical-radial pulse is taken by simultaneously counting apical and radial beats—the rhythm and amplitude by noting the pattern and force of the beats. If you detect an irregularity, repeat the count, *because pulse irregularities are important signs.* Note if the irregularity occurs in a pattern or randomly. If doubt remains, take an apical pulse.

### Taking an apical pulse
• Help the patient to a supine position and drape him if necessary.
• Warm the diaphragm or bell of the stethoscope in your hand before applying it to the patient's chest. *Placing a cold stethoscope against the skin may startle the patient and momentarily increase the heart rate.* Keep in mind that the stethoscope's bell transmits low-pitched sounds more effectively than its diaphragm.
• Place the diaphragm or bell of the stethoscope over the apex of the heart, which normally is located at the fifth intercostal space left of the midclavicular line. Then insert the earpieces into your ears. Count the beats for 60 seconds (or count for 30 seconds and multiply by 2) and note their rhythm and force. Also evaluate the intensity, or loudness, of heart sounds.
• Remove the stethoscope and make the patient comfortable.

### Taking an apical-radial pulse
• Two nurses work together to obtain the apical-radial pulse; one of you palpates the radial pulse while the other auscultates the apical pulse with a stethoscope. You should both use synchronized watches when counting beats.
• Help the patient to a supine position and drape him if necessary.
• Locate the apical and radial pulses.
• Determine a time to begin counting. Then each nurse should count beats for 60 seconds.

### Special considerations
When the peripheral pulse is irregular, take an apical pulse to measure the heart beat more directly. If the pulse is faint or weak, use a Doppler ultrasound stethoscope if available.

## Documenting pulse amplitude

> To document pulse amplitude, you may use a numerical scale or a descriptive term. Numerical scales differ slightly from hospital to hospital, but the one shown here is among the most commonly used.
>
> **+3** = bounding pulse (readily palpable, forceful, not easily obliterated by finger pressure)
> **+2** = normal pulse (easily palpable and obliterated only by strong finger pressure)
> **+1** = weak or thready pulse (hard to feel and easily obliterated by slight finger pressure)
> **0** = absent pulse (not palpable)

If a second nurse isn't available to help take an apical-radial pulse, you can hold the stethoscope in place with the hand that holds the watch while palpating the radial pulse with the other hand. You can then feel any discrepancies between the apical and radial pulses.

### Documentation
Record pulse rate, rhythm, amplitude, and the time of measurement. "Full" or "bounding" describes a pulse with an increased force; "weak" or "thready," decreased force. (See *Documenting pulse amplitude.*) When recording an apical pulse, include the intensity of heart sounds. When recording an apical-radial pulse, chart the rate according to the pulse site—for example, A/R pulse of 80/76.

## Respiration monitoring
Controlled by the respiratory center in the lateral medulla oblongata, respiration is the exchange of oxygen and carbon dioxide in the lungs (external respiration) and in the tissues (internal respiration). External respiration, or breathing, is accomplished by the diaphragm and chest muscles and delivers oxygen to the lower respiratory tract and alveoli. Internal respiration occurs only through diffusion.

## Identifying respiratory patterns

| TYPE | CHARACTERISTICS | PATTERN | POSSIBLE CAUSES |
|------|-----------------|---------|-----------------|
| Apnea | Periodic absence of breathing | | • Mechanical airway obstruction<br>• Conditions affecting the brain's respiratory center in the lateral medulla oblongata |
| Apneustic | Prolonged, gasping inspiration, followed by extremely short, inefficient expiration | | • Lesions of the respiratory center |
| Bradypnea | Slow, regular respirations of equal depth | | • Normal pattern during sleep<br>• Conditions affecting the respiratory center: tumors, metabolic disorders, respiratory decompensation; use of opiates and alcohol |
| Cheyne-Stokes | Fast, deep respirations of 30 to 170 seconds punctuated by periods of apnea lasting 20 to 60 seconds | | • Increased intracranial pressure, severe congestive heart failure, renal failure, meningitis, drug overdose, cerebral anoxia |
| Eupnea | Normal rate and rhythm | | • Normal respiration |
| Kussmaul's | Fast (over 20 breaths/minute), deep (resembling sighs), labored respirations without pause | | • Renal failure or metabolic acidosis, particularly diabetic ketoacidosis |
| Tachypnea | Rapid respirations. Rate rises with body temperature—about 4 breaths/minute for every 1° F above normal | | • Pneumonia, compensatory respiratory alkalosis, respiratory insufficiency, lesions of the respiratory center, and salicylate poisoning |

Four measures of respiration—rate, rhythm, depth, and sound—reflect the body's metabolic and neurologic state, diaphragm and chest-muscle condition, and airway patency. Respiratory rate is recorded as the number of cycles (with inspiration and expiration comprising one cycle) per minute; rhythm, as the regularity of these cycles; depth, as the volume of air inhaled and exhaled with each respiration; and sound, as the audible digression from normal, effortless breathing.

### Equipment
Watch with second hand.

## Implementation
• The best time to assess your patient's respirations is immediately after taking the pulse rate. Keep your fingertips over the radial artery, and don't tell the patient you're counting respirations. If you tell him, *he'll become conscious of his respirations and the rate may change.*
• Count respirations by observing the rise and fall of the patient's chest as he breathes. Or position the patient's opposite arm across his chest and count respirations by feeling its rise and fall. Consider one rise and one fall as one respiration.
• Count respirations for 30 seconds and multiply by 2 or count for 60 seconds if respirations are irregular *to account for variations in respiratory rate and pattern.* As you count respirations, be alert for and record such audible breath sounds as stertor, stridor, wheezing, and expiratory grunting. *Stertor* is a snoring sound resulting from secretions in the trachea and large bronchi. Listen for it in patients with neurologic disorders and in those who are comatose. *Stridor* is an inspiratory crowing sound that occurs with upper airway obstruction in laryngitis, croup, or the presence of a foreign body. When listening for stridor in infants and children with croup, also observe for sternal, substernal, or intercostal retractions. *Wheezing* is caused by partial obstruction of the smaller bronchi and bronchioles. This high-pitched, musical sound is common in patients with emphysema or asthma. In infants, *expiratory grunting* indicates imminent respiratory distress. In older patients, it may result from partial airway obstruction or neuromuscular reflex.
• To detect other breath sounds — such as crackles and rhonchi — or the lack of sound in the lungs, you will need a stethoscope.
• Observe chest movements for depth of respiration. If the patient inhales a small volume of air, record this as shallow; if he inhales a large volume, record this as deep.

• Watch chest movements and listen to breathing *to determine the rhythm and sound of respiration.* (See *Identifying respiratory patterns.*)

## Special considerations
Respiratory rates below 8 and above 40 breaths/minute usually are considered abnormal; report the sudden onset of such rates promptly. Observe for signs of dyspnea, such as an anxious facial expression, flaring nostrils, a heaving chest wall, and cyanosis. To detect cyanosis, look for characteristic bluish discoloration of the nail beds, the lips, tongue, or buccal mucosa, or the conjunctiva.

In assessing the patient's respiratory status, consider his personal and family history. Ask if he smokes and, if so, for how many years and how many packs a day.

A child's respiratory rate may double in response to exercise, illness, or emotion. Normally, the rate for newborns is 30 to 80 breaths/minute; for toddlers, 20 to 40; and for children of school age and older, 15 to 25. Children usually reach the adult rate (12 to 20) at about age 15.

## Documentation
Record the rate, depth, rhythm, and sound of the patient's respirations.

# Blood pressure monitoring
Defined as the lateral force exerted by blood on the arterial walls, blood pressure depends on the force of ventricular contractions, arterial wall elasticity, peripheral vascular resistance, and blood volume and viscosity. Systolic, or maximum, pressure occurs during left ventricular contraction and reflects the integrity of the heart, arteries, and arterioles. Diastolic, or minimum, pressure occurs during left ventricular relaxation and directly indicates blood vessel resistance.

Pulse pressure, the difference between systolic and diastolic pressures, varies inversely with arterial elasticity. Rigid vessels, incapable of distention and recoil, produce high systolic pressure and low diastolic pressure. Normally, systolic pressure exceeds diastolic pressure by about 40 mm Hg. Narrowed pulse pressure—a difference of less than 30 mm Hg—occurs when systolic pressure falls and diastolic pressure remains constant, when diastolic pressure rises and systolic pressure stays constant, or when systolic pressure falls and diastolic pressure rises. These changes reflect reduced stroke volume, increased peripheral resistance, or both. Widened pulse pressure—a difference of more than 50 mm Hg between systolic and diastolic blood pressures—occurs when systolic pressure rises and diastolic pressure remains constant, when diastolic pressure falls and systolic pressure remains constant, or when systolic pressure rises and diastolic pressure falls. These changes reflect increased stroke volume, decreased peripheral resistance, or both.

Blood pressure is measured in millimeters of mercury with a sphygmomanometer and a stethoscope, usually at the brachial artery (less often at the popliteal or radial artery). Lowest in the neonate, blood pressure rises with age, weight gain, prolonged stress, anxiety, and some disease processes. In a 16-year-old patient, blood pressure normally falls in the range from 104 to 108 mm Hg systolic and 60 to 92 mm Hg diastolic; in an adult, from 95 to 140 mm Hg systolic and 60 to 90 mm Hg diastolic; in an older adult, 140 to 160 mm Hg systolic and 70 to 90 mm Hg diastolic.

Frequent blood pressure measurement is critical after serious injury, surgery, or anesthesia and during any illness or condition that threatens cardiovascular stability. (This may be done with an automated vital signs monitor.) Regular measurement is indicated for patients with a history of hypertension or hypotension, and yearly screening is recommended for all adults.

## Equipment

Mercury or aneroid sphygmomanometer ▪ stethoscope ▪ alcohol sponge ▪ automated vital signs monitor if available.

The sphygmomanometer consists of an inflatable compression cuff linked to a manual air pump and a mercury manometer or an aneroid gauge. The mercury sphygmomanometer is more accurate and requires calibration less frequently than the aneroid model but is larger and heavier. To obtain an accurate reading with the mercury manometer, you must rest its gauge on a level surface and view the meniscus at eye level; you can rest an aneroid gauge in any position but must view it directly from the front. Some mercury manometers have specially designed cases that open to form a level surface; others must be attached to a wall or to a base unit that stands on the floor.

Hook, bandage, snap, or Velcro cuffs come in six standard sizes ranging from newborn to extra-large adult. Disposable cuffs are available.

The automated vital signs monitor is a noninvasive device that measures pulse rate, systolic and diastolic pressures, and mean arterial pressure at preset intervals. (See *Using an electronic vital signs monitor.*)

## Preparation of equipment

Carefully choose a cuff of appropriate size for the patient. *An excessively narrow cuff may cause a falsely high pressure reading; an excessively wide one, a falsely low reading.* If you're not using your own stethoscope, disinfect the earpieces with an alcohol sponge before placing them in your ears *to avoid cross-contamination.*

To use an automated vital signs monitor, collect the monitor, dual air hose, and pressure cuff. Then make sure the monitor unit is firmly positioned near the patient's bed.

# Using an electronic vital signs monitor

An electronic vital signs monitor allows you to track a patient's vital signs continually, without having to reapply a blood pressure cuff each time. What's more, the patient won't need an invasive arterial line to gather similar data. The machine shown here is a Dinamap VS Monitor 8100, but these steps can be followed with most other monitors.

Some automated vital signs monitors, such as the Dinamap, are lightweight and battery-operated, and can be attached to an I.V. pole for continual monitoring, even during patient transfers. Make sure you know the capacity of the monitor's battery, and plug the machine in whenever possible to keep it charged.

Before using any monitor, check its accuracy. Determine the patient's pulse rate and blood pressure manually, using the same arm you'll use for the monitor cuff. Compare your results with initial readings taken using the monitor. If the results differ, call your supply department or the manufacturer's representative.

## Preparing the device
• Explain the procedure to the patient. Describe the alarm system *so he won't be frightened if it's triggered.*
• Make sure the power switch is off. Then plug the monitor into a properly grounded wall outlet. Next, secure the dual air hose to the front of the monitor.
• Connect the pressure cuff's tubing into the other ends of the dual air hose, and tighten connections *to prevent air leaks.* Keep the air hose away from the patient *to avoid accidental dislodgment.*
• Squeeze all air from the cuff, and wrap it loosely around the patient's arm or leg, allowing 2 fingerbreadths between cuff and arm or leg. Never apply the cuff to a limb that has an I.V. line in place. Position the cuff's "artery" arrow over the palpated brachial or popliteal artery. Then secure the cuff for a snug fit.

## Selecting parameters
• When you turn on the monitor, it will default to a manual mode. (In this mode, you can obtain vital signs yourself before switching to the automatic mode.) Press the "auto/manual" button to select the automatic mode. The monitor will give you baseline data for the pulse rate, systolic and diastolic pressures, and mean arterial pressure.
• Compare your previous manual results with these baseline data. If they match, you're ready to set the arm parameters. Press the "select" button to blank all displays except systolic pressure.

• Use the "high" and "low" limit buttons to set the specific parameters for systolic pressure. (These limits range from a high of 240 to a low of 0 mm Hg.) You'll also do this three more times for mean arterial pressure, pulse rate, and diastolic pressure. After you've set the parameters for diastolic pressure, press the "select" button again to display all current data. Even if you forget to do this last step, the monitor will automatically display current data 10 seconds after you set the last parameters.

## Collecting data
• You'll also need to tell the monitor how often to obtain data. Press the "set" button until you reach the desired time interval in minutes. If you've chosen the automatic mode, the monitor will display a default cycle time of 3 minutes. You can override the default cycle time to set the interval you prefer.
• You can obtain a set of vital signs at any time by pressing the "start" button. Also, pressing the "cancel" button will stop the interval and deflate the cuff. You can retrieve stored data by pressing the "prior data" button. The monitor will display the last data obtained along with the time elapsed since then. Scrolling backward, you can retrieve data from the previous 99 minutes.

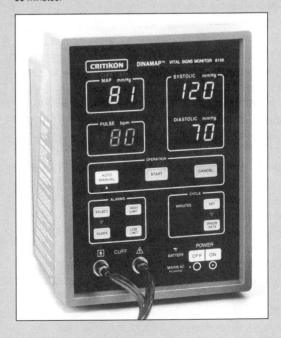

## Implementation

- Tell the patient that you're going to take his blood pressure.
- The patient can lie supine or sit erect during blood pressure measurement. His arm should be extended at heart level and be well supported. *If the artery is below heart level, the blood pressure may read falsely high.* Make sure the patient is relaxed and comfortable when you take his blood pressure *so it stays at its normal level.*
- Wrap the deflated cuff snugly around the upper arm.
- If necessary, connect the appropriate tube to the rubber bulb of the air pump and the other tube to the manometer. Then insert the stethoscope earpieces into your ears.
- Locate the brachial artery by palpation. Center the bell of the stethoscope over the part of the artery where you detect the strongest beats, and hold it in place with one hand. *The bell of the stethoscope transmits low-pitched arterial blood sounds more effectively than the diaphragm.*
- Using the thumb and index finger of your other hand, turn the thumbscrew on the rubber bulb of the air pump clockwise to close the valve.
- Then pump air into the cuff while auscultating the sound over the brachial artery *to compress and, eventually, occlude arterial blood flow.* Pump air until the mercury column or aneroid gauge registers 160 mm Hg or at least 10 mm Hg above the level of the last audible sound.
- Carefully open the valve of the air pump and slowly deflate the cuff — no faster than 5 mm Hg/second. While releasing air, watch the mercury column or aneroid gauge and auscultate the sound over the artery.
- When you hear the first beat or clear tapping sound, note the pressure on the column or gauge. This is the systolic pressure. (The beat or tapping sound is the first of five Korotkoff sounds. The second sound resembles a murmur or swish; the third sound, crisp tapping; the fourth sound, a soft, muffled tone and the fifth, the last sound heard.)

- Continue to release air gradually while auscultating the sound over the artery.
- Note the diastolic pressure — the fourth Korotkoff sound. If you continue to hear sounds as the column or gauge falls to zero (common in children), record the pressure at the beginning of the fourth sound *because, in some patients, a distinct fifth sound is absent.*
- Rapidly deflate the cuff. Record the pressure, wait 15 to 30 seconds, and then repeat the procedure and record the pressures *to confirm your original findings.* After doing so, remove and fold the cuff, and return it to storage.

## Special considerations

If you can't auscultate blood pressure, you may estimate systolic pressure. (For specific instructions, see *Alternative methods for auscultating blood pressure.*)

Palpation of systolic blood pressure also may be important *to avoid underestimating blood pressure in patients with an auscultatory gap.* This gap is a loss of sound between the first and second Korotkoff sounds that may be as great as 40 mm Hg. You may find this in patients with venous congestion or hypotension.

If your patient is crying or anxious, delay blood pressure measurement, if possible, until the patient becomes calm *to avoid falsely elevated readings.*

If your hospital considers the fourth and fifth Korotkoff sounds as the first and second diastolic pressures, record both pressures.

Remember that malfunction in an aneroid sphygmomanometer can be identified only by checking it against a mercury manometer of known accuracy. Be sure to check your aneroid manometer this way periodically. Malfunction in a mercury manometer is evident when the mercury column behaves abnormally. Don't attempt to repair either type of sphygmomanometer yourself; instead, send it to the appropriate service department.

Occasionally, blood pressure must be measured in both arms or with the patient in two different positions (such as lying and standing, or sitting and standing). In such cases, observe and record any significant difference between the two readings, and record the blood pressure, the extremity, and the position used.

## Complications

Don't take blood pressure in the arm on the affected side of a mastectomy *because it may decrease already compromised lymphatic circulation, worsen edema, and damage the arm.* Likewise, don't take blood pressure on an arm with an arteriovenous fistula or a hemodialysis shunt *because blood flow through the vascular device may be compromised.*

## Documentation

On the patient's chart, record blood pressure as systolic over diastolic pressures, such as 120/78 mm Hg; if necessary, record systolic over the two diastolic pressures, such as 120/78/20 mm Hg. Chart an auscultatory gap if present. If required by your hospital, chart blood pressures on a graph, using dots or check marks. Also document the extremity used and the patient's position.

# Pulse amplitude monitoring

Determining the presence and strength of peripheral pulses, an essential part of cardiovascular assessment, helps you to evaluate the adequacy of peripheral perfusion. A pulse amplitude monitor simplifies this procedure. A sensor taped to the patient's skin over a pulse point sends signals to a monitor that measures the amplitude of the pulse and displays it as a waveform on a screen. The system continuously monitors the patient's peripheral pulse so that you can perform other patient care duties.

The pulse amplitude monitor can be used after peripheral vascular reconstruction on the upper or lower extremities or after percutaneous transluminal peripheral or coronary angioplasty (ei-

## Alternative methods for auscultating blood pressure

Besides auscultation, alternative methods of monitoring blood pressure include palpation; return-to-flow, oscillatory, and Doppler methods; and automated systems. You must use reliable equipment and proper technique to ensure accurate, reproducible findings.

**Palpation method**
To palpate the arterial pulse using a blood pressure cuff, first inflate the cuff, and then deflate it slowly. When you detect the pulse, record the reading as systolic pressure.

**Return-to-flow method**
Inflate a blood pressure cuff to a measurement above the patient's anticipated or previously recorded systolic pressure. Then slowly deflate the cuff until you establish return of blood flow, such as by palpating the pulse or checking the manometer. The manometer reading at return to flow corresponds to approximate systolic blood pressure. You may also verify return to flow by using a Doppler ultrasound stethoscope or, if an arterial line is in place, watching for a waveform on the bedside monitor.

**Oscillatory method**
Inflate the blood pressure cuff and then deflate it slowly. Record systolic pressure when you observe oscillation of the mercury column or needle gauge. Record mean arterial pressure when maximum oscillation occurs.

**Doppler method**
Inflate the blood pressure cuff and then deflate it slowly. Record systolic pressure when the Doppler ultrasound stethoscope detects Korotkoff sounds.

**Automated systems**
Many types of automated systems are available. Some use oscillation, others detect sound or vessel wall movement (such as with a Doppler ultrasound stethoscope), and still others use a microcomputer to interpret Korotkoff sounds.

ther with the sheaths in place or after they've been removed.)

Because the sensor monitors only relatively flat pulse points, it can't be used for the posterior tibial pulse point. Also, movement will distort the waveform, so the patient must stay as still

## Identifying a normal pulse amplitude waveform

If your patient has adequate peripheral perfusion, the pulse amplitude monitor will usually display a normal waveform, like the one shown here. This waveform resembles the waveform seen when a patient has an arterial line.

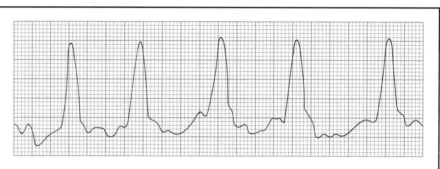

as possible during monitoring. The patient shouldn't have lesions on the skin where the pulse will be monitored because the sensor must be placed directly on this site (usually the foot). The sensor and tape could irritate the lesion, or the lesion could impair transmission of the pulse amplitude.

### Equipment
Pulse amplitude display monitor and a sensor. (This is a fairly new piece of equipment and may not be available in many hospitals.)

### Preparation of equipment
Plug the monitor into a grounded outlet. Although the monitor has battery power for up to 24 hours, it should be plugged in when the battery isn't needed.

Turn on the monitor and allow it to warm up, which may take up to 10 seconds. Plug the sensor cable into the monitor; then tap the sensor gently. If tapping causes interference on the display screen, you can assume the sensor-monitor connection is functioning properly.

### Implementation
• Tell the patient you're going to measure the strength of his pulse, and explain how the pulse amplitude monitor works. Mention that you'll

tape the sensor to the site you've selected, usually the foot.
• Locate the pulse that you want to monitor.
• Place the sensor over the strongest point of the pulse you're going to monitor. While observing the display screen, move the sensor until you see a strong upright waveform.
• Without moving the sensor from this site, peel off the adhesive strips and affix the sensor securely to the patient's foot. *The sensor must maintain proper skin contact, so be sure to tape it firmly.*
• Adjust the height of the pulse wave signal to half the height of the display screen. *This will give the waveform room to fluctuate as the pulse amplitude increases and decreases.*
• Set the low and high waveform amplitude alarms *so that you'll be alerted to any waveform changes.*
• To discontinue monitor use, peel the sensor tapes from the patient's skin. Turn the machine off but keep it plugged in. Discard the sensor and, if necessary, wipe the monitor with a mild soap solution.

### Special considerations
If the patient has a strong peripheral pulse, you'll see an adequate waveform. (See *Identifying a normal pulse amplitude waveform.*)

If the sensor doesn't pick up an adequate signal, suspect a weak pulse or significant vessel calcification. If waveform amplitude decreases, assess the patient's leg for capillary refill time, temperature, color, and sensation. The amplitude change may stem from a malfunction in the monitor itself (such as a low battery) or from a thrombus, hematoma, or significant change in the patient's hemodynamic status.

If the display screen is blank when you turn on the machine, check whether the monitor is plugged in. If it's plugged in but the screen remains blank, the screen may need repair. If the screen is functioning but no waveform appears on it, first check the sensor-monitor connection. Then check the sensor by gently tapping it to see if interference appears on the screen. If the sensor is working properly, relocate the peripheral pulse on the patient's foot and reapply the sensor. If your interventions don't work, the screen may need servicing.

Don't apply much pressure on the pulse sensor film or press on it with a sharp object *because such stress may warp or destroy the sensor.* Also never place the sensor over an open wound or ulcerated skin.

Be aware that although the waveform displayed by a pulse amplitude monitor may resemble an electrocardiograph or blood pressure waveform, it's not the same.

## Documentation

Print out a strip of the patient's waveform, and place the strip in the patient's chart during every shift and whenever you note a change in the waveform or the patient's condition. Along the left side of the strip, you'll see a reference scale used to measure pulse amplitude height. This scale should be included in your documentation.

# Arterial pressure monitoring

An invasive technique, arterial pressure monitoring provides continuous and accurate arterial pressure readings through a transducer that converts blood pressure into electrical impulses. These impulses are displayed on a monitor screen and recorded on paper tape. A visible and audible alarm sounds when the pressure exceeds preset limits.

The information obtained from arterial pressure monitoring is used to evaluate and guide therapies related to tissue perfusion and oxygenation. This technique also allows procurement of arterial blood samples.

Arterial pressure monitoring requires insertion of an arterial catheter through a large artery, usually the radial or femoral artery. (See *Arterial pressure monitoring setup,* page 16.)

## Equipment

Preassembled arterial pressure tubing with flush device and disposable transducer ■ monitoring equipment ■ pressure module, if necessary ■ patient cable ■ heparin flush solution (typically 500 or 1,000 units/500 ml of 0.9% sodium chloride solution as ordered or according to hospital policy) ■ pressure bag ■ I.V. pole ■ sterile gloves ■ hypoallergenic tape ■ antimicrobial ointment (if in accordance with hospital protocol) ■ dry, sterile dressing ■ labels.

If you'll need to obtain a blood sample from an arterial line, also assemble: 5-ml syringe ■ 5- to 10-ml syringe (depending on the amount of blood to be drawn) ■ two sterile 4″ × 4″ gauze pads ■ optional: blood collection tubes, dead-end caps.

Note that special tubing is now available for blood sampling from arterial lines. This tubing, placed between the transducer and the stopcock to the catheter, contains two ports. One port allows the aspiration of heparinized blood and fluid with a special syringe. Then, after the arterial blood sample is withdrawn from the second port, the flushing device returns the heparinized blood and fluid to the patient.

For *arterial line* removal, gather the following: gloves ■ mask ■ gown ■ protective eyewear ■ two sterile 4″ × 4″ gauze pads ■ sheet protector ■ sterile suture removal set ■ dressing ■ alcohol swabs ■ hypoallergenic tape. For *femoral line* removal, gather: additional sterile 4″ × 4″ gauze

## Arterial pressure monitoring setup

After insertion of an arterial catheter through a large artery, the catheter is connected to a flush device and a transducer. These are attached to a monitoring system that transforms electrical impulses into an arterial pressure waveform.

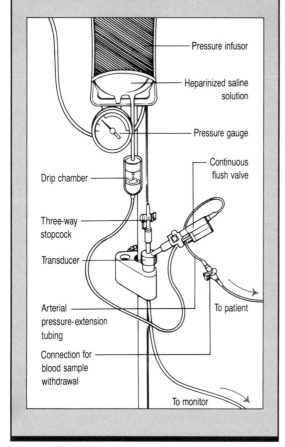

Pressure infusor

Heparinized saline solution

Pressure gauge

Continuous flush valve

Drip chamber

Three-way stopcock

Transducer

Arterial pressure-extension tubing

To patient

Connection for blood sample withdrawal

To monitor

pads ▪ small sandbag (which you may wrap in a towel or place in a pillowcase) ▪ adhesive bandage. If the doctor has ordered a *catheter tip culture,* also gather sterile scissors and a sterile container.

### Preparation of equipment

Wash your hands. Maintain sterile technique as you prepare the equipment. If necessary, turn on the monitor to warm it up. (Make sure that the pressure module is in the monitor if one isn't built in.) Insert the arterial line tubing spike into the bag of heparin flush solution. Make sure that the roller clamp is closed.

To remove air from the bag, invert it. Squeeze the air out through the tubing, or insert a needle into the injection port and squeeze air out through the needle.

If necessary, place the transducer in the pole mount on the I.V. pole. (Some transducers don't need to be mounted; they can be laid on the bed.)

Insert the bag of heparin flush solution inside the pressure bag. Inflate the bag to approximately 50 mm Hg. Then gently squeeze the drip chamber until it's about half full. Open the roller clamp. Prime the tubing by activating the flush device. (Follow the manufacturer's directions for flushing the transducer. Many transducers need to be inverted during flushing *so that no air becomes trapped.*) As you flush each vented stopcock, replace it with a sterile dead-end cap. Verify that no air remains in the tubing. Then inflate the pressure bag to 300 mm Hg, which will create a flow rate of 2 to 3 ml/hour. Connect the monitor cable to the transducer.

If you have a reusable transducer and transducer dome, follow the manufacturer's directions for attaching the dome to the transducer and to the preassembled pressure tubing and flush system. (You may need to place several drops of sterile 0.9% sodium chloride solution or bacteriostatic water on the transducer's surface before attaching the dome.)

Follow the manufacturer's directions to calibrate and zero the equipment if the machine doesn't automatically calibrate. Label the tubing with the date, the time, and your initials.

### Implementation

• Describe the procedure to the patient and explain its purpose.

## Locating the phlebostatic axis

The intersection of two imaginary lines approximates the location of the phlebostatic axis, the point where the right atrium and vena cava meet. The tip of the monitoring catheter should rest within the body at this point.

The anterior view shows the vertical line passing from the fourth intercostal space at the right side of the sternum. The lateral view shows the horizontal line passing through the fourth intercostal space, midway between the outermost part of the chest's anterior and posterior surfaces.

**Anterior view**

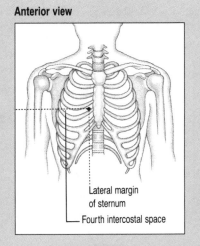

Lateral margin of sternum

Fourth intercostal space

**Lateral view**

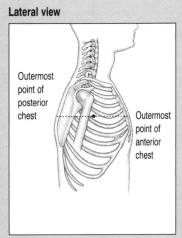

Outermost point of posterior chest

Outermost point of anterior chest

### Inserting an arterial line
• Prepare the tubing as explained previously. Wash your hands and put on sterile gloves.
• After the doctor positions the arterial catheter, attach the tubing to it, securing the tubing to the catheter with a slight twisting motion. Secure the catheter with hypoallergenic tape or a transparent dressing or, alternatively, the doctor may suture the catheter in place. Unless you've already applied a transparent dressing, apply antimicrobial ointment and a dry, sterile dressing to the site, according to hospital protocol. Label the dressing with the date, the time, and your initials.
• Level the transducer to the phlebostatic axis, located at the fourth intercostal space in the midaxillary line at the level of the right atrium. You may use a carpenter's level to do so. (See *Locating the phlebostatic axis.*) Zero the transducer according to the manufacturer's directions.
• Select the scale on the arterial pressure monitor that makes the waveform clearly visible.
• Flush the arterial pressure monitoring setup.

• Obtain pressure readings. (See *Interpreting arterial pressure waveforms,* pages 18 and 19.)
• Set alarms between 10 and 20 mm Hg above and below the patient's blood pressure.

### Changing arterial line tubing
• Prepare the tubing as explained previously. Wash your hands and put on sterile gloves.
• Determine the length of tubing to be changed. (The tubing to the catheter, to the hub, or to the stopcock closest to the patient may be changed.)
• Turn off or suspend the alarms.
• Clamp the tubing being changed before disconnecting it. Disconnect the old segment of tubing and immediately replace it with new tubing.
• Activate the flush device to clear blood from the line and catheter. Clean any blood from the tubing or catheter, and apply a dry, sterile dressing (if the tubing to the catheter was changed).
• Level the transducer, zero the equipment, and set the alarms (as described above).

*(Text continues on page 20.)*

## Interpreting arterial pressure waveforms

Arterial waveforms reflect changes in left ventricular function and pressure and resistance in the systemic arterial tree. By observing the waveform, you may detect such conditions as aortic stenosis, atrial fibrillation, pulsus alternans, and pulsus paradoxus.

### Normal waveform

A normal arterial waveform has four distinct components. *Peak systolic pressure* reflects pressure in the left ventricle during systole, which starts with the opening of the aortic valve. When aortic pressure exceeds left ventricular pressure, the aortic valve closes. On the waveform, the *dicrotic notch* indicates aortic valve closure. *Diastolic pressure* reflects vessel recoil, or the degree of arterial vasoconstriction. The *anacrotic notch,* indicating the first phase of ventricular systole (isovolumetric contraction), precedes aortic valve opening. (With peripheral arterial monitoring, the anacrotic notch normally doesn't appear.)

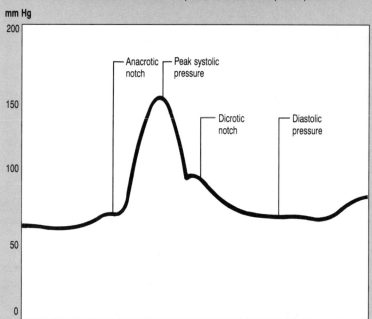

### Aortic stenosis

In *aortic stenosis*, you'll see a small pulse wave with delayed peak systolic pressure. This lower systolic pressure results from slowed ventricular ejection through the stenotic aortic valve. Frequently, the dicrotic notch is not well-defined because of the abnormal closure of the valve leaflets. Because the systolic pressure is lower, these patients have a narrow pulse pressure.

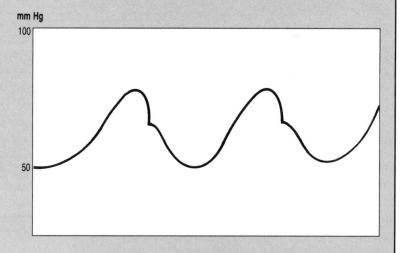

## Interpreting arterial pressure waveforms *(continued)*

### Atrial fibrillation

In *atrial fibrillation*, the amplitude varies because of the characteristic irregular rhythm.

### Pulsus alternans

In *pulsus alternans*, the waveform shows regular, alternating amplitudes of peak systolic pressure. These waveforms reflect an increased pooling of blood in the pulmonary vasculature, due to low intrathoracic pressure during inspiration, which is indicated by lower systolic pressure. Upon expiration, the higher systolic pressure results from a shunting of the pooled blood in the pulmonary bed to the left side of the heart.

### Pulsus paradoxus

In *pulsus paradoxus*, systolic pressure varies by more than 10 mm Hg from inspiration to expiration. This usually results from alterations in venous return to the right side of the heart and changes in intrathoracic or intrapericardial pressures.

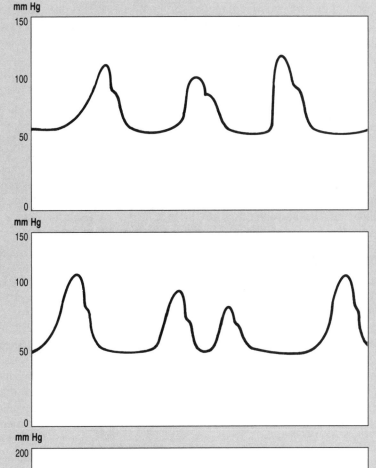

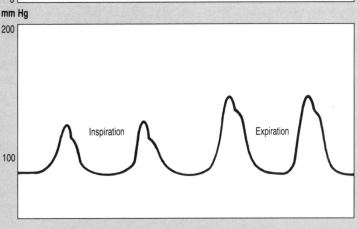

### Obtaining a blood sample from an arterial line

• Assemble the equipment, wash your hands, and put on sterile gloves.
• Turn off or suspend the alarms.
• Open one package of sterile 4″ × 4″ gauze pads, and position one near the arterial line. Remove the dead-end cap from the stopcock closest to the patient and place it on a sterile gauze pad *to keep the dead-end cap clean.*
• Insert the 5-ml syringe into the stopcock. Turn off the stopcock to the flush solution. Slowly withdraw 3 to 5 ml of blood from the line; this will be discarded. Turn the stopcock halfway back to the open position, *which closes the system in all directions.* Remove the discard syringe, and replace it with the 5- to 10-ml specimen syringe.
• Turn off the stopcock to the flush solution. Using the specimen syringe, slowly withdraw the required amount of blood from the line. Turn the stopcock to the original position. Remove the syringe.
• Activate the flush device *to clear blood from the tubing.* Turn off the stopcock to the patient, and flush the stopcock port until the solution runs clear. Return the stopcock to the original position. *This opens the flush system to the catheter.* Replace the dead-end cap or apply a new one. Zero the transducer, reflush the system, and turn on the alarms. Transfer the blood to the appropriate tubes, and send the specimens to the laboratory.

### Removing an arterial line

• Consult hospital policy to determine if you are permitted to perform this procedure.
• Explain the procedure to the patient.
• Assemble all equipment. Wash your hands. Observe universal precautions, including wearing personal protective equipment, for this procedure.
• Document the systolic, diastolic, and mean blood pressures. If a manual, indirect blood pressure has not been assessed recently, obtain one now to establish a new baseline.

• Turn off the monitor alarms. Then turn off the flow clamp to the flush solution.
• Carefully remove the dressing over the insertion site. Remove any sutures, using the suture removal kit, and then carefully check that all sutures have been removed.
• Withdraw the catheter using a gentle, steady motion. Keep the catheter parallel to the artery during withdrawal to reduce the risk of traumatic injury.
• Immediately after withdrawing the catheter, apply pressure to the site with a sterile 4″ × 4″ gauze pad. Maintain pressure for at least 10 minutes (longer if bleeding or oozing persists). Apply additional pressure to a femoral site or if the patient has coagulopathy or is receiving anticoagulants.
• Cover the site with an appropriate dressing and secure the dressing with tape. If stipulated by hospital policy, make a pressure dressing for a femoral site by folding in half four sterile 4″ × 4″ gauze pads, and apply the dressing. Cover the dressing with a tight adhesive bandage; then cover the bandage with a sandbag. Maintain the patient on bed rest for 6 hours with the sandbag in place.
• If the doctor has ordered a culture of the catheter tip (to diagnose a suspected infection), gently place the catheter tip on a 4″ × 4″ sterile gauze pad. Once the patient's bleeding is under control, hold the catheter over the sterile container. Using sterile scissors, cut the tip so it falls into the sterile container. Label the specimen and send it to the laboratory.
• Observe the site for bleeding. Evaluate circulation in the extremity distal to the site by assessing color, pulses, and sensation. Repeat this assessment every 15 minutes for the first 4 hours, every 30 minutes for the next 2 hours, then hourly for the next 6 hours.

### Special considerations

Always use sterile technique and maintain electrical safety when working with arterial lines. Note that many factors can alter pressure readings and waveforms, including air in the tubing, the transducer, or both; an inappropriate transducer level; loose connections; cracks or leaks in the system; a clot in the catheter; or the catheter tip resting against the vessel wall.

Level and zero the system at the beginning of each shift and after any manipulation of the patient or system. Mark the level of the phlebostatic axis *to maintain consistency and accuracy.* Check the patient's blood pressure with a cuff for comparison every 4 to 8 hours, depending on hospital policy. Change the dressing and tubing every 24 to 72 hours.

Monitor the patient frequently. *Considerable blood can be lost quickly if the system becomes disconnected.* Keep alarms on at all times, except when replacing tubing, as noted.

Bear in mind that pressure tubing is made of stiff, nondistensible plastic. *Inaccurate arterial pressure measurements will result if you use conventional I.V. tubing below the level of the transducer.*

## Documentation

Document the date and time of the insertion and the dressing and tubing changes. Record the patient's blood pressure as indicated. Observe the shape of the arterial waveform and note any changes.

# MONITORING CARDIOVASCULAR STATUS

## Introduction

Cardiovascular disorders, the leading cause of death in the United States, affect millions of Americans each year. The responsibility of caring for patients with these disorders pervades nearly every aspect of nursing practice. As a result, cardiovascular care ranks as one of the most rapidly growing areas of nursing. What's more, it's one of the most rapidly changing fields, with the continuing proliferation of new diagnostic tests, new drug and other treatments, and sophisticated monitoring equipment. Consequently, nurses face a constant challenge to keep up with the latest developments. To assist you, this chapter reviews cardiac anatomy and physiology and covers heart sounds monitoring, electrocardiogram (ECG) and other cardiac monitoring, ST-segment monitoring, and pulmonary artery pressure (PAP) monitoring. You'll also learn about central venous pressure (CVP) monitoring, cardiac output monitoring, and intra-aortic balloon counterpulsation (IABC) monitoring.

Cardiac and hemodynamic monitoring represent critical cardiovascular care responsibilities. Cardiac monitoring uses either hardwire or telemetric systems to continuously record the patient's cardiac activity. Continuous monitoring is useful not only for assessing cardiac rhythm, but also for gauging a patient's response to drug therapy and for preventing complications associated with diagnostic and therapeutic procedures. Once used only in critical care areas, cardiac monitoring is now performed in general medical, pediatric, and transplantation departments, and in high-risk obstetric departments.

Similarly, hemodynamic monitoring has become more widely used since its inception in the 1970s. Its invasive techniques measure pressure, flow, and resistance within the cardiovascular system. Obtained with a pulmonary artery (PA) catheter, these measurements are used to guide therapy. Hemodynamic monitoring includes PAP monitoring, cardiac output measurements, right ventricular ejection fraction and volume measurements, and continuous evaluation of mixed venous oxygen saturation.

## Anatomy and physiology review

The cardiovascular system performs two basic functions: It delivers oxygenated blood to body tissues and removes waste substances through the action of the heart. The average person's heart beats 60 to 100 times/minute, pumping 4 to 6 liters of blood in that time.

Controlled by the autonomic nervous system, the heart pumps blood through the entire body. The vascular network that carries blood throughout the body consists of high-pressure arteries, which deliver the blood, and low-pressure veins, which return it to the heart. This complex network keeps the pumping heart filled with blood and maintains blood pressure.

A muscular organ, the heart accounts for about 0.5% of a person's total body weight and is about the size of a closed fist. It lies obliquely in the chest, with two-thirds located to the left of the sternum. The base of the heart (the superior portion) corresponds to the level of the third costal cartilage. The apex of the heart (the inferior portion) is normally located at the fifth left intercostal space at the midclavicular line.

### Heart chambers

The heart contains four chambers — two atria and two ventricles — encircled by a thin outer sac called the pericardium. Located in the superior portion of the heart, the atria function as receptacles for blood during ventricular contraction or systole. The larger ventricles lie below and receive blood from the atria and eject it into the pulmonary system and systemic circulation.

### *Atria*

The right atrium receives venous blood returning from the systemic circulation by way of the inferior and superior venae cavae. The left atrium receives oxygenated blood from the pulmonary system by way of the pulmonary veins (the only veins that carry oxygenated blood). During ventricular diastole, the atria allow the blood to pass into the corresponding right and left ventricles.

### Ventricles

During ventricular diastole, the right ventricle receives unoxygenated blood from the right atrium by way of the tricuspid valve. The left ventricle receives oxygenated blood from the left atrium by way of the mitral valve.

During ventricular systole, the right ventricle ejects blood through the pulmonic valve into the pulmonary system by way of the pulmonary artery (the only artery to carry deoxygenated blood). The left ventricle expels blood through the aortic valve into the aorta and, eventually, the systemic circulation.

The ventricles consist of three layers of muscle tissue. The outer layer, called the epicardium, contains nerve fibers, coronary blood vessels, and large flattened cells called mesothelia. The middle layer, called the myocardium, is thick, muscular, and rich in nerve and sensory fibers. The endocardium is the smooth inner layer. The myocardium of the left ventricle is two to three times thicker than that of the right ventricle. The reason: Much higher pressure is required to eject blood into the systemic circulation than to eject blood into the pulmonary system.

### Heart valves

The heart has four valves — the mitral, tricuspid, aortic, and pulmonic — which ensure that blood moves in the right direction without backflow (or regurgitation). Each valve consists of cusps (or leaflets) that open with pressure from downstream and close with pressure from upstream.

The two atrioventricular valves are the tricuspid valve, which normally has three leaflets, and the mitral valve, which normally has two. The tricuspid valve separates the right atrium from the right ventricle; the mitral valve separates the left atrium from the left ventricle.

Both atrioventricular valves are attached to the chambers by complex interconnected structures. The papillary muscles, which arise from the ventricular wall, are connected to the valve leaflets by the chordae tendineae, a series of fibrous cords that cause the valve leaflets to close during ventricular systole.

The two semilunar valves are the pulmonic valve, which separates the right ventricle from the pulmonary artery, and the aortic valve, which separates the left ventricle from the aorta. These valves have three cusps that open during ventricular systole, allowing blood to pass into the pulmonary system and the systemic circulation. During ventricular diastole, the valve cusps close, preventing regurgitation of blood into the ventricles. (See *Reviewing the heart's structure.*)

## Heart sounds monitoring

Most normal heart sounds result from vibrations created by the opening and closing of the heart valves. When valves close, they suddenly terminate the motion of blood; when valves open, they accelerate the motion of blood. This sudden acceleration or deceleration is responsible for producing heart sounds. (See *Events in the cardiac cycle,* page 26.) Auscultation sites don't lie directly over the valves, but over the pathways the blood takes as it flows through chambers and valves.

Auscultating for heart sounds reveals a great deal of information about a patient's cardiac function. Differentiating between normal and abnormal heart sounds, however, requires practice. Therefore, first gain experience identifying normal heart sounds, rates, and rhythms. Then auscultate patients with known abnormal sounds, seeking help from experts to identify findings.

Also keep in mind that the auscultation of heart sounds can be difficult. Even with a stethoscope, you will find that the amount of tissue between the source of the sound and the outer chest wall can affect which sounds you can hear.

## Reviewing the heart's structure

This cross-sectional view shows the heart's major structures.

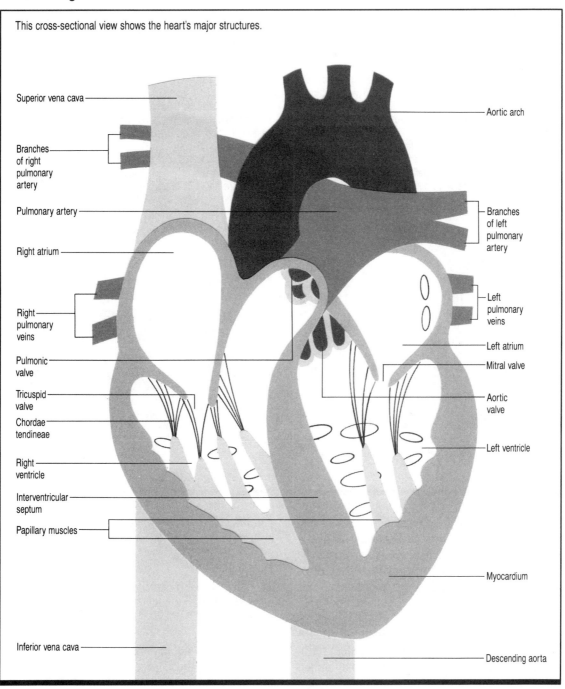

## Events in the cardiac cycle

Basically, the cardiac cycle has two phases: systole, when the ventricles contract, ejecting blood into the aorta and the pulmonary artery; and diastole, when the ventricles relax and the atria contract.

At the beginning of systole, increasing ventricular pressure forces the mitral and tricuspid valves to shut. The closing of these atrioventricular (AV) valves produces the first heart sound, known as $S_1$ or the *lub* of *lub-dub*. The ventricular pressure builds until it exceeds that in the pulmonary artery and aorta. Then the aortic and pulmonic semilunar valves open and the ventricles eject blood into the arteries.

As the ventricles empty and relax, ventricular pressure falls below that in the pulmonary artery and the aorta. The

semilunar valves close, producing the second heart sound, $S_2$ or the *dub* of *lub-dub,* and marking the end of systole. As the ventricles relax during diastole, the pressure in the ventricles is less than that in the atria. The AV valves open and blood begins to flow into the ventricles from the atria. When the ventricles become full near the end of diastole, the atria contract to send the rest of the blood to the ventricles. Ventricular pressure is now greater than atrial pressure. The AV valves close, marking the beginning of systole and repetition of the cardiac cycle.

Events on the right side of the heart occur a fraction of a second after events on the left side because the pressure is lower on the right side of the heart.

**Systole**

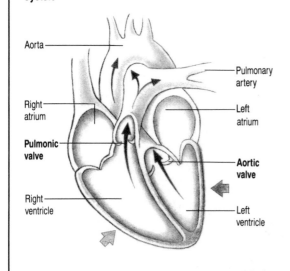

Aorta
Pulmonary artery
Right atrium
Left atrium
**Pulmonic valve**
**Aortic valve**
Right ventricle
Left ventricle

**Diastole**

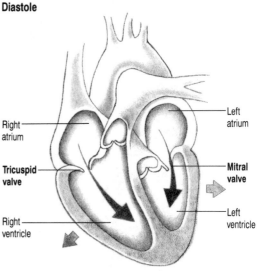

Right atrium
Left atrium
**Tricuspid valve**
**Mitral valve**
Right ventricle
Left ventricle

Fat, muscle, and air tend to reduce sound transmission. Thus, if a patient is obese or has a muscular chest wall or hyperinflated lungs, the sounds may seem more distant and difficult to hear. These natural limitations will require you to control the environment as much as possible during auscultation.

When auscultating heart sounds, you'll use the diaphragm of the stethoscope to detect high-pitched sounds and the bell to detect low-pitched

sounds and murmurs. The first and second heart sounds are termed $S_1$ and $S_2$.

### Equipment

Stethoscope with chestpiece size appropriate for patient's chest ■ pediatric chestpiece for thin adult.

### Preparation of equipment

Warm the stethoscope chestpiece by rubbing it between your hands.

## Auscultation sites

When auscultating for heart sounds, place the stethoscope over four different sites. Follow the same auscultation sequence during every cardiovascular assessment.

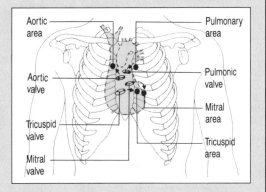

• Place the stethoscope in the second intercostal space along the right sternal border, as shown. In the aortic area, blood moves from the left ventricle during systole, crossing the aortic valve and flowing through the aortic arch.
• Move to the pulmonary area, located in the second intercostal space at the left sternal border. In the pulmonary area, blood ejected from the right ventricle during systole crosses the pulmonic valve and flows through the main pulmonary artery.
• Assess in the third auscultation site, the tricuspid area, which lies in the fifth intercostal space along the left sternal border. In the tricuspid area, sounds reflect blood movement from the right atrium across the tricuspid valve, filling the right ventricle during diastole.
• Finally, listen in the mitral area, located in the fifth intercostal space near the midclavicular line. (If the patient's heart is enlarged, the mitral area may be closer to the anterior axillary line.) In the mitral, or apical, area, sounds represent blood flow across the mitral valve and left ventricular filling during diastole.

## Implementation

• Explain the procedure to the patient, and instruct him to breathe normally, inhaling through the nose and exhaling through the mouth.
• Help the patient into a supine position, either flat or at a comfortable elevation. If you're right-handed, stand at the patient's right side. *This allows you to manipulate the stethoscope with your dominant hand.* Use alternative positions, as needed, *to improve heart sound auscultation.*
• Open the front of the patient's gown and drape the patient appropriately. *Clothing and surgical dressings will muffle heart sounds or render them inaudible.*
• Move the stethoscope slowly and methodically over the four main auscultation sites, listening selectively for each cardiac cycle component. (See *Auscultation sites.*)
• Concentrate *to hear these relatively quiet sounds.* Closing your eyes while you listen may help. Noise from stethoscope movement, especially over chest hair, or patient movement or shivering, will interfere with hearing sounds clearly. So keep your hand steady, and ask the patient to remain as still as possible.
• Begin by listening for a few cycles to become accustomed to the rate and rhythm of the sounds. The first and second heart sounds ($S_1$ and $S_2$) are relatively high pitched and are separated by a silent period.
• At each auscultation site, use the diaphragm to listen closely to $S_1$ and $S_2$ and compare them. Next, listen to the systolic period and the diastolic period. Then, auscultate again using the bell of the stethoscope. If you hear any sounds during the diastolic or systolic period, or any variations in $S_1$ and $S_2$, note the characteristics of the sound. Note the auscultation site and the part of the cardiac cycle during which it occurred.

### Special considerations

To aid in auscultation, make sure that the room remains as quiet as possible. If the patient has special equipment, such as an oxygen nebulizer or suction device, perform auscultation with equipment off, if possible.

The timing of heart sounds in relation to the cardiac cycle is particularly important. Normal heart sounds last only a fraction of a second, followed by slightly longer periods of silence.

$S_1$ is louder in the mitral and tricuspid listening areas *(LUB-dub)* and softer in the aortic and pulmonary areas *(lub-DUB)*. The mitral valve actually closes slightly before the tricuspid valve. An experienced examiner may be able to discriminate the corresponding sound (split $S_1$), which sounds somewhat like *li-lub*. However, an inexperienced examiner may confuse a split $S_1$ with an abnormal extra sound occurring just before $S_1$.

$S_2$ is louder in the aortic and pulmonary areas of the chest. At these sites, the sequence sounds like *lub-DUB*. At normal rates, the diastolic pause between $S_2$ and the next $S_1$ exceeds the systolic pause between $S_1$ and $S_2$.

During auscultation, $S_2$ may have a split sound, like that of a broken syllable. This may occur normally when aortic and pulmonic valves don't close at exactly the same time. Split $S_2$ commonly occurs in healthy children and young adults.

Comparing the loudness of the normal heart sounds at each site will help you differentiate systole from diastole. Learning to identify phases of the cardiac cycle will enable you to time abnormal sounds.

## Documentation
Record all characteristics of the patient's heart sounds, including their pitch (frequency), intensity (loudness), duration, quality (such as musical or harsh), location, and radiation.

# ECG monitoring
One of the most valuable and frequently used diagnostic tools, ECG measures the heart's electrical activity as waveforms. Impulses moving through the heart's conduction system create electric currents that can be monitored on the body's surface. Electrodes attached to the skin can detect these electric currents and transmit them to an instrument that produces a record (the electrocardiogram) of cardiac activity.

The standard 12-lead ECG uses a series of electrodes placed on the extremities and the chest wall to assess the heart from 12 different views (leads). The 12 leads consist of 3 standard bipolar limb leads (designated I, II, III), 3 unipolar augmented leads ($aV_R$, $aV_L$, $aV_F$), and 6 unipolar precordial leads ($V_1$ to $V_6$). The limb leads and augmented leads reveal the heart's functioning from the frontal plane. The precordial leads show the heart from the horizontal plane.

The ECG device measures and averages the differences between the electrical potential of the electrode sites for each lead and graphs them over time. This creates the standard ECG complex, called P-QRS-T. The P wave represents atrial depolarization; the QRS complex, ventricular depolarization; and the T wave, ventricular repolarization. (See *Reviewing ECG waveform components.*)

You can use a multichannel or a single-channel method to do ECG monitoring. With the multichannel method, you attach all electrodes to the patient at once and the machine prints a simultaneous view of all leads. With the single-channel method you must systematically attach and remove selected electrodes — stopping and starting the tracing each time.

## Equipment
ECG machine ▪ recording paper ▪ disposable pregelled electrodes or reusable electrodes with suction bulbs, electrode gel, and rubber straps ▪ 4″ × 4″ gauze pads ▪ moist cloth towel ▪ sterile drape ▪ optional: shaving supplies, marking pen.

## Preparation of equipment
Before using the ECG machine, check the date of its last inspection by the hospital's engineering department. If the period for authorized use has elapsed, avoid using the machine *because even a miniscule leakage of electric current (10 microamperes) may put the patient at risk for life-threatening arrhythmias.*

## Reviewing ECG waveform components

An electrocardiogram (ECG) waveform has three basic components: a P wave, a QRS complex, and a T wave. These elements can be further divided into a PR interval, a J point, an ST segment, a U wave, and a QT interval.

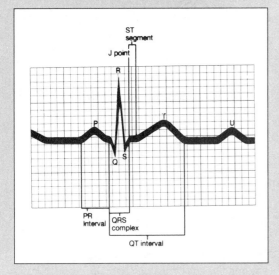

### P wave and PR interval
The P wave represents atrial depolarization. The PR interval represents the time it takes an impulse to travel from the atria

through the atrioventricular node and bundle of His. The PR interval measures from the beginning of the P wave to the beginning of the QRS complex.

### QRS complex
The QRS complex represents ventricular depolarization (the time it takes for the impulse to travel through the bundle branches to the Purkinje fibers). The Q wave appears as the first negative deflection in the QRS complex; the R wave, as the first positive deflection. The S wave appears as the second negative deflection or the first negative deflection after the R wave.

### J point and ST segment
Marking the end of the QRS complex, the J point also indicates the beginning of the ST segment. The ST segment represents part of ventricular repolarization.

### T wave and U wave
Usually following the same deflection pattern as the P wave, the T wave represents ventricular repolarization. The U wave follows the T wave, but isn't always seen.

### QT interval
The QT interval represents ventricular depolarization and repolarization. It extends from the beginning of the QRS complex to the end of the T wave.

## Implementation
• Explain the procedure to the patient *to allay his fears and promote cooperation.* Inform him that no special preparation is required and that the procedure takes no longer than 15 minutes. Instruct him to relax, lie still, and breathe normally. Advise him not to talk during the procedure *because the movement of his muscles may distort the ECG tracing.*
• Check the patient's history for cardiac medications, and note any current therapy on the test request form.
• Place the patient in the supine position. If he can't tolerate lying flat, help him to assume semi-Fowler's position.

• Instruct the patient to expose his chest, both ankles, and both wrists for electrode placement. Drape the female patient's chest until chest leads are applied.
• Turn on the machine *to warm up the stylus mechanism.* Check the paper supply.

### Recording a multichannel ECG
• Place electrodes on the inner aspect of the wrists, the medial aspect of the lower legs, and the chest. (See *Positioning precordial electrodes,* page 30.) If using disposable electrodes, remove the paper backing before positioning. Then connect the leadwires after all electrodes are in place. For reusable electrodes, apply electrode gel and affix the electrodes with suction bulbs.

## Positioning precordial electrodes

The precordial leads – $V_1$ through $V_6$ – complement the limb leads, providing a complete view of the heart by reflecting the current moving through the horizontal plane. The electrodes on the chest represent the positive poles. To record the precordial leads, place the electrodes as follows:

$V_1$ – fourth intercostal space, right sternal border
$V_2$ – fourth intercostal space, left sternal border
$V_3$ – midway between $V_2$ and $V_4$
$V_4$ – fifth intercostal space, left midclavicular line
$V_5$ – fifth intercostal space, left anterior axillary line
$V_6$ – fifth intercostal space, left midaxillary line

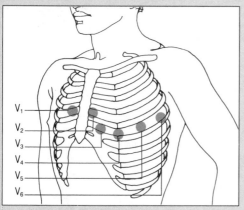

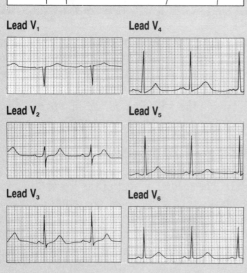

Lead $V_1$

Lead $V_4$

Lead $V_2$

Lead $V_5$

Lead $V_3$

Lead $V_6$

Secure the limb electrodes with rubber straps, but avoid tightening them *to prevent circulatory impairment and distortion on the recording.*

• If frequent ECGs will be necessary, use a marking pen to indicate lead positions on the patient's chest *to ensure consistent placement.*

• Set the paper speed to 25 mm/second or as ordered. Calibrate the machine by adjusting the sensitivity to normal and checking the quality and baseline position of the tracing.

• Press the start button and the machine will produce a printout showing all 12 leads simultaneously on thermal or pressure-sensitive recording paper.

• As the machine records the ECG, check to make sure that all leads are represented in the tracing. If not, determine which one has come loose, reattach it, and restart the tracing. Check for interference (often called "artifact") in the tracing.

• Also observe to be sure that the wave doesn't peak beyond the top edge of the recording grid. If it does, adjust the machine to bring the wave inside the boundaries.

• When the machine finishes the tracing, remove the electrodes and reposition the patient's gown and bedcovers.

### Recording a single-channel ECG

• Apply either disposable or standard electrodes to the inner aspects of the wrists and medial aspects of the lower legs.

• Connect each leadwire to the corresponding electrode by inserting the wire prong into the terminal post and tightening the screw.

• Set the paper speed to 25 mm/second or as ordered. Calibrate the machine by adjusting the sensitivity to normal and checking the quality and baseline position of the tracing. Recalibrate the machine after running each lead *to provide a consistent test standard.*

• Turn the lead selector to I. Then mark the lead by writing "I" on the paper strip or by depressing the marking button on the machine (some machines do this automatically). Record for 3 to 6 seconds and then return the machine to the standby mode. Repeat this procedure for leads II, III, $aV_R$, $aV_L$, and $aV_F$.

• Determine proper placement for the chest electrodes. If frequent ECGs are necessary, use a marking pen to indicate lead positions on the patient's chest *to ensure consistent placement.*

• Connect the chest leadwire to the suction bulb in the same manner as you connected the limb electrodes. Apply gel to each of the six chest positions; then firmly press the suction bulb to attach the chest lead to the $V_1$ position. Mark the strips as before. Then turn the lead selector to V and record $V_1$ for 3 to 6 seconds. Return the lead selector to standby. Reposition the electrode and repeat the procedure for $V_2$ to $V_6$.

• After completing $V_6$, run a rhythm strip on lead II for at least 6 seconds.

• Assess the quality of the tracings and repeat any that are unclear.

• Disconnect the equipment, remove the electrodes, and wipe the gel from the patient with a moist cloth towel. Wash the gel from the electrodes and dry them thoroughly.

### Special considerations

In place of the electrodes and straps on the extremities, suction bulbs may be used *to enhance baseline stability.*

Small areas of hair on the patient's chest or extremities may be shaved, but this usually isn't necessary.

If the patient's skin is exceptionally oily, scaly, or diaphoretic, rub the electrode site with a dry $4'' \times 4''$ gauze pad before applying the electrode *to help reduce interference in the tracing.* During the procedure, ask the patient to breathe normally. If his respirations distort the recording, ask him to hold his breath briefly *to reduce baseline wander in the tracing.*

If the patient has a pacemaker, you can perform ECG with or without a magnet. Be sure to note on the strip the presence of a pacemaker and the use of the magnet to turn on the pacemaker.

### Documentation

Label the ECG recording with the patient's name, room number, and hospital identification number. If you're sending the ECG to another department for interpretation and mounting, complete all information on the request form. Document in your notes the date, the time the test was performed, and any significant responses.

## Cardiac monitoring

Because it allows continuous observation of the heart's electrical activity, cardiac monitoring is used in patients with conduction disturbances or in those at risk for life-threatening arrhythmias. It's also used to evaluate the effects of therapy.

Like other forms of ECG, cardiac monitoring uses electrodes placed on the patient's chest to transmit electrical signals that are converted into a tracing of cardiac rhythm on an oscilloscope.

Two types of monitoring exist: hardwire or telemetry. In *hardwire monitoring,* you connect the patient to a monitor at bedside. The rhythm display appears at bedside, but it may also be transmitted to a console at a remote location. *Telemetry* uses a small transmitter connected to the ambulatory patient to send electrical signals to another location where they're displayed on a monitor screen. (See *Setting up for telemetry,* page 32.)

Regardless of type, cardiac monitors can display the patient's rhythm and heart rate; produce a printed record of cardiac rhythm; and sound an alarm if the patient's heart rate rises above or falls below specified limits. Some monitors can also recognize and count abnormal heartbeats and trigger an alarm if the heartbeats exceed a set limit.

### Equipment

Cardiac monitor ▪ leadwires ▪ patient cable ▪ disposable pregelled electrodes (the number of electrodes varies from three to five, depending on

## Setting up for telemetry

Telemetry detects arrhythmias that occur during sleep, or when the patient is resting, performing mild exercise, or undergoing stress. It's especially useful for the ambulatory patient because it permits greater freedom than hardwire monitoring and avoids electrical hazards by isolating the monitor system from leakage and accidental shock. To set up a telemetry monitor, follow these steps.

• Insert a battery in the telemetry transmitter, matching the polarity markings on the transmitter case with those on the battery.

• Test the battery's charge by observing the oscilloscope screen, which registers no cardiac activity if the battery is low. In some models, check the battery by pushing the test-light button on the back of the transmitter. If the test light fails to go on, replace the battery. Make sure the leadwire cable is securely attached to the transmitter.

• Show the transmitter to the patient and explain how it works. Before proceeding, answer any questions he may have.

• Place the transmitter in the pouch provided by the manufacturer or hospital. Tie the pouch strings around the patient's neck and waist. Make sure the pouch fits snugly without making the patient uncomfortable. If no pouch is available, place the transmitter in the patient's bathrobe pocket.

• After locating the patient's telemetry monitor in the central console, calibrate it and adjust the heart rate alarms as you would a hardwire monitor.

• Some units have a button that can be pushed if the patient has symptoms. This causes the central console to print a rhythm strip. Tell the patient how and when to use this button.

• Tell the patient to remove the transmitter if he takes a shower or bath.

the manufacturer) ■ alcohol sponges ■ 4″ × 4″ gauze pads ■ optional: shaving supplies, washcloth.

### Preparation of equipment

Plug the monitor into an electrical outlet and turn it on *to warm up the unit while you prepare the equipment and the patient.* Insert the cable into the appropriate socket in the monitor.

Connect the leadwires to the cable. In some systems, the leadwires are permanently secured to the cable. Each leadwire should indicate the location for attachment to the patient: right arm (RA), left arm (LA), right leg (RL), left leg (LL), and ground (C or V). This designation should appear on the leadwire—if it's permanently connected—or at the connection of the leadwires and cable to the patient. Then connect an electrode to each of the leadwires, carefully checking that each leadwire is in its correct outlet.

### Implementation

• Explain the procedure to the patient, provide privacy, and ask the patient to expose his chest. Wash your hands.

• Determine electrode positions on the patient's chest, based on the system and lead you're using. (See *Understanding lead placement,* pages 34 and 35.)

• If the leadwires and patient cable aren't permanently attached, verify that the electrode placement corresponds to the label on the patient cable.

• If necessary, shave an area about 4″ (10 cm) in diameter around each electrode site. Clean the area with an alcohol sponge and dry it completely *to remove skin secretions that may interfere with electrode function.* Gently abrade the dried area by rubbing it briskly until it reddens *to remove dead skin cells and to promote better electrical contact with living cells.* (Some electrodes have a small, rough patch for abrading the skin; if yours don't, use a dry washcloth or a dry gauze pad.)

• Remove the backing from the pregelled electrode. Check the gel for moistness. If the gel is dry, discard it and replace it with a fresh electrode.

• Apply the electrode to the site and press firmly *to ensure a tight seal.* Repeat with the remaining electrodes.

• When all the electrodes are in place, check for a tracing on the cardiac monitor. Assess the quality of the ECG. *To verify that each beat is being detected by the monitor,* compare the digital heart rate display with your count of the patient's heart rate.

• If necessary, use the gain control to adjust the size of the rhythm tracing, and the position control *to adjust the waveform position on the recording paper.*

• Set the upper and lower limits of the heart rate alarm, based on hospital policy. Turn the alarm on.

### Special considerations
Make sure that all electrical equipment and outlets are grounded *to avoid electric shock and interference.* Also ensure that the patient is clean and dry *to prevent electric shock.*

Avoid opening the electrode packages until just before using *to prevent the gel from drying out.*

Avoid placing the electrodes on bony prominences, hairy areas, areas where defibrillator pads will be placed, or areas for chest compression.

If the patient's skin is exceptionally oily, scaly, or diaphoretic, rub the electrode site with a dry 4″ × 4″ gauze pad before applying the electrode *to help reduce interference in the tracing.* During the procedure, ask the patient to breathe normally. If his respirations distort the recording, ask him to hold his breath briefly *to reduce baseline wander in the tracing.*

Assess skin integrity, and reposition the electrodes every 24 hours or as necessary.

### Documentation
Record the date and time that monitoring begins and the monitoring lead used in your notes. Document a rhythm strip at least every 8 hours with any changes in the patient's condition (or as stated by hospital policy). Label the rhythm strip with the patient's name, his room number, the date, and the time.

If cardiac monitoring will continue after the patient's discharge, ensure that all caregivers have some knowledge of rhythm interpretation and cardiopulmonary resuscitation. Also discuss troubleshooting techniques to use if the monitor malfunctions. As needed, contact the monitor supplier to help in discharge planning.

## ST-segment monitoring
ST-segment monitoring helps detect myocardial ischemia, electrolyte imbalances, coronary artery spasm, and hypoxic events. The ST segment represents early ventricular repolarization, and any changes in this waveform component reflect alterations in myocardial oxygenation. Any monitoring lead that views an ischemic heart region will reveal ST-segment changes. A deviation of more than 1 mm from the original baseline tracing is considered significant and may indicate myocardial ischemia.

Current equipment used for ST-segment monitoring can analyze two, three, or four leads chosen from any of the standard 12 ECG leads, as well as the right-side chest leads $V_{3R}$, $V_{4R}$, and $V_{5R}$. Depending on how the monitor has been programmed, it may display one or more leads. (Monitors that display up to 12 leads are available.)

The monitor software establishes a template of the patient's normal QRST pattern from the selected leads, and then displays ST-segment changes. Some monitors display such changes continuously, others only on command. With some models, the changes appear over the original template; with other models, the template and the ST-segment changes appear side by side. (See *ST-segment recording,* page 36.)

ST-segment monitoring is especially useful for patients at risk for silent ischemia because it allows prompt assessment and immediate treatment that can prevent myocardial necrosis. The technique also helps caregivers evaluate the effectiveness of specific treatments in returning the ST segment to baseline.

Candidates for continuous ST-segment monitoring include patients with coronary artery disease, those who've undergone percutaneous transluminal coronary angioplasty, intraoperative and postoperative patients at high risk for

## Understanding lead placement

You'll have several leads and electrodes to place depending on the cardiac monitoring system you're using. The most typical system is the three-electrode system, which uses standard limb leads and a modified version of standard chest leads. To increase monitoring capability, you may need to use the four- or five-electrode system. Review the manufacturer's instructions for your particular system and use the following guidelines to place the leads precisely.

### Three-electrode system
In this system, the most commonly used limb lead is lead II, and typically used modified chest leads are MCL₁ and MCL₆ (modified versions of V₁ and V₆). In general, a three-electrode monitoring system has one positive lead and one negative lead. A third lead serves as a ground.

### Lead II
For lead II, you'll place the right arm (RA) or white electrode below the right clavicle, the left arm (LA) or black electrode below the left clavicle, and the left leg (LL) or red electrode on the left lower anterior rib cage.

Lead II measures the electrical flow from the negative RA electrode to the positive LL electrode, producing good QRS complexes, which reflect ventricular activity, and positive P waves, which show atrial activity.

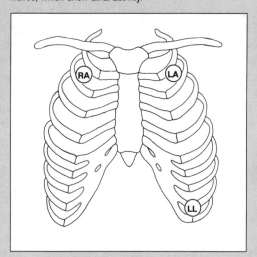

### Lead MCL₁
Using MCL₁, position the RA on the right side of the patient's chest just below the right clavicle. Position the LL on the right sternal border at the fourth intercostal space, and the LA electrode on the left side of the chest just below the clavicle.

Lead MCL₁ records the sequence of ventricular depolarization better than lead MCL₆ does, so it's used to differentiate between right or left bundle-branch heart block. It is also used when monitoring a patient with supraventricular impulses, atrial hypertrophy, and ventricular ectopy. Note that in MCL₁, you position the LL directly over the right ventricle.

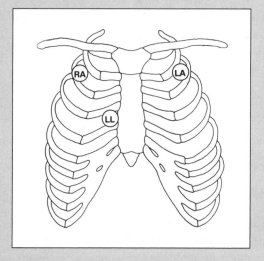

### Lead MCL₆
With lead MCL₆, position the RA just below the right clavicle, the LA just below the left clavicle, and the LL over the fifth intercostal space on the midaxillary line.

Lead MCL₆ is useful when you're monitoring a patient with a myocardial injury or infarction. It allows you to easily see tall QRS complexes so that you can identify right bundle-branch heart block and ST-segment and T-wave changes. In MCL₆, the LL lies over the apex of the left ventricle.

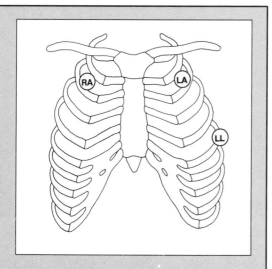

**Four- and five-electrode systems**
In a four-electrode system, a right leg (RL) or green electrode is added to provide a permanent ground for all leads used in the three-electrode system. Place this electrode on the right lower anterior rib cage.

A five-electrode system uses an additional exploratory chest electrode (C or V). This lets the examiner obtain any of the six modified chest leads and the standard limb leads as well. In this illustration, the chest electrode is in the V, position, but you can place this leadwire in any of the six chest lead positions.

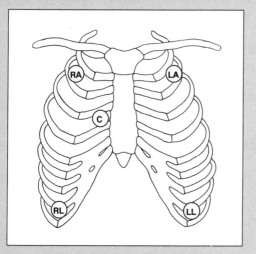

myocardial injury, and those who've received thrombolytic therapy. ST-segment monitoring also may be indicated for patients with head injury, chest trauma, major vascular trauma, bundle-branch heart block, pacemaker rhythms, electrolyte imbalances, pericarditis, hypothermia, or pulmonary infarction. Patients who are undergoing suctioning or receiving drugs such as vasopressors, potassium supplements, and digitalis glycosides also may benefit from ST-segment monitoring.

## Equipment
ST-segment software and computer ▪ cardiac monitor ▪ leadwires ▪ patient cable ▪ disposable pregelled electrodes (the number of electrodes varies from three to five, depending on the manufacturer) ▪ alcohol sponges ▪ $4'' \times 4''$ gauze pads ▪ optional: shaving supplies, washcloth.

## Preparation of equipment
Follow the manufacturer's recommendations to prepare the equipment. Use the primary channel to monitor for specific arrhythmias or heart blocks to which the patient is predisposed. Use the second channel to detect ischemic changes.

The specific leads you'll use depend on the patient's needs and clinical status. Research shows that leads $V_2$ and $V_3$ can best detect ST-segment elevation during occlusion of the left anterior descending coronary artery. Lead III is recommended for detecting occlusion of the left circumflex coronary artery, and lead II or $aV_F$, for detecting right coronary artery occlusion. Use lead $V_{4R}$ or lead $V_{6R}$ to monitor for right ventricular ischemia.

## Implementation
• If necessary, explain the purpose of ST-segment monitoring to the patient and his family. Emphasize why such monitoring is important to the patient's treatment regimen.
• Prepare the patient's skin by shaving any excess hair and thoroughly cleaning the sites where the electrodes will be placed. (See *Placing leads*

## ST-segment recording

This waveform, produced by ST-segment monitoring, displays ST-segment changes as an overlay on (or beside) the patient's normal pattern. The numbers beneath the waveform denote millimeters of ST depression or elevation.

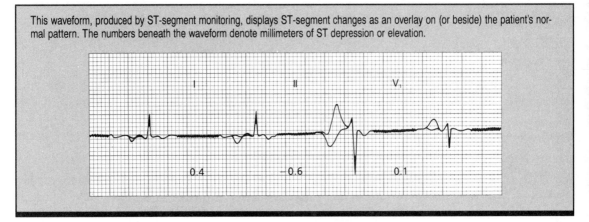

*for ST-segment monitoring,* page 37.) Dry the skin completely before placing the electrodes. *To promote better contact between the skin and electrodes,* rub the skin briskly.

• Apply the electrodes to the patient as appropriate for the selected leads. Be sure to position the electrodes precisely *to allow accurate detection of ST-segment changes.*

• Obtain rhythm strips at least every 8 to 12 hours, and place them in the patient's chart. You should also obtain rhythm strips whenever you note ST-segment changes, during interventions, and after each intervention to document its result.

• The doctor will tell you when to discontinue ST-segment monitoring.

### Special considerations

Closely observe the monitoring system to detect subtle changes in the patient's ST segment that may be precursors to major changes in his condition.

The monitoring system analyzes each ST segment for changes. Some systems analyze a block of ECG complexes, whereas others analyze individual complexes. Most systems compare ST segments with baseline data. Be sure to find out how the system you're using analyzes ST seg-

ments. Also find out how often it updates baseline data, how it's affected by interference, and how you can adjust it to get the most accurate analysis.

Monitoring systems that analyze trends in ST-segment changes can be especially valuable in coordinating nursing and patient self-care activities. You can determine, for example, how long the patient can be active before the ST segment changes. Be sure you understand how the software performs trend analysis *so you can interpret findings accurately.*

Assess electrode skin sites regularly for signs of an allergic reaction (such as redness and blisters) to the conduction gel or electrode patch, and switch to different types of gel or electrode patches if necessary. You should also note if the patient complains of any itching or irritation.

Change the electrode patches according to the manufacturer's recommendations or your hospital's policy.

## PAP and PAWP monitoring

Continuous PAP monitoring and intermittent pulmonary artery wedge pressure (PAWP) measurements provide important information about left ventricular function and preload. You can

## Placing leads for ST-segment monitoring

To ensure accuracy, you must place leads precisely for ST-segment monitoring. The first illustration shows where to place the four limb leads. The second illustration shows where to place the chest or precordial (V) leads. You may place the positive electrode at any V-lead position.

**Limb leads**

**V leads**

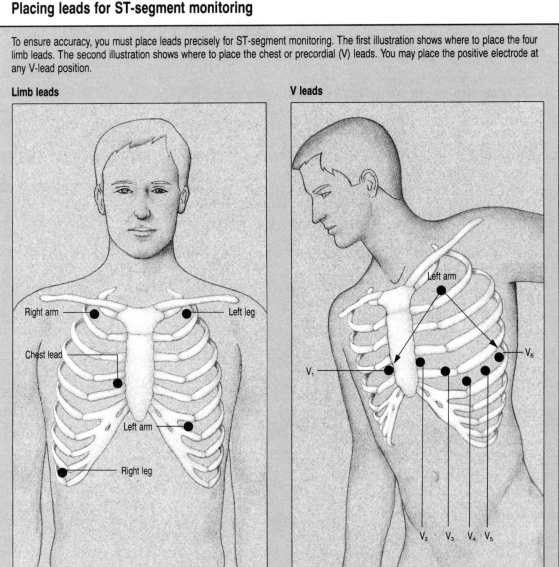

use this information not only for monitoring but also for aiding diagnosis, refining your assessment, guiding interventions, and projecting patient outcome.

Nearly all acutely ill patients are candidates for PAP monitoring—especially those who are hemodynamically unstable, who need fluid management or continuous cardiopulmonary assessment, or who are receiving multiple or frequently

## A look at the pulmonary artery catheter

The pulmonary artery catheter is made of pliable radiopaque polyvinylchloride and may contain two to six lumens.

When connected to a transducer, the distal lumen measures pulmonary artery pressure; during balloon inflation, it measures pulmonary artery wedge pressure (PAWP). It also permits drawing of mixed venous blood samples.

The proximal lumen measures central venous pressure. The balloon inflation lumen inflates the balloon at the distal tip of the catheter for PAWP measurement.

Other lumens may provide a port for pacemaker electrodes or a fiber-optic filament (an Opticath catheter) for measurement of mixed venous oxygen saturation ($S\bar{v}O_2$).

The latest six-lumen (right ventricular ejection fraction-volumetric fast-response thermistor) catheter is shown below. It incorporates intracardiac electrodes, which can be used with the thermistor to determine the right ventricular ejection fraction and systolic and end-diastolic right ventricular volumes.

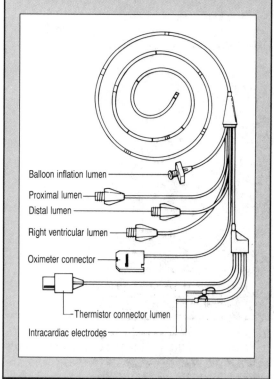

Balloon inflation lumen
Proximal lumen
Distal lumen
Right ventricular lumen
Oximeter connector
Thermistor connector lumen
Intracardiac electrodes

administered cardioactive drugs. PAP monitoring also is crucial for patients with shock, trauma, pulmonary or cardiac disease, or multiorgan disease.

The original PAP monitoring catheter, which had two lumens, was invented by two doctors, Swan and Ganz. The device still bears their name but is commonly referred to as a PA catheter. Current versions have up to six lumens, allowing you to gather additional hemodynamic information. (See *A look at the pulmonary artery catheter.*)

Fluoroscopy usually isn't required during catheter insertion because the catheter is flow directed, following venous blood flow from the right heart chambers into the pulmonary artery. Also, the pulmonary artery, right atrium, and right ventricle produce characteristic pressures and waveforms that can be observed on the monitor to help track catheter tip location. Marks on the catheter shaft, with 10-cm gradations, assist tracking by showing how far the catheter has been inserted.

The doctor inserts the PA catheter either percutaneously into the subclavian, jugular, or femoral vein or through a venous cutdown in the antecubital fossa. He then threads the catheter into the heart's right side with the distal tip lying in the pulmonary artery. Left-sided pressures can be assessed indirectly.

During ventricular systole, the tricuspid and mitral valves are closed and the pulmonic and aortic valves are open. The higher pressure generated by the right ventricle during contraction is transmitted to the catheter tip. With the balloon deflated, the catheter records pulmonary artery systolic pressure, which reflects right ventricular systolic pressure.

During ventricular diastole, the tricuspid and mitral valves are open, the ventricles are filling with blood from their respective atria, and the pulmonic and aortic valves are closed. With the balloon still deflated, pulmonary artery diastolic pressure (PADP) is recorded.

After the pulmonic valve closes, the right ventricle continues to relax, causing a lower diastolic pressure in the right ventricle than in the pulmonary artery. Right ventricular end-diastolic pressure (RVEDP) is less than PADP. The proximal lumen of the catheter exits in the right atrium or vena cava. During this phase, with a competent tricuspid valve, the RVEDP is reflected back to the right atrium. Therefore, right atrial pressure (RAP) is equal to RVEDP.

Because no obstruction normally exists between the pulmonary artery and the left atrium, the pressure recorded during diastole is virtually the same as left atrial pressure (LAP). With a pressure range of 6 to 20 mm Hg, this pressure is nearly the same as left ventricular end-diastolic pressure (LVEDP). PADP, LAP, and LVEDP are thus roughly equal, with PADP slightly higher than LAP by 1 to 4 mm Hg.

When the balloon is inflated, the catheter floats downstream into a more distal branch of the pulmonary artery. Once the balloon lodges, the catheter is wedged. Because of the absence of valves between the pulmonic and mitral valves, and because the pulmonary capillary bed is a compliant system, an unrestricted vascular channel now exists between the catheter tip in the pulmonary artery through the pulmonary vascular bed, the pulmonary vein, the left atrium, the open mitral valve, and into the left ventricle. The distal lumen is now monitoring left ventricular filling pressure, or LVEDP, more closely.

This pressure—usually referred to as PAWP—is also known as left atrial filling pressure, pulmonary capillary wedge pressure, pulmonary artery occlusion pressure, or the wedge. The importance of PAWP is that normally it closely approximates the pressure in the left ventricle during end diastole and provides a means of measuring left ventricular preload.

No specific contraindications for PAP monitoring exist. However, some patients undergoing PAP monitoring require special precautions. These include older patients with pulmonary hypertension, those with left bundle-branch heart block, and those for whom a systemic infection would be life-threatening.

## Equipment

Pressure cuff ▪ balloon-tipped, flow-directed PA catheter ▪ bag of heparin flush solution (usually 500 ml of 0.9% sodium chloride solution with 500 or 1,000 units of heparin) ▪ alcohol sponges ▪ medication-added label ▪ preassembled disposable pressure tubing with flush device and disposable transducer ▪ monitor and monitor cable ▪ I.V. pole with transducer mount ▪ emergency resuscitation equipment ▪ ECG monitor ▪ ECG electrodes ▪ arm board (for antecubital insertion) ▪ lead aprons (if fluoroscope is used during insertion) ▪ sutures ▪ sterile 4″ × 4″ gauze pads or other dry, occlusive dressing material ▪ prepackaged introducer kit ▪ optional: dextrose 5% in water ($D_5W$), shaving materials (if a femoral insertion site is used).

If a prepackaged introducer kit is unavailable, obtain the following: introducer (one size larger than catheter) ▪ sterile tray containing instruments for procedure ▪ masks ▪ sterile gowns ▪ sterile gloves ▪ povidone-iodine ointment ▪ sutures ▪ two 10-ml syringes ▪ local anesthetic (1% to 2% lidocaine) ▪ one 5-ml syringe ▪ 25G ½″ needle ▪ 1″ and 3″ tape.

## Preparation of equipment

You'll need to obtain at least one single-channel transducer and flush system for PAP and PAWP readings. The number of other systems needed will depend on the catheter inserted and specific monitoring requirements.

Turn on the monitor *to allow it to warm up.* Make sure the pressure module is in the monitor if one isn't built in. Wash your hands and maintain sterile technique as you prepare the equipment.

Insert a tubing spike into the bag of heparin flush solution. Withdraw air from the bag by inserting a large-gauge needle into the bag's injection port and squeezing the bag gently until no air remains. Or, *to decrease the number of entries into the bag and minimize the risk of contamination,* invert the I.V. bag to allow air to move to the top, and squeeze air into the drip chamber. Make sure the roller clamp is closed.

If necessary, place the transducer in the pole mount on the I.V. pole. (Some transducers don't need to be mounted; they can be laid on the bed.)

Squeeze the drip chamber until it's half full. Open the roller clamp and prime the tubing by activating the flush device. (Follow the manufacturer's directions for flushing the transducer and tubing. Many transducers need to be inverted so that air isn't trapped during flushing.) As you flush, replace each vented stopcock with a sterile dead-end cap.

Verify that no air remains in the tubing. Then insert the heparin flush bag into the pressure bag and inflate it to 300 mm Hg. This will create a flow rate between 2 and 5 ml/hour. (Some hospitals recommend inflating the bag with less pressure before insertion, believing that the transducer may be damaged if it's pressurized before insertion.) Connect the monitor cable to the transducer.

If you have a reusable transducer and transducer dome, follow the manufacturer's directions for attaching the dome to the transducer and to the preassembled pressure tubing and flush system. (You may need to place several drops of sterile sodium chloride solution or bacteriostatic water on the transducer's surface before attaching the dome.)

## Implementation

• Explain the procedure to the patient *to allay his fears and promote cooperation.* Make sure he understands and has signed a consent form.

• Place the ECG electrodes on the patient, if they're not already in place, and connect them to the cardiac monitor. For subclavian catheter insertion, keep the chest electrodes on the side opposite the insertion site.

• Bring the equipment to the same side of the patient as the insertion site. Connect the monitor

cable to the transducer, and plug it into the monitor.

### Zeroing and calibrating the system

• Position the transducer level with the right atrium by locating the fourth intercostal space at the midaxillary line, the phlebostatic axis. Adjust the transducer to the proper level.

• Remove the dead-end cap, and open the stopcock closest to the transducer (or follow the manufacturer's guidelines) *to open the transducer to air.*

• Zero and calibrate it according to the manufacturer's directions. (Some monitors calibrate automatically.) Then replace the dead-end cap, and close the stopcock to this port.

### Assisting with catheter insertion

• Make sure you have emergency resuscitation equipment available.

• Maintaining sterile technique, open the tray containing the equipment for insertion.

• Position the patient supine or in a slight Trendelenburg position with the insertion site exposed.

• Put on a mask and goggles, and help the doctor to put on a sterile gown, mask, goggles, and gloves. If catheter placement will be guided by fluoroscopy, the doctor must wear a lead apron under the sterile gown. You should also put one on. Place a mask over the patient's nose and mouth, if desired.

• Open the supplies as ordered, or assist with the opening of the prepackaged introducer material, maintaining sterile technique.

• Clean the top of the local anesthetic bottle with an alcohol sponge, and invert it *so the doctor can insert the syringe and withdraw the drug.*

• Connect the pressure tubing to the proximal and distal catheter lumens as ordered. Using the pressure tubing fast-flush device, flush each lumen. The doctor will inflate the balloon and verify its integrity before catheter insertion.

• Once all lines are prepared, the doctor will insert the catheter via the introducer. The balloon is inflated intermittently *to allow normal blood flow and to aid catheter insertion.*

• As the doctor advances the catheter, monitor pressure in each chamber and ECG tracings *to help locate the catheter if it accidentally moves backward from the pulmonary artery (especially into the right ventricle, which may cause arrhythmias).* (See *Monitoring pressure tracings,* page 42.)

• After the doctor sutures the catheter, put on sterile gloves and apply povidone-iodine ointment to the insertion site (if in accordance with hospital policy).

• Apply a dry, occlusive dressing — either sterile gauze or a transparent dressing — to the site. Then use tape to secure the catheter to the dressing *to prevent accidental dislodgment.*

• If the line was inserted into the antecubital fossa, apply a padded arm board *to keep the arm from bending.*

• Write the date, the time, and your initials on a piece of tape and place it on the dressing.

• Remove all used or unnecessary equipment from the room, and properly discard all disposable equipment. Send reusable equipment for sterilization.

• Arrange for a chest X-ray at the patient's bedside *to verify correct catheter placement.*

### Taking a PAP reading

• Make sure all the stopcocks are set properly.

• Observe the monitor for pulmonary artery systolic and diastolic waveforms, and obtain waveform strips *for documentation and baseline reference and to accurately plot PAP values.*

• Record the systolic and diastolic waveform and mean values. Some monitors record these continuously; some require manual setting.

### Taking a PAWP reading

• Make sure the machine is set to monitor mean pressure.

(Some monitors automatically change to mean during wedging.)

• To the balloon port, attach a syringe (of the size specified on the catheter shaft) filled with the maximum amount of air (usually 1.0 to 1.5 cc). Some catheter kits contain a syringe with a gauge that prevents larger amounts of air from being injected.

• Slowly inject the air from the syringe into the balloon while observing the monitor screen. Inject only until the PAP waveform changes to the PAWP waveform. *The PAWP waveform often occurs before the maximum amount of air is injected — depending on the size of the pulmonary artery and the position of the PA catheter.*

• Record the mean pressure.

• Remove the syringe and leave the port lock in the open position *to allow air to escape and to prevent the balloon from accidentally remaining inflated.*

• Check the waveform on the monitor screen *to verify that the catheter has returned to a pulmonary artery position.*

• According to hospital policy, activate the fast-flush release to flush the catheter, *which helps reposition the catheter tip.*

• Set the high and low alarms as required by hospital policy.

### Special considerations

Use sterile technique throughout the procedure *to avoid infection.* Prevent exsanguination from a disconnection in the system by using luer-locks or other positive locks at all connections, keeping the catheter and all parts of the system unobscured, and making sure the monitor and alarms are on at all times. Always observe electrical-hazard precautions. (For further information, see *Identifying hemodynamic pressure monitoring problems,* pages 43 and 44.)

Activate the fast-flush release at intervals specified by the hospital's policy *to prevent thrombus formation.*

Frequently check the involved extremity, if applicable, for pulse, color, temperature, and sensation. Notify the doctor of any changes.

Change the catheter dressing at each tubing change, when it becomes wet or soiled, or at intervals specified by hospital policy.

*(Text continues on page 44.)*

# Monitoring pressure tracings

Characteristic waveforms appear on the cardiac monitor as the pulmonary artery (PA) catheter is passed through the heart.

### Right atrial pressure
When the catheter tip reaches the right atrium from the superior vena cava, the waveform looks like the one shown below. The doctor then inflates the balloon. This carries the tip through the tricuspid valve and into the right ventricle.

**Normal range**
Mean: 3 to 6 mm Hg

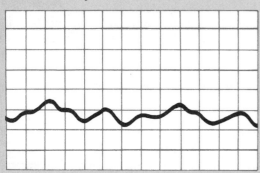

### Right ventricular pressure
When the catheter tip reaches the right ventricle, the waveform looks like the one shown below.

**Normal range**
Systolic: 17 to 22 mm Hg
Diastolic: 1 to 7 mm Hg

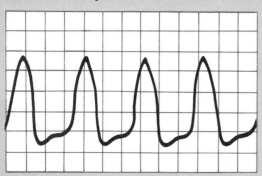

### Pulmonary artery pressure (PAP)
The waveform below appears when the catheter tip has moved through the pulmonic valve and into the pulmonary artery.

**Normal range**
Systolic: 17 to 32 mm Hg
Diastolic: 4 to 13 mm Hg
Mean: 9 to 19 mm Hg

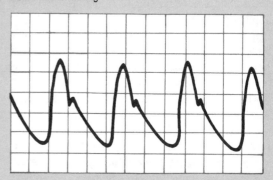

### Pulmonary artery wedge pressure
The waveform below appears once the PA catheter's balloon, carried by the circulation, becomes wedged in a small vessel. At this point the doctor will deflate the balloon, which causes the catheter tip to slip back into the main branch of the pulmonary artery. The PAP waveform then reappears.

**Normal range**
Mean: 8 to 12 mm Hg

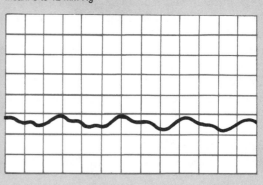

## Identifying hemodynamic pressure monitoring problems

| PROBLEM | POSSIBLE CAUSES | INTERVENTIONS |
|---|---|---|
| No waveform | • Power supply turned off<br>• Monitor screen pressure range set too low<br><br>• Loose connection in line<br>• Transducer not connected to amplifier<br>• Stopcock off to patient<br>• Catheter occluded or out of blood vessel | • Check power supply.<br>• Raise monitor screen pressure range, if necessary.<br>• Rebalance and recalibrate equipment.<br>• Tighten loose connections.<br>• Check and tighten connection.<br>• Position stopcock correctly.<br>• Use fast-flush valve to flush line, or try to aspirate blood from catheter. If line remains blocked, notify doctor and prepare to replace line. |
| Drifting waveforms | • Improper warm-up<br><br>• Electrical cable kinked or compressed<br><br>• Temperature change in room air or I.V. flush solution | • Allow monitor and transducer to warm up for 10 to 15 minutes.<br>• Place monitor's cable where it can't be stepped on or compressed.<br>• Routinely zero and calibrate equipment 30 minutes after setting it up to allow I.V. fluid to warm to room temperature. |
| Line fails to flush | • Stopcocks positioned incorrectly<br>• Inadequate pressure from pressure bag<br>• Kink in pressure tubing<br>• Blood clot in catheter | • Make sure stopcocks are positioned correctly.<br>• Make sure pressure bag gauge reads 300 mm Hg.<br>• Check pressure tubing for kinks.<br>• Try to aspirate clot with a syringe. If line still won't flush, notify doctor and prepare to replace line, if necessary. *Important:* Never use a syringe to flush a hemodynamic line. |
| Waveform interference | • Patient movement<br>• Electrical interference<br><br>• Catheter fling (tip of pulmonary artery catheter moving rapidly in large blood vessel or heart chamber) | • Wait until patient is quiet before taking a reading.<br>• Make sure electrical equipment is connected and grounded correctly.<br>• Notify doctor. He may try to reposition catheter. |
| False-high readings | • Transducer balancing port positioned below patient's right atrium<br>• Flush solution flow rate too fast<br><br>• Air in system<br>• Catheter fling (tip of pulmonary artery catheter moving rapidly in large blood vessel or heart chamber) | • Position balancing port level with patient's right atrium.<br>• Check flush solution flow rate. Maintain it at 3 to 4 ml/hour.<br>• Remove air from lines and transducer.<br>• Notify doctor, who may try to reposition catheter. |
| False-low readings | • Transducer balancing port positioned above right atrium<br>• Transducer imbalance<br><br>• Loose connection | • Position balancing port level with patient's right atrium.<br>• Make sure transducer's flow system isn't kinked or occluded and rebalance and recalibrate equipment.<br>• Tighten loose connections. |

*(continued)*

## Identifying hemodynamic pressure monitoring problems *(continued)*

| PROBLEM | POSSIBLE CAUSES | INTERVENTIONS |
|---|---|---|
| Damped waveform | • Air bubbles | • Secure all connections.<br>• Remove air from lines and transducer.<br>• Check for and replace cracked equipment. |
| | • Blood clot in catheter | • Refer to "Line fails to flush" (this chart). |
| | • Blood flashback in line | • Make sure stopcock positions are correct; tighten loose connections and replace cracked equipment; flush line with fast-flush valve; replace transducer dome if blood backs up into it. |
| | • Transducer position | • Make sure transducer is kept at level of patient's right atrium at all times. Improper levels give false-high or false-low pressure readings. |
| | • Arterial catheter out of blood vessel or pressed against vessel wall | • Reposition if catheter is against vessel wall.<br>• Try to aspirate blood to confirm proper placement in vessel. If you can't aspirate blood, notify doctor and prepare to replace line. *Note:* Bloody drainage at insertion site may indicate catheter displacement. Notify doctor immediately. |
| Pulmonary artery wedge pressure tracing unobtainable | • Ruptured balloon | • If you feel no resistance when injecting air, or if you see blood leaking from balloon inflation lumen, stop injecting air and notify doctor. If catheter is left in, label inflation lumen with warning not to inflate. |
| | • Incorrect amount of air in balloon | • Deflate balloon. Check label on catheter for correct volume. Reinflate slowly with correct amount. To avoid rupturing balloon, never use more than stated volume. |
| | • Catheter malpositioned | • Notify doctor. Obtain chest X-ray. |

Take PAP and PAWP readings at the end of expiration. To do this, assess the patient's chest, noting when he completely exhales because *when he inhales, intrathoracic pressure drops, causing a decline in cardiac pressures.* When he exhales, intrathoracic pressure rises causing a slight elevation of cardiac pressures. Because of this, the pressure at the end of expiration is the best indicator of normal cardiac pressures without respiratory interference.

*To prevent infection,* change tubing, stopcocks, continuous flush devices, and fluid for infusion every 24 to 72 hours, depending on hospital policy.

Besides monitoring arterial pressures, you can also monitor central venous pressure (CVP), if ordered. Set the stopcocks to allow direct communication between the proximal lumen and the transducer, set the monitor to mean, observe the waveform, and record the CVP measurement. Return the stopcocks to their original positions.

Positive pressure ventilation may alter the patient's reading in any direction. Pressures should be recorded with the patient on the ventilator.

$D_5W$ is sometimes used as the I.V. solution *because it's not a plasma expander and doesn't conduct electric current.* However, the dextrose also provides a medium for bacteria growth.

*Nursing alert:* During catheter insertion, alert the doctor immediately if the patient experiences arrhythmias, dyspnea, tachypnea, hemoptysis, stridor, or drastic changes in vital signs or pressure readings. *These may indicate cardiac perforation, pulmonary artery rupture, hemorrhage, pneumothorax, or hemothorax.*

Note the volume of air needed to achieve a wedge. If the volume of air needed is significantly below that indicated on the catheter, notify the doctor *because the catheter may have migrated distally.* Also notify the doctor if the volume of air needed is close to the maxiumum of 1.5 cc *because the catheter may need to be advanced.* You should feel resistance when inflating the balloon. If you don't, notify the doctor immediately — *the balloon may have ruptured.*

*Nursing alert:* Never introduce air into a balloon if you suspect it's ruptured; *this can cause an air embolus.* Prevent balloon rupture by knowing the maximum volume of the balloon, and avoid overinflating the balloon or aspirating from it. Don't leave the balloon wedged for more than 15 to 30 seconds. *Air in the flush system can also cause an embolus.*

If the waveform won't return to PAP from PAWP, or if it's damping with low numbers and a decreased pulmonary artery systolic-diastolic differential, check for equipment problems. Then check the patient's blood pressure and pulse rate. If these aren't changed, the catheter is probably wedged. *Because a permanent wedge can cause pulmonary infarct and necrosis,* flush the PAP port *to push the catheter tip away from a vessel wall.* (Don't activate the fast-flush release, which could rupture capillaries.) Then check for a slowed drip rate and increased pressure readings — signs that the catheter is still wedged. If it is, turn the patient on his right side, and instruct him to cough as you flush the line. If the waveform doesn't return to the PAP area, turn the patient onto his left side and repeat the procedure. If there's still no change, notify the doctor immediately.

Also, closely monitor the PA waveform, remaining alert for spontaneous wedging. Spontaneous wedging may occur if the PA catheter migrates into a small branch of the pulmonary artery. If this happens, follow the steps listed in the preceding paragraph.

Avoid administering large volumes of fluid and drugs through the distal port *because vessel spasm or rupture may result.*

## Complications

Various complications can occur during hemodynamic monitoring. These include infection, air embolism, pulmonary artery perforation, ventricular arrhythmias, tricuspid or pulmonic valve damage, and tension pneumothorax, which may occur during insertion.

## Documentation

Record the time, size, and type of catheter inserted, insertion site, vital signs, administration of drugs (if any), initial PAP and PAWP readings and tracings, and patient's tolerance of the procedure. Start a flowchart of PAP readings and tracings, noting any changes.

# CVP monitoring

Measurements of CVP are monitored with a manometer or pressure transducer system connected to a catheter that's threaded through the subclavian or jugular vein (or through the basilic, cephalic, or saphenous veins) and placed in or near the right atrium. This procedure accurately determines RAP, which reflects RVEDP and the pumping ability of the right side of the heart. CVP is also used to assess blood volume and vascular tone.

Because CVP rises only after significant changes have occurred in the left heart or pulmonary venous system, CVP monitoring has been replaced in most hospitals by PA catheterization for assessing rapidly changing cardiovascular status. PA catheterization uses PAP and PAWP measurements to detect cardiovascular changes.

## Interpreting CVP findings

To interpret pressure readings correctly, establish a normal central venous pressure (CVP) for the patient. The average CVP may range from 2 to 4 cm $H_2O$ or 3 to 8 mm Hg, but it varies from patient to patient. To establish a normal range, measure CVP at 15-, 30-, and 60-minute intervals.

**What to do if readings vary**
If a reading differs from the established range by more than 2 cm $H_2O$, double-check it by taking vital signs and assessing the patient's cardiopulmonary status.
If these appear stable, check the I.V. line for patency and review the measurement procedure. Remember, a blocked line can cause a false-low reading. Notify the doctor if you're sure the abnormal reading reflects actual CVP and if CVP deviates from the range set for the patient.

**Why CVP measurements are important**
Don't rely on vital signs to reflect stable cardiovascular states; regular CVP measurements can detect disorders before changes in vital signs are apparent. For example, a high CVP reading may signal congestive heart failure, hypervolemia, vasoconstriction, or early-stage cardiac tamponade; a low reading may signal peripheral blood pooling, hypovolemia, vasoconstriction, or vasodilation.
If the CVP changes significantly, the doctor will probably order a chest X-ray to detect possible disorders or to detect possible migration of the catheter tip.

CVP measurements can be obtained directly from the PA catheter.

CVP is measured in millimeters of mercury or centimeters of water. The normal range varies with the patient's size, position, and hydration state. CVP readings may be obtained continuously, through the use of a transducer, or intermittently, through the use of a manometer. (See *Interpreting CVP findings*.)

## Equipment
### For intermittent monitoring
Disposable CVP manometer set with stopcock, extension tubing, and leveling rod or yardstick ▪ additional stopcock ▪ I.V. pole ▪ I.V. solution, as ordered ▪ I.V. tubing ▪ tape ▪ marking pen ▪ optional: extension tubing, dressing materials.

### For continuous monitoring
Pressure monitoring kit with disposable pressure transducer ▪ leveling device ▪ bedside pressure module with oscilloscope ▪ bag of heparin flush solution (usually 500 ml of 0.9% sodium chloride solution with 500 or 1,000 units of heparin) ▪ pressure bag.

If you'll need to obtain a blood sample from a CVP line, also assemble: 5-ml syringe ▪ 5- to 10-ml syringe (depending upon the amount of blood to be drawn) ▪ stopcock or heparin lock device ▪ optional: blood collection tubes.

If you'll be removing a CVP line, gather: suture removal kit ▪ sterile $4'' \times 4''$ gauze pads ▪ antimicrobial ointment ▪ dry, sterile dressing ▪ hypoallergenic tape.

## Preparation of equipment
Gather the appropriate equipment and wash your hands.

### For intermittent CVP monitoring
Clamp the manometer to the I.V. pole, spike the I.V. container, and hang it 30" to 36" (76 to 91 cm) above the insertion site *to prevent blood from backing up in the catheter.*

Now examine the stopcock *to learn the proper operating positions.* (See *Stopcock positoning and operation.*)

Next, insert the distal end of the tubing into the left side of the stopcock. Turn the stopcock to the container-to-patient position, open the flow clamp, and flush the tubing. Then turn the stopcock to the container-to-manometer position. Make sure the tubing doesn't contain an in-line filter, which can distort pressure readings. Fill the manometer column with I.V. solution (about 20 to 25 cm $H_2O$ or about 10 cm $H_2O$ higher than the expected CVP value). Then close the flow clamp on the tubing. Avoid overfilling the manometer *to prevent inactivation of the filter and increased risk of contamination; also, if a small*

## Stopcock positioning and operation

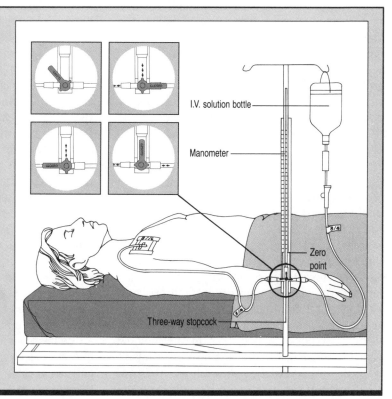

To ensure accurate central venous pressure readings, the base of the manometer must be aligned with the right atrium. For this reason, the manometer set usually contains a leveling rod to allow you to determine quickly that the base of the manometer is level with the previously determined zero reference point.

After adjusting the manometer's position, examine the three-way stopcock. By turning it to any position shown, you can control the direction of fluid flow. Four-way stopcocks are also available; the fourth position blocks all openings.

I.V. solution bottle

Manometer

Zero point

Three-way stopcock

---

*plastic ball is used to indicate fluid level in the manometer, it may be forced from the tube and rendered useless.*

### For continuous CVP monitoring

Make sure that the central line or the proximal lumen of a PA catheter is attached to the system. (If the patient has a central line with multiple lumens, one lumen may be dedicated to continuous CVP monitoring and the other lumens to administering fluids.) In this instance, use the distal port, which terminates in the right atrium, for CVP monitoring. Then set up a pressure transducer system as you would for monitoring PAP. Connect noncompliant pressure tubing from the CVP catheter hub to the transducer. Then

connect the flush solution container to a flush device.

### Implementation

• Explain the procedure to the patient *to allay his fears and promote cooperation.*

### Performing intermittent CVP monitoring

• Loosen the protective cover on the distal end of the extension tubing (from the stopcock to the patient), and ask the patient to perform Valsalva's maneuver *to avoid formation of an air embolus.* Quickly disconnect the existing I.V. tubing, remove the protective covering from the new tubing, and connect it to the patient's catheter.

• If the patient is unconscious, wait until he inhales fully, and then quickly connect the tubing.

Lowering the head of the bed also helps prevent an air embolus in a patient unable to cooperate. If the patient is intubated, maintain full inflation as you connect the tubing. Finally, adjust the flow clamp to the desired infusion rate.

• Place the patient in a supine position (his head can be slightly raised). He doesn't need to be kept flat. *Studies show this to be unnecessary for accurate monitoring as long as the zero mark on the manometer remains at the zero reference point and the patient's position stays the same for each reading.*

• Adjust the position of the manometer so that the stopcock aligns horizontally with the right atrium.

• *To find the position of the right atrium,* locate the fourth intercostal space at the midaxillary line (phlebostatic axis). This site becomes the zero reference point—the location for all subsequent readings. Mark this area on the patient's skin.

• If the manometer has a leveling rod, extend it between the zero reference point and the zero mark at the bottom of the manometer scale. If the rod has a small viewing window, a bubble will appear between two lines in the window when the rod is horizontal. If a leveling rod isn't available, use a yardstick with a level attached. With this, you can also watch the bubble on the level to determine when the yardstick is horizontal.

• When the stopcock of the manometer is level with the right atrium, tape the manometer set to the I.V. pole *to secure its position.* Recheck the level before each pressure reading. If an adjustment is required, first raise or lower the bed and then readjust the manometer on the I.V. pole as necessary *to maintain alignment with the atrium.*

• Check the patency of the line by briefly increasing the infusion rate. If the line isn't patent, notify the doctor. Never irrigate a clogged CVP line *because doing so could release a thrombus.* If the line is patent, proceed.

• Turn the stopcock to the container-to-manometer position *to slowly fill the manometer with I.V. solution,* as before.

• Turn the stopcock to the manometer-to-patient position; the fluid level then falls with inspiration, as intrathoracic pressure decreases, and rises slightly with expiration.

• When the fluid column stabilizes, tap the manometer lightly *to dislodge air bubbles that may distort pressure readings.* Then position yourself so that the top of the fluid column is at eye level. Expect the column to rise and fall slightly as the patient breathes. Note the lowest level the fluid reaches, and take your reading from the base of the meniscus. If the manometer has a small ball floating on the fluid surface, take the reading from the ball's midline. If the fluid fails to fluctuate during the patient's breathing, the end of the catheter may be pressed against the vein wall. Ask the patient to cough *to change the catheter's position slightly.*

• Maintain catheter patency by returning the stopcock to the container-to-patient position as soon as you take the reading. Then check for blood backflow.

• Readjust the infusion rate and make sure that all connections are secure *to minimize the risk of hemorrhage or an air embolus.* (Some hospital policies recommend taping all connections for these reasons.)

• Return the patient to a comfortable position.

### Performing continuous CVP monitoring

• Position the patient flat. If he can't tolerate this position, use semi-Fowler's position. Locate the level of the right atrium by identifying the phlebostatic axis.

• Zero the transducer, leveling the transducer air-fluid interface stopcock with the right atrium.

• Read the CVP value from the digital display on the monitor and note the waveform. Both the numerical value and the waveform provide valuable information about the patient's status. If possible, obtain a printout of the patient's CVP waveform to correlate with the ECG waveform.

• Document the patient's position during the CVP reading and then use this same position for all subsequent readings.

### Obtaining blood samples through a CV line

• Wash your hands and maintain sterile technique throughout the procedure.

• If the catheter was inserted using a superior approach (such as through the jugular or subclavian vein), position the patient flat *to prevent entry of air into the bloodstream.*

• As appropriate, attach a stopcock to the end of the catheter or use a heparin lock device.

• Attach a 5-ml syringe to the stopcock or heparin lock device. Then withdraw and discard approximately 5 ml of blood from the catheter. This removes I.V. solution from the inner lumen of the catheter and helps ensure accurate laboratory values. Dispose of the sample according to hospital policy.

• For the laboratory samples, withdraw blood from the stopcock or heparin lock attachment. The amount to withdraw depends on the test ordered.

• After withdrawing blood, flush the CV line with I.V. solution and restart the infusion. If using a heparin lock device, flush the line by attaching a separate syringe of sterile solution (usually 0.9% sodium chloride solution). As ordered, add heparin to the solution to prevent clotting of the catheter lumen.

• Alternatively, you may use a closed system to obtain blood samples through a CVP line. (See *Understanding the closed blood sampling system,* page 50.)

### Removing a CV line

• Assist the doctor in removing a CV line. (In some states, you may remove the catheter with a doctor's order or when acting under advanced collaborative standards of practice.)

• If the head of the bed is elevated, take measures to minimize the risk of air embolism during catheter removal. For instance, place the patient in Trendelenburg's position if the line was inserted using a superior approach. If the patient can't tolerate this position, position him flat.

• Turn the patient's head to the side opposite the catheter insertion site. The doctor or nurse removes the dressing and exposes the insertion site. If sutures are in place, the doctor will remove them carefully.

• Turn the I.V. solution off.

• The doctor or nurse pulls the catheter out in a slow, smooth motion and then applies pressure to the insertion site for at least 2 minutes.

• Clean the insertion site with gauze pads, apply antimicrobial ointment, and cover it with a sterile dressing, as ordered.

• Assess the patient for bleeding at the insertion site or for signs of respiratory distress, which may indicate air embolism.

• Document the date and time of catheter removal, the type of dressing applied, and the patient's tolerance for the procedure.

### Special considerations

If the patient is connected to a ventilator and is receiving positive end-expiratory pressure, you may obtain variable CVP readings. *To detect significant changes,* record all pressure readings while the patient is connected to the ventilator, and take readings at end-expiration before the next inspiration begins.

Report any deviations from the prescribed CVP range to the doctor. Avoid making pressure observations when the patient is sitting up *because this position causes false-low measurements if the patient has been put in a sitting position within 3 minutes of your manometer reading.* Remember that the patient with chronic obstructive pulmonary disease usually has a high CVP.

### Documentation

Record the time, date, and pressure reading. If the patient was placed in a special position, note this on the nursing Kardex to ensure consistent readings.

## Cardiac output monitoring

Measuring cardiac output—the amount of blood ejected from the heart—helps evaluate cardiac function. Normal output is 4 to 8 liters/minute.

## Understanding the closed blood sampling system

Unlike an open blood sampling system, a closed system has a reservoir that doesn't allow air to enter the system during blood collection. It eliminates the use of needles and permits reinfusion of unused but collected blood.

After the reservoir has been filled with blood, a syringe with an attached cannula is connected to the blood sampling site. Blood is withdrawn into the syringe. Once the syringe and cannula have been removed, the blood in the reservoir can be slowly reinfused.

The illustration shows the closed sampling system.

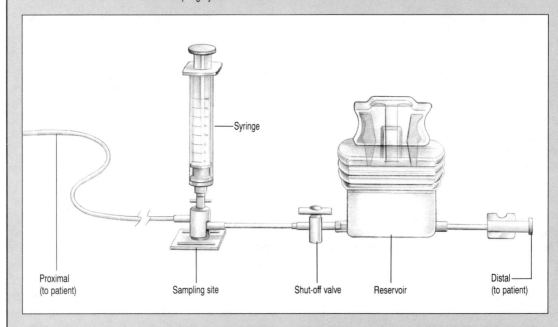

Low cardiac output can be caused by decreased myocardial contractility from myocardial infarction, drug effects, acidosis, or hypoxia. Other possible causes include decreased left ventricular filling pressure from fluid depletion or increased systemic tension. Output can also fall below normal as a result of decreased blood flow from the ventricles in valvular heart disease.

High cardiac output can occur with some arteriovenous shunts and from decreased vascular resistance (for example, in septic shock), or it can be unusually high but still normal (for example, in well-conditioned athletes).

Cardiac output is measured indirectly by the thermodilution method. Other methods include the Fick method and the indicator-dilution test, although these are usually confined to research projects or the cardiac catheterization laboratory. (See *Determining cardiac output using the Fick and indicator-dilution methods*.)

In the thermodilution method, a balloon-tipped, flow-directed catheter is inserted into a large vein, advanced to the right side of the heart, and positioned in the pulmonary artery. A solution is injected into the proximal or right atrium port of the PA catheter. A computer then calculates the cardiac output from the temperature changes in the injected solution in the proximal lumen and the temperature of the pulmonary

## Determining cardiac output using the Fick and indicator-dilution methods

Besides bolus thermodilution, two other techniques can be used to measure cardiac output: the Fick method and the indicator-dilution method. Although these two older methods may be highly accurate, their use is usually confined to research projects or the cardiac catheterization laboratory.

### Fick method
Often used as a standard by which other cardiac output measurement methods are evaluated, the Fick method measures the blood's oxygen content before and after it passes through the lungs.

By determining the amount of oxygen taken up from every 100 ml of blood during one passage through the tissues and the total volume of oxygen taken up by the body during a period of time (the body's oxygen consumption), you can calculate the number of 100-ml increments that passed through the body during that time.

For example, if 5 cc of oxygen is taken up from 100 ml of blood, and 300 cc of oxygen is taken up in 1 minute, then 60 increments of 5 cc of oxygen must have flowed through the tissues during that minute, indicating a cardiac output of 6 liters/minute.

Measuring cardiac output by the Fick method requires venous and arterial blood samples to determine the arterial and venous oxygen difference. Oxygen consumption – the amount of air entering the lungs each minute – is calculated using a spirometer. Next, cardiac output is calculated:

$$\text{cardiac output} = \frac{\text{oxygen consumption (cc/min)}}{\text{arterial oxygen}\atop\text{content (cc/min)} - {\text{venous oxygen}\atop\text{content (cc/min)}}}$$

### Indicator-dilution method
In this method, dye is injected into the right superior vena cava or right atrium. A blood sample is then taken from a peripheral arterial site to measure the concentration of the dye. Cardiac output is calculated by dividing the quantity of the dye injected in the blood by the mean concentration of dye in the blood and time in minutes.

This method is particularly helpful in detecting intracardiac shunts and valvular insufficiency, but measurements aren't accurate if these conditions are already present. The indicator-dilution method is more accurate in high cardiac output states.

---

artery. (See *Closed cardiac output systems,* page 52.)

## Equipment
Cardiac output machine (portable or within the monitoring system ▪ 500-ml bag of D₅W ▪ closed injection system ▪ 10-ml syringe ▪ stopcocks ▪ optional: styrofoam container, crushed ice, and water for icing injectant.

## Preparation of equipment
Gather all the equipment and bring it to the patient's bedside. Insert the closed injection system tubing into the 500-ml bag of I.V. solution. Connect the 10-ml syringe to the system tubing and prime the tubing with I.V. solution until it's free of air. Then clamp the tubing. The steps that follow differ, depending on whether you're using an iced or room-temperature injectant.

### For an iced injectant
Place the coiled segment into the styrofoam container and add crushed ice and water to cover the entire coil. Let the solution cool for 15 to 20 minutes. Next, connect the primed system to the stopcock of the proximal injection lumen of the PA catheter. Then connect the temperature probe from the cardiac output computer to the closed injection system's flow-through housing device. Connect the cardiac output computer cable to the thermistor connector on the PA catheter and verify the blood temperature reading. Finally, turn on the cardiac output computer and enter the correct computation constant, as provided by the catheter's manufacturer. The constant is determined by the volume and temperature of the injectant as well as the size and type of catheter. (With children, you'll need to adjust the computation constant to reflect a smaller volume and a smaller catheter size.)

## Closed cardiac output systems

This illustration shows the equipment needed to measure cardiac output, using a closed injection delivery system. First, an iced or room-temperature solution is injected into the proximal or right atrium port of the pulmonary artery catheter.

A computer then calculates the cardiac output from temperature changes in the injectant in the proximal lumen and the temperature at the pulmonary artery. The thermistor on the catheter tip measures the temperature at the pulmonary artery. The computer displays the cardiac output as a digital readout.

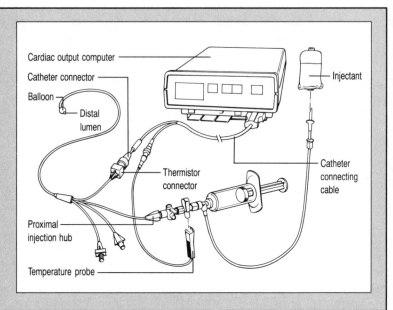

### For a room-temperature injectant
Connect the primed system to the stopcock of the proximal injection lumen of the PA catheter. Then connect the temperature probe from the cardiac output computer to the closed injection system's flow-through housing device. Connect the cardiac output computer cable to the thermistor connector on the PA catheter and verify the blood temperature reading. Finally, turn on the cardiac output computer and enter the correct computation constant, as provided by the catheter's manufacturer. The constant is determined by the volume and temperature of the injectant as well as the size and type of catheter.

### Implementation
• Wash your hands. Explain the procedure to the patient. Tell him that you'll be injecting a solution into the catheter in his heart. Tell him that this will help determine how well his heart is pumping. Assure him that he won't feel any discomfort. Advise him not to move during the procedure, *because movement can cause error in measurement.*
• Place the patient in the supine position (his head can be slightly elevated.)

### Determining cardiac output using iced injectant
• Unclamp the I.V. tubing and withdraw 5 ml of solution into the syringe. (With children, use 3 ml or less.)
• Inject the solution until it flows past the temperature sensor while you observe the injectant temperature that registers on the computer. Verify that the injectant temperature is between 43° F and 54° F (6° C and 12° C).
• Verify a PA waveform on the cardiac monitor.
• Withdraw exactly 10 ml of cooled solution before reclamping the tubing.
• Turn the stopcock at the catheter injection hub to open a fluid path between the injection lumen of the PA catheter and syringe.
• Press the START button on the cardiac output computer or wait for the INJECT message to flash.

• Inject the solution smoothly within 4 seconds, making sure that it doesn't leak at the connectors.

• If a strip chart recorder is available, analyze the contour of the thermodilution washout curve for a rapid upstroke and a gradual, smooth return to baseline.

• Wait 1 minute between injections and repeat the procedure until three values are within 10% to 15% of the median value. Compute the average and record the patient's cardiac output.

• Return the stopcock to its original position and make sure the injection delivery system tubing is clamped.

• Verify the presence of a PA waveform on the cardiac monitor.

### Determining cardiac output using room-temperature injectant

• Verify the presence of a PA waveform on the cardiac monitor.

• Unclamp the I.V. tubing and withdraw exactly 10 ml of solution. Reclamp the tubing.

• Turn the stopcock at the catheter injection hub to open a fluid path between the injection lumen of the PA catheter and the syringe.

• Press the START button on the cardiac output computer or wait for an INJECT message to flash.

• Then inject the solution smoothly within 4 seconds, making sure that the solution does not leak at the connectors.

• If a strip chart recorder is available, analyze the contour of the thermodilution washout curve for a rapid upstroke and a gradual, smooth return to the baseline.

• Repeat these steps until three values are within 10% to 15% of the median value. Compute the average and record the patient's cardiac output.

• Then return the stopcock to its original position and make sure that the injection delivery system tubing is clamped.

• Verify a PA waveform on the cardiac monitor.

## Special considerations

Monitor the patient for signs or symptoms of inadequate perfusion, including restlessness, fatigue, changes in level of consciousness, decreased capillary refill time, diminished peripheral pulses, oliguria, and pale, cool skin.

If ordered, calculate the cardiac index—divide cardiac output by body surface area. This is a more specific measurement than cardiac output alone. The cardiac index normally ranges from 2.5 to 4.2 liters/minute.

Many experts recommend injecting boluses at a fixed point in the respiratory cycle, such as at end expiration. This ensures a more stable baseline blood temperature before each injection, yielding less variation in repeated measurements. However, others believe that injections shouldn't be timed with respiration because the practice can affect the measurement.

*Because accurate cardiac output measurement requires a stable baseline pulmonary artery temperature before injection,* avoid giving bolus injections of fluid or medications just before measuring cardiac output. Concomitant infusions given at a continuous rate should not affect measurement accuracy.

Measure cardiac output as often as necessary, depending on your patient's condition. You may need to provide hourly assessments for postoperative cardiac or myocardial infarction (MI) patients, whereas stable patients may only require cardiac output measurements every 4 to 8 hours. Cardiac output should be measured after significant changes in heart rate, preload, afterload, or contractility, or after the patient has been given drugs.

PA catheters are usually removed after 72 hours *because the incidence of infection increases significantly with longer indwelling times.* For patients who still need hemodynamic monitoring, you can insert a new catheter in a new site for another 72 hours. Injection delivery systems and I.V. solutions should be changed according to your hospital's policy.

Discontinue cardiac output measurements when the patient is hemodynamically stable and weaned from his vasoactive and inotropic medications. You can leave the PA catheter inserted for pressure measurements. Simply disconnect and discard the injection delivery system and the I.V. bag. Cover any exposed stopcocks with dead-end caps.

When monitoring any patient parameter, make sure you evaluate trends rather than isolated values. For example, an hourly decrease in cardiac output by 0.1 liter/minute may seem insignificant from hour to hour. However, at the end of 24 hours, the cardiac output would have fallen by 2.4 liters/minute, which is a significant change in any patient.

Add the fluid volume injected for cardiac output determinations to the total intake for the patient. Injectate delivery of 30 ml/hour will contribute 720 ml to the patient's 24-hour intake.

After cardiac output measurement, make sure the clamp on the injection bag is secured *to prevent inadvertent delivery of the injectant to the patient.*

## Documentation

Record the average cardiac output and related calculations. Document the amount and type of injectant used on the intake and output record. Also note the patient's tolerance for the procedure.

# IABC monitoring

The IABC device consists of a single-chamber or multichamber polyurethane balloon attached to an external pump console by a large-lumen catheter. A surgeon advances the balloon catheter up the patient's descending thoracic aorta to a point just distal to the left subclavian artery. The pumping console inflates the balloon with helium or carbon dioxide during diastole and deflates it during systole.

This inflation-deflation cycle, called counterpulsation, is synchronized with the patient's ECG, which appears on the console's oscilloscope. IABC increases systemic circulation, improves coronary perfusion, and reduces left ventricular workload. (See *Understanding the balloon pump.*)

The balloon inflates early in diastole, just after the aortic valve closes. Normally, about 70% to 80% of coronary perfusion occurs during diastole. Balloon inflation forces blood toward the aortic valve, which increases pressure in the aortic root and augments diastolic pressure to enhance coronary perfusion. It also forces blood through the brachiocephalic, common carotid, and subclavian arteries arising from the aortic trunk, which improves peripheral circulation.

During systole, blood pressure in the left ventricle must exceed that in the aorta to allow the aortic valve to open and eject blood. The aortic resistance that must be overcome is called afterload. The balloon rapidly deflates just before systole, which reduces aortic volume and decreases aortic pressure and afterload. Because aortic pressure is diminished, the left ventricle doesn't need to work as hard to open the aortic valve. This decreased workload reduces the heart's oxygen requirement and, combined with the more efficient myocardial perfusion provided by the IABC, prevents or reduces myocardial ischemia.

The IABC console can be preset to assist the heart at intervals—for example, it can inflate and deflate every one to four beats, depending on the patient's need and the type of machine used. Inflation and deflation of the balloon is inhibited by certain ventricular arrhythmias.

The balloon catheter can be inserted percutaneously at bedside, in the operating room, or in a cardiac catheterization laboratory. If insertion is performed in the unit, strict sterile technique must be followed. In some hospitals, technicians help the doctor insert and remove the catheter and troubleshoot problems. You'll

## Understanding the balloon pump

An intra-aortic balloon counterpulsation (IABC) device (also called a *balloon pump*) consists of either a multichambered polyurethane balloon or a single-chambered balloon attached to an external pump console by means of a large-lumen catheter.

This external pump works in precise counterpoint to the left ventricle, inflating the balloon with helium or carbon dioxide early in diastole and deflating it just before systole. Balloon inflation forces blood toward the aortic valve, augmenting diastolic pressure and improving cardiac perfusion.

Balloon deflation, which occurs quickly after diastole, reduces aortic volume and pressure and the workload of the left ventricle in opening the aortic valve. These reductions, together with the improved perfusion, help control myocardial ischemia by lessening the heart's need for oxygen.

IABC can be synchronized with the electrocardiogram (ECG) or the arterial waveform.

In the ECG mode, the R wave triggers balloon deflation (as shown); inflation can occur on the T wave's downslope or after a specific delay following the R wave. (The R wave corresponds to systole; the T wave corresponds to aortic valve closure.)

The arterial wave is a useful alternative when the ECG triggers inconsistent counterpulsation. In the arterial wave mode, deflation is triggered by systolic ejection and inflation is triggered by the dicrotic notch, which corresponds to aortic valve closure and the onset of diastole. For the arterial mode to work two criteria must be satisfied: the patient must have a pulse pressure greater than 20 mm Hg, and his arterial waveform must have a steep upstroke.

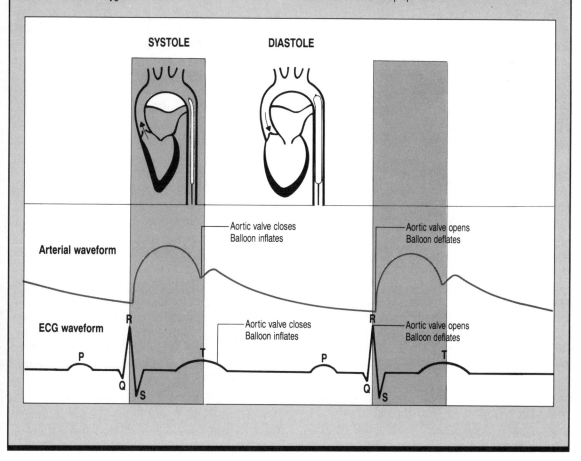

usually be responsible for patient assessment and management.

Before insertion of the balloon catheter, a PA catheter, an indwelling urinary catheter, and an arterial line should be inserted. A peripheral I.V. or subclavian line should also be in place for administering fluids and medications as needed. A transducer connected to the IABC console projects a visible arterial pressure waveform on the oscilloscope. A separate monitor and transducer may be required to display PAPs.

Common indications for IABC monitoring include left ventricular failure and cardiogenic shock caused by acute MI, unstable or preinfarction angina, and high-risk cardiac surgery. IABC monitoring may also be used to provide preoperative support to the patient undergoing cardiac catheterization.

Use of IABC monitoring is contraindicated in patients with atherosclerotic vessels that prevent catheter placement and in patients with irreversible brain damage, incompetent aortic valve, dissecting aortic aneurysm, or ventricular fibrillation.

## Equipment

IABC console and balloon catheters ▪ Dacron graft (for surgically inserted balloon) ▪ ECG electrodes ▪ I.V. solution and infusion set ▪ sedative ▪ pain medication ▪ arterial line catheter ▪ heparin flush solution, transducer, and flush setup ▪ PA catheter setup ▪ temporary pacemaker setup ▪ sterile drape ▪ sterile gloves ▪ suture material ▪ povidone-iodine solution and sodium chloride solution or sterile water for irrigation and suction setup ▪ oxygen setup and respirator, if necessary ▪ defibrillator and emergency drugs ▪ ECG monitor ▪ fluoroscope ▪ indwelling urinary catheter ▪ urimeter ▪ arterial blood gas (ABG) kits and tubes for laboratory studies ▪ povidone-iodine swabs and ointment ▪ dressing materials ▪ 4″ × 4″ gauze pads ▪ shaving supplies ▪ optional: atropine, I.V. heparin, low-molecular-weight dextran.

## Preparation of equipment

The doctor tests the balloon catheter for leaks before insertion. The pump console's pressure transducer must be balanced, and the oscilloscope monitor on the pump console must be calibrated for accuracy. Depending on hospital policy, you or another specially trained member of the health care team may balance the pressure transducer and calibrate the monitor.

IABC setup and operation vary with the manufacturer. Consult the manufacturer's instructions for additional information.

## Implementation

• Explain the procedure to the patient. Inform him that the balloon catheter temporarily reduces the heart's workload to promote rapid healing of the ventricular muscle. Tell him that it will be removed after his heart can resume an adequate workload again.

### Preparing for intra-aortic balloon insertion

• Make sure the patient or responsible family member understands and signs a consent form. Ensure that the form is on the patient's chart.
• Obtain baseline vital signs, including PAPs if the line is already inserted. Obtain a baseline ECG.
• Apply chest electrodes in a standard lead II position or in whatever position produces the largest R wave on the oscilloscope. *The R wave triggers the inflation-deflation cycle.*
• Assess the patient's respiratory status and administer oxygen as necessary.
• Prepare and insert a peripheral I.V. line *to deliver medications as ordered.*
• Prepare for and assist with insertion of an arterial line, as indicated, *to allow arterial pressure monitoring.* The augmented pressure waveform demonstrates elevated diastolic and lowered systolic pressure and allows you to check proper timing of the inflation-deflation cycle. (Remember, the balloon should inflate during diastole and deflate during systole.)

• If bradycardia occurs, give atropine or prepare the patient for pacemaker insertion, as ordered. The balloon pump is ineffective if the patient has bradycardia.

• Obtain specimens for preoperative laboratory tests, as ordered. These tests usually include blood typing and crossmatching, serum electrolyte levels, and coagulation studies.

• Insert an indwelling urinary catheter *to allow accurate measurement of urinary output and assessment of fluid balance and renal function.*

• Shave or clip the patient's hair from the lower abdomen to the lower thigh bilaterally, including the pubic area, *to reduce the risk of infection.* Although the catheter is usually inserted in the left side, it may be inserted in the right side if the left artery is diseased.

• Attach another set of ECG monitoring electrodes to the patient unless the ECG pattern is being transmitted from the patient's monitor to the balloon pump monitor.

• Administer a sedative, as ordered.

### Inserting the intra-aortic balloon

• The surgeon may insert a special intra-aortic balloon catheter percutaneously through the femoral artery into the descending thoracic aorta. This simplified procedure may be performed in the unit or in a cardiac catheterization laboratory.

• If the surgeon chooses not to insert the catheter percutaneously, he performs a femoral arteriotomy to insert the balloon. This procedure is best performed in an operating room.

• After making the incision and isolating the artery, the surgeon attaches a Dacron graft to a small opening in the arterial wall, passes the catheter through this graft, and, with optional fluoroscopic guidance, advances it up the descending thoracic aorta and positions the catheter tip between the left subclavian artery and the renal arteries. The surgeon then sews the Dacron graft around the catheter at the insertion point and connects the other end of the catheter to the pumping console.

### Monitoring the patient after balloon insertion

• Obtain a chest X-ray *to determine correct balloon placement.*

• Observe the arterial pressure pattern every 30 minutes for diastolic augmentation *to verify correctly timed counterpulsation.* (See *Interpreting intra-aortic balloon waveforms*, pages 58 and 59.)

• Measure blood pressure every 15 minutes to 1 hour *to determine the effectiveness of therapy and anticipate the need for vasopressors or vasodilators, such as dopamine or nitroprusside.*

• Take an apical pulse rate at least every hour, noting rate and rhythm. *Increased or decreased pulse rate alters the effectiveness of the pump and may require drugs, such as atropine, or pacemaker therapy.*

• Check the patient's temperature every hour. If it's elevated, obtain blood samples for culture, send them to the laboratory immediately, and notify the doctor.

• Measure intake and output hourly.

• Observe for ischemia in the limbs — especially the affected limb — every hour. Be alert for changes in pulse rate, color, temperature, and sensation. Explain to the patient the importance of keeping the affected extremity straight.

• Watch for pump interruptions, which may result from loose ECG electrodes or broken wires, static or 60-cycle interference, kinked catheters, and improper body alignment. Elevate the head of the bed no more than 45 degrees, keeping the patient's leg unflexed at the groin *to prevent catheter kinking or forward displacement causing trauma or injury to the aorta.*

• Observe for optimal timing. Balloon inflation should begin when the aortic valve closes or at the dicrotic notch on the arterial waveform. Deflation should occur just before systole. Improper timing includes late inflation, which reduces coronary artery perfusion, and prolonged inflation, which dangerously increases the resistance against which the left ventricle must pump. In both situations, readjust timing according to the manufacturer's guidelines, or notify the person responsible for the balloon pump adjustments.

# Interpreting intra-aortic balloon waveforms

During intra-aortic balloon counterpulsation (IABC), you can use electrocardiogram and arterial pressure waveforms to determine whether the balloon pump is functioning properly.

## Normal inflation-deflation timing

Balloon inflation usually occurs after aortic valve closure; deflation, during isovolumetric contraction, just before the aortic valve opens. In a properly timed waveform, like the one shown at right, the inflation point lies at or slightly above the dicrotic notch on the waveform. Both inflation and deflation cause a sharp V. Peak diastolic pressure exceeds peak systolic pressure, peak systolic pressure exceeds assisted peak systolic pressure, and patient aortic end-diastolic pressure is 5 to 15 mm Hg higher than balloon aortic end-diastolic pressure.

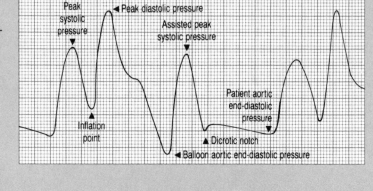

## Early inflation

With *early inflation,* the inflation point lies before the dicrotic notch on the waveform. Early inflation dangerously increases myocardial stress and decreases cardiac output.

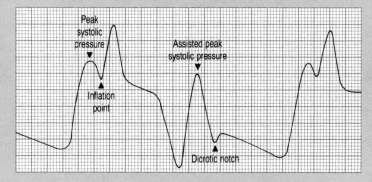

## Early deflation

With *early deflation,* a U shape appears and peak systolic pressure is less than or equal to assisted peak systolic pressure. Early deflation will not decrease afterload or myocardial oxygen consumption.

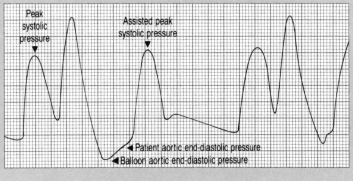

## Interpreting intra-aortic balloon waveforms *(continued)*

### Late inflation

With *late inflation*, the dicrotic notch precedes the inflation point on the waveform, and the notch and the inflation point create a W shape. Late inflation can reduce peak diastolic pressure, coronary and systemic perfusion augmentation time, and augmented coronary perfusion pressure.

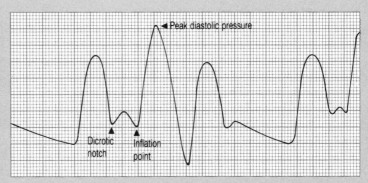

### Late deflation

With *late deflation*, peak systolic pressure exceeds assisted peak systolic pressure. Late deflation threatens the patient by increasing afterload, myocardial oxygen consumption, cardiac workload, and preload. It occurs when the balloon has been inflated for too long.

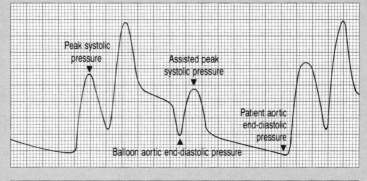

### Proper timing with reduced augmentation

Sometimes, inflation and deflation are properly timed but the balloon doesn't inflate enough. When this happens, peak diastolic pressure equals or drops below peak systolic pressure. You'll need to evaluate the patient's condition to determine the cause of reduced augmentation.

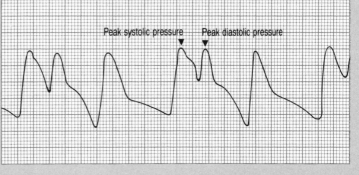

• If the IABC device is inadvertently shut off for more than 5 minutes, notify the doctor immediately *to determine the need for heparinization before restarting the balloon. Resuming pumping without adequate anticoagulant precipitates emboli.*

• Check for gas leaks from the catheter or the balloon. Such leaks may be indicated by an alarm on the pump console. If the balloon ruptures, blood will appear in the catheter. If this happens, shut off the pump console and notify the doctor.

• If you suspect balloon rupture, promptly place the patient in Trendelenburg's position *to prevent the gas embolus from reaching the brain.*

• If the patient isn't receiving anticoagulants, the doctor may order I.V. heparin or low-molecular-weight dextran *to prevent platelet aggregation on the quiescent balloon.*

• Measure PAP and PAWP every 1 to 2 hours, or as ordered. A rising PAWP indicates increased ventricular pressure and workload; notify the doctor if this occurs. Some patients require the administration of I.V. nitroprusside in addition to the IABC *to reduce preload and afterload.*

• Obtain arterial samples for ABG analysis, as ordered. If the patient is connected to a ventilator, perform ventilation checks, suctioning, and respiratory assessment.

• Monitor electrolyte levels as ordered, especially sodium *to assess fluid balance* and potassium *to prevent cardiac arrhythmias.*

• Monitor hematologic status. Blood products are usually used to maintain the hematocrit at 30%. Platelets may be required if the platelet count drops. Observe for bleeding gums, blood in urine or stool, or petechiae.

• Monitor the results of clotting tests. As ordered, administer heparin through a pressure infusion to maintain the activated partial thromboplastin time at 1½ to 2 times the normal value.

• Turn and position the patient every 2 hours, keeping the affected extremity straight. Provide oral hygiene at least every 4 hours. Give pain medication *for insertion site discomfort,* as ordered.

• Re-dress the balloon site, as ordered, and observe for signs of inflammation or excessive bleeding. Apply pressure *to control bleeding.*

• Prevent constipation *to avoid strain on the patient's heart.*

• If angina occurs, notify the doctor immediately *because the IABC device is not effective.*

• Watch for signs and symptoms of a dissecting aortic aneurysm, such as a difference in blood pressure between arms; elevated blood pressure; pain in the chest, abdomen, or back; syncope; pallor; diaphoresis; dyspnea; throbbing abdominal mass; and a reduced red blood cell count with an elevated white blood cell count. If you suspect an aortic aneurysm, notify the doctor.

### Weaning the patient from the intra-aortic balloon

• Assess cardiac index, systemic blood pressure, and PAWP *to evaluate readiness for weaning,* which usually begins about 24 hours after balloon insertion.

• To begin weaning, gradually decrease the frequency of balloon augmentation (per patient heartbeat) to 1:2, 1:4, and 1:8 as ordered, and measure the cardiac index at each ratio. (Output is frequently measured both on and off the machine.) Some doctors prefer to wean the patient by diminishing balloon volume; however, this must be done cautiously *to avoid reducing volume so much that the balloon can't inflate and deflate forcibly enough to repel platelets.* The increased risk of emboli with this method makes it controversial; when using it, some doctors choose to administer I.V. heparin or low-molecular-weight dextran.

• Avoid leaving the patient on a low augmentation setting for more than 2 hours *to skirt the risk of embolus formation.* Check your hospital policy.

### Removing the intra-aortic balloon

• The surgeon removes the balloon catheter when augmentation is no longer necessary (for example, when cardiac output improves during weaning). He also removes it if circulation to the limb is seriously compromised, if the patient's condition is considered inoperable during cardiac catheterization, or if the patient's condition deteriorates beyond recovery. Then he closes the Dacron graft and sutures the insertion site. If a percutaneous catheter is in place, the surgeon usually removes it. Pressure must be applied to the site for 15 to 30 minutes or until bleeding stops; in some hospitals, this is the doctor's responsibility.

• After removal of an IABC device, provide necessary wound care, according to hospital policy.

## Complications
Aortic or femoral artery dissection or perforation may occur during balloon insertion. Ischemia or loss of pulses may occur in extremities (especially the legs) from compromised circulation. Thrombi may form on the balloon, predisposing the patient to emboli. Platelets are destroyed during balloon pumping, causing a decrease in circulating platelets (thrombocytopenia). A gas embolus can occur from balloon rupture. Infection may occur at the balloon insertion site.

## Documentation
Document all aspects of patient assessment and management. If you're responsible for the IABC device, document all routine checks, problems, and troubleshooting measures. If a technician is responsible for the IABC device, record only when and why the technician was notified, as well as the result of his actions on the patient, if any. Document any teaching of the patient, family, or close friends, as well as responses to therapy and teaching.

# 3 MONITORING RESPIRATORY STATUS

## Introduction

By supplying body cells with oxygen and eliminating excess carbon dioxide, gas exchange plays an essential role in sustaining life and promoting growth. Unfortunately, all hospital patients are at risk for altered gas exchange, an abnormality that can impede recovery from illness or injury and even cause death.

To monitor your patient's gas exchange, you must know how to set up various monitoring systems and interpret the results. This chapter provides the up-to-date information you need. It reviews the factors that affect gas exchange, including respiratory control, oxygen transport and delivery, and lung ventilation and perfusion. You'll also learn the monitoring techniques that provide important data about your patient's oxygenation status: pulse oximetry, transcutaneous oxygen ($TcPO_2$) and transcutaneous carbon dioxide ($TcPCO_2$) monitoring, end-tidal carbon dioxide ($ETCO_2$) monitoring, mixed venous oxygen saturation monitoring ($S\bar{v}O_2$), bedside pulmonary function monitoring, arterial blood gas (ABG) monitoring, and apnea monitoring. For each technique, you'll discover how the equipment works, how to prepare for and carry out the procedure, and how to interpret the values supplied by the monitor.

# Physiology review

Gas exchange—the addition of oxygen and removal of carbon dioxide from pulmonary capillary blood—occurs during breathing, or ventilation. Breathing has two phases—*inspiration*, which moves air into the lungs, and *expiration*, which moves air out of the lungs.

## Respiratory control

The brain, nerves, and various chemical and physical factors interact to regulate breathing and maintain ventilatory homeostasis.

### Respiratory centers

Respiratory centers in the brain stem control respiratory rate and depth, adjust ventilation to meet the body's metabolic demands, innervate the diaphragm, and contain chemoreceptors that affect ventilation.

The *medullary respiratory center* controls respiratory rate and depth through the interaction of inspiration and expiration. These neurons also react to other impulses from the *pons*. Regulating respiratory rhythm, the pons harmonizes the transition from inspiration to expiration through its interaction with the medullary respiratory center. The *apneustic center* within the pons stimulates inspiratory neurons in the medulla to trigger inspiration. These neurons, in turn, induce the *pneumotaxic center* (also in the pons) to inhibit the apneustic center and trigger expiration.

### Receptors

Various receptors contribute to ventilation. *Chemoreceptors* in the medullary respiratory center help regulate respiratory rate and depth in response to changes in oxygen, carbon dioxide, and pH in the blood. The *central chemoreceptor*, or carbon dioxide sensor, responds to carbon dioxide changes affecting hydrogen ion concentration in the cerebrospinal fluid (CSF). When CSF acidity rises, the central chemoreceptor stimulates the respiratory centers to increase respiratory rate and depth until the carbon dioxide level returns to normal. Conversely, lowered CSF acidity triggers the central chemoreceptor to decrease respiratory rate and depth until cellular metabolism produces more carbon dioxide.

*Peripheral chemoreceptors* in the carotid and aortic bodies stimulate respiratory centers in the brain stem to increase ventilation if the partial pressure of arterial oxygen ($PaO_2$) decreases. Ventilation normally increases when the $PaO_2$ falls below 50 mm Hg.

### Reflex responses

The Hering-Breuer reflex, a protective mechanism, limits lung expansion. When the lungs expand, stretch receptors in the alveolar ducts trigger the flow of inhibitory messages to the respiratory center. In response, the diaphragm and intercostal muscles relax, allowing passive expiration.

Changes in arterial blood pressure also cause reflex respiratory responses by stimulating pressoreceptors in the aortic and carotid bodies. For instance, respirations reflexively slow when blood pressure suddenly rises and speed up when blood pressure suddenly falls.

### Other stimuli

Fever may trigger the respiratory center to increase respirations, whereas a reduced temperature may lead to a decreased respiratory rate. Airway irritation causes receptors to induce coughing or sneezing. Sensory stimulation, such as sudden heat or cold, may cause a reaction—for example, a gasp—that affects respirations.

### Physical factors

Physical factors, including resistance and compliance, also affect gas exchange.

**Resistance.** The three types of resistance—elastic, nonelastic, and airway—can challenge effective gas exchange and must be overcome to avoid compromising the patient's breathing.

*Elastic resistance,* the result of elastic lung fibers and the surface tension between alveolar air and the alveolar sac lining, allows the lungs to contract during expiration. Certain factors counteract lung elasticity—chest wall rigidity; negative intrathoracic pressure, which allows the lungs to expand with the chest wall; and surfactant, a lipoprotein that prevents alveolar collapse.

*Nonelastic resistance* results from forces that interfere with normal chest expansion. For instance, obesity, pregnancy, weight gain, and restrictive dressings inhibit downward thoracic expansion. These conditions compromise inspiration by increasing the work of breathing.

*Airway resistance* refers to the force that must be overcome for air to flow through the airway. The greater the airway resistance, the more pressure is needed to move air into and out of the lungs. Airway resistance depends on airway radius, length, and flow rate. A 50% reduction in radius (such as from accumulated secretions) increases airway resistance 16-fold. Even a slight reduction in radius (such as from mucus or airway edema) may seriously impede airflow, particularly in neonatal and pediatric patients.

Airway resistance increases with airway length: the longer the airway, the higher the resistance. Long endotracheal tubes and breathing circuit tubing can elevate airway resistance and reduce airflow to the alveoli, increasing the work of breathing.

The airflow rate influences airway resistance by affecting the airflow pattern. Turbulence, caused by a high flow rate, increases resistance, whereas laminar airflow, a linear pattern occurring at low flow rates, decreases resistance. However, an extremely low flow rate may prevent adequate alveolar ventilation. Ideally, the flow rate is low enough to produce a laminar airflow while effectively ventilating the alveoli.

**Compliance.** A measure of how easily the lung and chest wall expand during inspiration, compliance also affects the work of breathing. Changes in the lung's elastic and collagen fibers can increase or decrease lung compliance. Aging and such lung diseases as emphysema increase compliance, making the lungs easier to inflate. Other diseases, such as interstitial fibrosis, diminish compliance, making the lungs harder to inflate. Lung compliance relates inversely to airway resistance: As resistance increases, lung compliance decreases.

## Gas exchange

The exchange of oxygen and carbon dioxide takes place at the alveolocapillary membrane, where the alveolus and pulmonary capillary meet. Gas exchange occurs by *diffusion*, a process in which gases move from an area of higher pressure to an area of lower pressure.

### Partial pressures of gases

To understand how oxygen and carbon dioxide diffuse, you must be familiar with the concept of the partial pressure of gases. *Partial pressure,* or tension, refers to the pressure exerted by any one gas in a mixture of gases or in a liquid. Dalton's law states that the pressure exerted by a particular gas in a mixture of gases (such as the air that enters the lungs) corresponds to the sum of the partial pressures of the separate components. Within the body, changes in the partial pressures of oxygen and carbon dioxide provide the driving force for diffusion.

The rate and extent of gas diffusion depend largely on the pressure gradient—the differential in partial pressures between the two sides of a semipermeable membrane. Gas moves from a high-pressure area to a low-pressure area until pressures are equalized. Diffusion slows as the pressure gradient diminishes and pressures on each side of the membrane approach equilibrium.

The rate of blood flow through pulmonary capillaries, the hemoglobin level, the surface area available for gas exchange, and gas solubility also affect diffusion. For instance, carbon dioxide diffuses across the alveolocapillary membrane about 20 times more easily than oxygen because it's more soluble.

# Breath sounds monitoring

Auscultating for breath sounds is a key component of assessing a patient's respiratory status. Auscultation helps you detect abnormal fluid or mucus as well as obstructed passages. You can also determine the condition of the alveoli

and surrounding pleura. (See *Auscultating normal breath sounds,* page 66.)

During auscultation, you'll hear four types of normal breath sounds: tracheal, bronchial, bronchovesicular, and vesicular. You'll hear tracheal breath sounds—harsh, discontinuous sounds—over the trachea. These sounds occur equally during inspiration and expiration. Bronchial breath sounds—high-pitched, discontinuous sounds that occur during expiration—can be heard over the manubrium of sternum. Bronchovesicular breath sounds—medium-pitched, continuous sounds that are equally audible during inspiration and expiration—occur over the upper third of the sternum anteriorly and in the interscapular area posteriorly. And vesicular breath sounds—low-pitched, continuous sounds that are prolonged during inspiration—can be heard over the peripheral lung fields. If you hear any of these four sounds in areas other than those described, you've detected an abnormal breath sound. Bronchial breath sounds over the peripheral lung fields, for instance, may indicate consolidation or atelectasis. (See *Auscultating adventitious breath sounds,* page 67.)

Differentiating between normal and abnormal breath sounds requires practice. Therefore, to gain confidence, practice auscultation on a normal chest.

## Equipment

Stethoscope with chestpiece size appropriate for patient's chest.

## Preparation of equipment

Warm the stethoscope chestpiece by rubbing it between your hands.

## Implementation

• Explain the procedure to the patient. Tell him that he'll need to take deep breaths and change position occasionally. Place the patient in a comfortable position and provide privacy.
• Open the front of the patient's gown because *clothing interferes with accurate auscultation,* and

## Auscultating normal breath sounds

The area in which you auscultate a particular breath sound will help you identify whether the sound is normal or adventitious. Study the illustrations below to learn the typical locations for auscultating normal breath sounds.

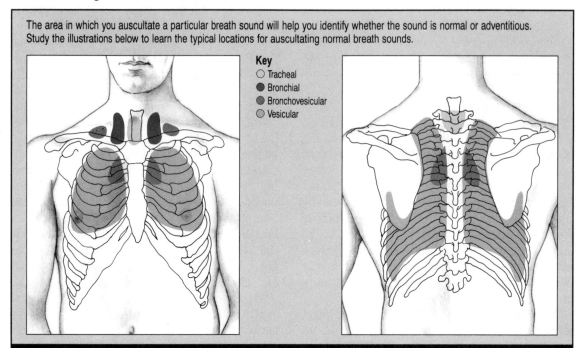

**Key**
○ Tracheal
● Bronchial
● Bronchovesicular
○ Vesicular

drape him appropriately. Note whether the patient has excess chest hair. If so, wet and mat it with a damp washcloth. That way, *the hair won't cause sounds that can be confused with crackles.*

• Instruct the patient to take full, slow breaths through his mouth. *(Nose breathing changes the pitch of the breath sounds.)*

• Using the diaphragm of the stethoscope, begin auscultating over the patient's trachea. Moving to the upper lobes of the lungs, auscultate a point on one side of the anterior chest and then on the other side. Be sure to work systematically, auscultating the anterior, lateral, and posterior chest over the intercostal spaces.

• Listen for one full inspiration and expiration before moving the stethoscope. Remember, a patient may try to accommodate you by breathing quickly and deeply with every movement of the stethoscope, which can cause hyperventilation.

If your patient becomes light-headed or dizzy, stop auscultation and allow him to breathe normally for a few minutes.

• Now, *to assess the middle lung lobes,* auscultate laterally at the level of the fourth to sixth intercostal spaces, following the lateral auscultation sequence.

• Now auscultate the patient's posterior chest in the same manner, comparing sounds on both sides before moving to the next area.

• As you auscultate, classify normal and abnormal breath sounds according to their location, intensity (amplitude), characteristic sound, pitch (tone), and duration. Also identify the inspiratory and expiratory phases of normal and abnormal breath sounds, and then determine whether the sound occurs during inspiration, expiration, or both.

## Auscultating adventitious breath sounds

These photographs show you where to auscultate to identify four adventitious breath sounds – crackles, wheezes, rhonchi and pleural friction rubs. By studying them, you can learn the typical locations for these adventitious breath sounds.

**Crackles**

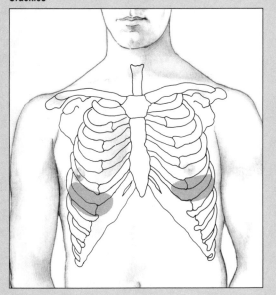

**Wheezes**

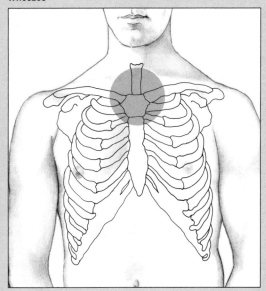

**Rhonchi**

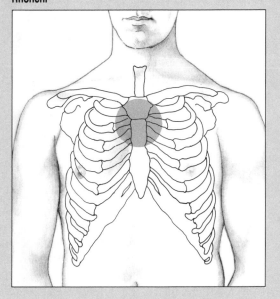

**Pleural friction rubs**

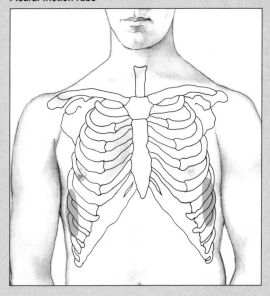

## Special considerations

Because solid tissue transmits sound better than air or fluid, breath sounds (as well as spoken and whispered sounds) will be louder than normal over an area of consolidation. However, if pus, fluid, or air fills the pleural space, breath sounds will be quieter than normal. If a foreign body or secretions obstruct a bronchus, breath sounds will be diminished or absent over distal lung tissue.

Diminished breath sounds may indicate an obstructed airway, partial or total lung collapse, thickening of the pleurae, emphysema, or chronic lung disease.

Absent breath sounds typically indicate loss of ventilation power. Underlying causes may include laryngospasm, bronchospasm, pneumonectomy, phrenic nerve palsy, pneumothorax, hemothorax, or a malpositioned endotracheal tube.

Adventitious breath sounds occur when air passes either through narrowed airways or through moisture, or when the membranes lining the chest cavity and the lungs become inflamed. Adventitious breath sounds include crackles, rhonchi, wheezes, and pleural friction rubs. Usually, these sounds indicate pulmonary disease.

## Documentation

After noting the date and time of the procedure, document the characteristics of the breath sounds, including location, intensity, pitch, and duration. Also document whether the sounds occurred before, during, or after inspiration or expiration. Document any other abnormal findings along with the nursing or medical interventions taken and the patient's response.

# Bedside spirometry monitoring

This procedure measures forced vital capacity (FVC) and forced expiratory volume (FEV), allowing calculation of other pulmonary function indices, such as timed forced expiratory flow rate. Depending on the type of spirometer used, bedside spirometry can also allow direct measurement of vital capacity and tidal volume (VT).

Bedside spirometry aids in diagnosing pulmonary dysfunction before it appears on an X-ray or physical examination, evaluating its severity, and determining the patient's response to therapy. By allowing assessment of the relationship of flow rate to vital capacity, it helps distinguish between obstructive and restrictive pulmonary disease. It's also useful for evaluating preoperative anesthesia risk. Because the required breathing patterns can aggravate conditions such as bronchospasm, use of the bedside spirometer requires a review of the patient's history and close observation during testing.

## Equipment

Spirometer ▪ disposable mouthpiece ▪ breathing tube, if required ▪ spirographic chart, if required ▪ chart and pen, if required ▪ noseclips ▪ optional: vital capacity predicted-values table.

## Preparation of equipment

Review the manufacturer's instructions for assembly and use of the spirometer. If necessary, firmly insert the breathing tube *to ensure a tight connection.* If the tube comes preconnected, check the seals for tightness and the tubing for leaks. Check the operation of the recording mechanism, and insert a chart and pen if necessary. Insert the disposable mouthpiece and make sure it's tightly sealed.

## Implementation

• Explain the procedure to the patient. Emphasize that his cooperation is essential *to ensure accurate results.*
• Instruct the patient to remove or loosen any constricting clothing, such as a bra, *to prevent alteration of test results from restricted thoracic expansion and abdominal mobility.* Instruct the patient to void *to prevent abdominal discomfort.* Don't perform pulmonary function tests immediately after a patient has eaten a large meal *because he'll experience abdominal discomfort.*

• If the patient wears dentures that fit poorly, remove them *to prevent incomplete closure of his mouth, which could allow air to leak around the mouthpiece.* If his dentures fit well, leave them in place *to promote a tight seal.*
• Plug in the spirometer and set the baseline time.
• If desired, allow the patient to practice the required breathing with the breathing tube unhooked. After practice, replace the tube and check the seal.
• Tell the patient not to breathe through his nose. If the patient has difficulty complying, apply noseclips.
• To measure vital capacity, instruct the patient to inhale as deeply as possible, and then insert the mouthpiece so that his lips are sealed tightly around it *to prevent air leakage and ensure an accurate digital readout or spirogram recording.* (See *Digital bedside spirometer.*)
• Tell him to exhale completely. Then remove the mouthpiece *to prevent recording his next inspiration.*
• Allow the patient to rest and repeat the procedure twice.
• *To measure FEV and FVC,* repeat this procedure with the chart or timer on, but instruct the patient to exhale as quickly and completely as possible. Tell him when to start, and turn on the recorder or timer at the same time.
• Allow the patient to rest. Then repeat the procedure twice more.
• After completing the procedure, discard the mouthpiece, remove the spirographic chart, and follow the manufacturer's instructions for cleaning and sterilizing.

## Special considerations

Encourage the patient during the test; *this may help him to exhale more forcefully, which can be significant.* If the patient coughs during expiration, wait until coughing subsides before repeating the measurement.

Read the vital capacity directly from the readout or spirogram chart. The FVC is the highest

## Digital bedside spirometer

Various models of bedside spirometers are commercially available. The instrument shown below has a digital readout. Other models display results on an individual chart record or on a roll of chart paper.

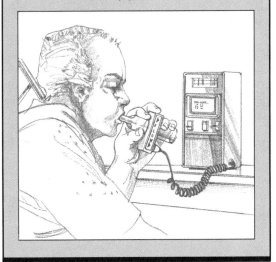

volume recorded on the curve. Of the three trials, accept the highest recorded exhalation as the vital capacity result.

To determine the percentage of predicted vital capacity, first determine the patient's predicted value from the vital capacity predicted-values table, then calculate the percentage by using the following formula:

$$\frac{\text{observed vital capacity}}{\text{predicted vital capacity}} \times 100 = \frac{\text{\% predicted}}{\text{vital capacity}}$$

To determine the FEV for a specified time, mark the point on the spirogram where it crosses the desired time, and draw a straight line from this point to the side of the chart, which indicates volume in liters. This measurement is usually calculated for 1, 2, and 3 seconds and reported as a percentage of vital capacity. A healthy patient will have exhaled 75%, 85%, and 95%, respectively, of his FVC. Calculate this percentage by using the following formula:

$$\frac{observed\ FEV}{observed\ vital\ capacity} \times 100 = \%\ vital\ capacity$$

## Complications
Forced exhalation can cause dizziness or lightheadedness, precipitate or worsen bronchospasm, rapidly increase exhaustion (possibly to where the patient will require mechanical support), and increase air trapping in the emphysemic patient.

## Documentation
Record the date and time of the procedure; the observed and calculated values, including FEV at 1, 2, and 3 seconds; any complications and the nursing action taken; and the patient's tolerance for the procedure.

# ABG monitoring

Obtaining an arterial blood sample requires percutaneous puncture of the brachial, radial, or femoral artery or withdrawal of a sample from an arterial line. Once drawn, the sample can be analyzed for ABGs.

ABG analysis evaluates ventilation by measuring blood pH, $PaO_2$, and partial pressure of arterial carbon dioxide ($PaCO_2$). Blood pH measurement reveals the blood's acid-base balance. $PaO_2$ indicates the amount of oxygen that the lungs deliver to the blood, and $PaCO_2$ indicates the lungs' capacity to eliminate carbon dioxide. ABG samples can also be analyzed for oxygen content and arterial oxygen saturation ($SaO_2$ and for bicarbonate values. (See *Interpreting ABG values.*)

ABG analysis is ordered commonly for patients who have chronic obstructive pulmonary disease (COPD), pulmonary edema, acute respiratory distress syndrome (ARDS), myocardial infarction, or pneumonia. It's also performed during episodes of shock and after coronary artery bypass surgery, resuscitation from cardiac arrest, changes in respiratory therapy or status, and prolonged anesthesia.

Most ABG samples can be drawn by a respiratory technician or specially trained nurse. Collection from the femoral artery, however, is usually performed by a doctor. Before attempting a radial puncture, perform Allen's test *to assess the adequacy of the blood supply to the patient's hand.* (See *Performing Allen's test,* page 72.)

## Equipment
10-ml glass syringe or plastic luer-lock syringe specially made for drawing blood gases ▪ 1-ml ampule of aqueous heparin (1:1,000) ▪ 20G 1¼" needle ▪ 22G 1" needle ▪ alcohol sponge ▪ povidone-iodine sponge ▪ two 2"×2" gauze pads ▪ gloves ▪ rubber cap for syringe hub or rubber stopper for needle ▪ ice-filled plastic bag ▪ label ▪ laboratory request form ▪ adhesive bandage ▪ optional: 1% lidocaine solution.

Many hospitals use a commercial ABG kit that contains all the equipment listed above (except the adhesive bandage and ice). If your hospital doesn't use such a kit, obtain a sterile syringe specially made for drawing blood gases, and use a clean emesis basin filled with ice instead of the plastic bag to transport the sample to the laboratory.

## Preparation of equipment
Prepare the collection equipment before entering the patient's room. Wash your hands thoroughly; then open the ABG kit and remove the specimen label and the plastic bag. Record on the label the patient's name and room number, the date and collection time, and the doctor's name. Fill the plastic bag with ice and set it aside.

*To heparinize the syringe,* first attach the 20G needle to the syringe. Then open the ampule of heparin. Draw all the heparin into the syringe *to prevent the sample from clotting.* Hold the syringe upright, and pull the plunger back slowly

## Interpreting ABG values

Arterial blood gas (ABG) values provide crucial information about the efficiency of your patient's gas exchange and acid-base balance. You can also use ABG values to monitor the effects of respiratory interventions.

Although ABG measurement requires blood sampling, an invasive procedure that sometimes causes pain (especially for patients without an arterial line), the information it provides allows thorough assessment of gas exchange. Here are normal ABG values:
• Blood pH: 7.35 to 7.45
• Partial pressure of oxygen in arterial blood ($PaO_2$): 80 to 100 mm Hg (decreases with age)
• Partial pressure of carbon dioxide in arterial blood ($PaCO_2$): 35 to 45 mm Hg
• Bicarbonate ($HCO_3^-$): 22 to 26 mEq/liter
• Arterial oxygen saturation ($SaO_2$): 95% to 100%.

### Evaluating acid-base balance

To interpret ABG results, start by evaluating acid-base balance. Suspect *alkalosis* as the primary or initiating disorder if the pH exceeds 7.45. Suspect *acidosis* if the pH is below 7.35. With normal pH, ABG values may be normal if a patient has compensated for his problem. For example, kidneys can compensate by retaining $HCO_3^-$ if the lungs can't eliminate enough carbon dioxide.

To determine the specific type of alkalosis or acidosis, analyze the $PaCO_2$ and $HCO_3^-$ values. If the former is abnormal but the latter normal, suspect acute respiratory alkalosis or acidosis without metabolic compensation by the kidneys. If the $HCO_3^-$ value is abnormal but the $PaCO_2$ value is normal, suspect metabolic alkalosis or acidosis.

A borderline high or low pH combined with an abnormal $PaCO_2$ or $HCO_3^-$ value indicates whether or not the acid-base disorder is compensated (pH has returned to normal). With compensated respiratory acidosis, pH is borderline low, $PaCO_2$ is high, and $HCO_3^-$ is high.

### Assessing oxygenation status

To assess your patient's oxygenation status, check the $PaO_2$ and $SaO_2$. Note the fraction of inspired oxygen he was receiving at the time the blood sample was drawn. Decreased $PaO_2$ and $SaO_2$ values may indicate hypoxemia.

Be sure to track serial ABG measurements, noting whether any significant changes followed medical or nursing interventions.

---

to about the 7-ml mark. Rotate the barrel while pulling the plunger back *to allow the heparin to coat the inside surface of the syringe.* Then, slowly force the heparin toward the hub of the syringe and expel all but about 0.1 ml of heparin.

*To heparinize the needle,* first replace the 20G needle with the 22G needle. Then, hold the syringe upright, tilt it slightly, and eject the remaining heparin. *Excess heparin in the syringe alters blood pH and $PaO_2$ values.*

## Implementation

• Tell the patient you need to collect an arterial blood sample, and explain the procedure *to help ease anxiety and promote cooperation.* Tell him that the needle stick will cause some discomfort but that he must remain still during the procedure.
• After washing your hands and donning gloves, place a rolled towel under the patient's wrist *for support.* Locate the artery and palpate it for a strong pulse.
• Clean the puncture site with a povidone-iodine sponge or with an alcohol sponge. Don't wipe off the povidone-iodine with alcohol *because alcohol cancels the effect of povidone-iodine.*
• Using a circular motion, clean the area, starting in the center of the site and spiraling outward *to avoid introducing potentially infectious skin flora into the vessel during the procedure.* If you use alcohol, apply it with friction for 30 seconds or until the final sponge comes away clean. Allow the skin to dry.
• Palpate the artery with the index and middle fingers of one hand while holding the syringe over the puncture site with the other hand.
• Hold the needle bevel up at a 30- to 45-degree angle. When puncturing the brachial artery, hold the needle at a 60-degree angle. (See *Arterial puncture technique,* page 73.)

## Performing Allen's test

Rest the patient's arm on the mattress or bedside stand. Have him clench his fist. Then, using your index and middle fingers, press on the radial and ulnar arteries. Hold this position for a few seconds.

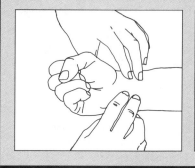

Without removing your fingers from the patient's arteries, ask him to unclench his fist and hold his hand in a relaxed position. The palm will be blanched because pressure from your fingers has impaired the normal blood flow.

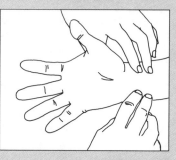

Release pressure on the patient's ulnar artery. If the hand becomes flushed, which indicates blood filling the vessels, you can safely proceed with the radial artery puncture. If the hand doesn't flush, perform the test on the other arm.

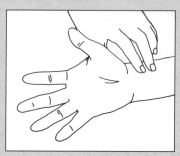

• Puncture the skin and the arterial wall in one motion, following the path of the artery.

• Watch for blood backflow in the syringe. Don't pull back on the plunger *because arterial blood should enter the syringe automatically.* Fill the syringe to the 5-ml mark.

• After collecting the sample, press a gauze pad firmly over the puncture site until bleeding stops — at least 5 minutes. If the patient is receiving anticoagulant therapy or has a blood dyscrasia, apply pressure for 10 to 15 minutes; if necessary, ask a coworker to hold the gauze pad in place while you prepare the sample for transport to the laboratory. Don't ask the patient to hold the pad. *If he fails to apply sufficient pressure, a large, painful hematoma may form, hindering future arterial punctures at that site.*

• Check the syringe for air bubbles *because these can alter PaO$_2$ values.* If air bubbles appear, remove them by holding the syringe upright and slowly ejecting some of the blood onto a 2″ × 2″ gauze pad.

• Insert the needle into a rubber stopper, or remove the needle and place a rubber cap directly on the needle hub. *This prevents the sample from leaking and keeps air out of the syringe.*

• Put the labeled sample in the ice-filled plastic bag or emesis basin. Attach a properly completed laboratory request form, and send the sample to the laboratory immediately.

• When the patient stops bleeding, apply a small adhesive bandage to the site.

• Monitor the patient's vital signs, and observe for signs of circulatory impairment, such as swelling, discoloration, pain, numbness, or tingling in the bandaged arm or leg. Watch for bleeding at the puncture site.

### Special considerations

If the patient is receiving oxygen, make sure that his therapy has been underway for at least 15 minutes before drawing arterial blood.

Unless ordered, don't turn off existing oxygen therapy before drawing arterial blood samples. However, be sure to indicate the amount and type of oxygen therapy the patient is receiving on the laboratory request form.

If the patient isn't receiving oxygen, indicate that he is breathing room air.

If the patient has just received a breathing treatment or nebulizer treatment, wait about 20 minutes before drawing the sample.

If necessary, you may anesthetize the puncture site with 1% lidocaine solution. Consider such use of lidocaine carefully *because it delays the procedure, the patient may be allergic to the drug, or the resulting vasoconstriction may prevent successful puncture.*

When filling out a laboratory request form for ABG analysis, be sure to include the following information *to help the laboratory staff calibrate the equipment and evaluate results correctly:* the patient's current temperature, most recent hemoglobin level, current respiratory rate, and fraction of inspired oxygen (FIO₂) and tidal volume (VT) if the patient is on a ventilator.

### Complications

If you use too much force when attempting to puncture the artery, the needle may touch the periosteum of the bone, causing the patient considerable pain; or you may advance the needle through the opposite wall of the artery. If this happens, slowly pull the needle back a short distance and check to see if there is a blood return. If blood still fails to enter the syringe, withdraw the needle completely and start with a fresh heparinized needle. Don't make more than two attempts to withdraw blood from the same site. *Probing the artery may injure it and the radial nerve. Also, hemolysis will alter test results.*

If arterial spasm occurs, blood won't flow into the syringe and you won't be able to collect the sample. If this happens, replace the needle with a smaller one and attempt the puncture again. *A smaller-bore needle is less likely to cause arterial spasm.*

### Documentation

Record the results of Allen's test, the time the sample was drawn, the patient's temperature, the site of the arterial puncture, the length of time pressure was applied to the site to control bleeding, and the type and amount of oxygen

## Arterial puncture technique

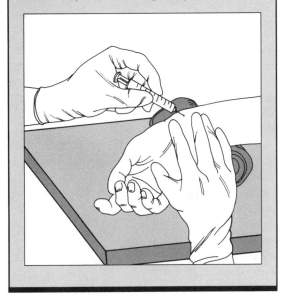

The angle of needle penetration in arterial blood gas sampling depends on the artery to be sampled. For the radial artery, which is used most commonly, the needle should enter bevel up at a 30- to 45-degree angle.

therapy the patient was receiving. Also document the patient's tolerance for the procedure along with any complications.

## S̄vO₂ monitoring

This procedure uses a fiber-optic thermodilution pulmonary artery (PA) catheter to continuously monitor changes in oxygen delivery to tissues and oxygen consumption by tissues. Monitoring of S̄vO₂ allows rapid detection of impaired oxygen delivery, such as from decreased cardiac output, hemoglobin level, or SaO₂. It also helps evaluate a patient's response to drug administration, endotracheal tube suctioning, ventilator setting changes, positive end-expiratory pressure, and FIO₂. S̄vO₂ usually ranges from 60% to 80%, with the normal value being 75%.

## Equipment
Fiber-optic PA catheter ▪ co-oximeter (monitor) ▪ optical module and cable ▪ gloves.

## Preparation of equipment
Review the manufacturer's instructions for assembly and use of the fiber-optic PA catheter. Connect the optical module and cable to the monitor. Next, peel back the wrapping covering the catheter just enough to uncover the fiber-optic connector. Attach the fiber-optic connector to the optical module, while allowing the rest of the catheter to remain in its sterile wrapping. Calibrate the fiber-optic catheter by following the manufacturer's instructions.

To prepare for the rest of the procedure, follow the instructions for PA catheter insertion, as described in "PAP and PAWP pressure monitoring," in Chapter 2. (See also *S$\bar{v}O_2$ monitoring equipment.*)

## Implementation
• Wash your hands and put on gloves.
• Explain the procedure to the patient *to allay his fears and promote cooperation.*
• Assist with the insertion of the fiber-optic catheter just as you would for a PA catheter.
• Once the catheter is inserted, set the intensity of the signal display *so that it's within normal limits.* Then calibrate the monitor.
• Observe the digital readout and record the baseline S$\bar{v}O_2$ on graph paper. Repeat readings at least once each hour *to monitor and document trends.*
• Set the machine alarms 10% above and 10% below the patient's current S$\bar{v}O_2$ reading.

### Recalibrating the monitor
• Draw a mixed venous blood sample from the distal port of the PA catheter. Send it to the laboratory for analysis *to compare the laboratory's S$\bar{v}O_2$ measurement with the measurement indicated by the fiber-optic catheter.*

• If the catheter values and the laboratory values differ by more than 4%, follow the manufacturer's instructions to enter the S$\bar{v}O_2$ value obtained by the laboratory into the co-oximeter.
• Recalibrate the monitor every 24 hours, or whenever the catheter has been disconnected from the optical module.

## Special considerations
• If the patient's S$\bar{v}O_2$ drops below 60%, or if it varies by more than 10% for 3 minutes or longer, reassess the patient. If the S$\bar{v}O_2$ doesn't return to the baseline value after appropriate nursing interventions, notify the doctor. A decreasing S$\bar{v}O_2$, or a value less than 60%, indicates impaired oxygen delivery, such as occurs during hemorrhage, hypoxia, shock, arrhythmias, or suctioning. S$\bar{v}O_2$ may also decrease as a result of increased oxygen demand from hyperthermia, shivering, or seizures, for example.
• If the intensity of the tracing is low, ensure that all connections between the catheter and co-oximeter are secure and that the catheter is patent and not kinked.
• If the tracing is damped or erratic, try to aspirate blood from the catheter *to check for patency.* If you can't aspirate blood, notify the patient's doctor *so that he can replace the catheter.* Also check the PA waveform *to determine whether the catheter has wedged.* If the catheter has wedged, attempt to flush the line. Also turn the patient from side to side and instruct him to cough. If the catheter remains wedged, notify the patient's doctor immediately.
• If the tracing shows a high intensity, the catheter may be pressing against a vessel wall. Flush the line. If the tracing doesn't return to normal, notify the doctor *so he can reposition the catheter.*

## Complications
Thrombosis can result from local irritation by the catheter; however, administering a heparin flush solution helps prevent this complication.

## SvO₂ monitoring equipment

The mixed venous saturation (SvO₂) monitoring system consists of a flow-directed pulmonary artery (PA) catheter with fiber-optic filaments, an optical module, and a co-oximeter. The co-oximeter displays a continuous digital SvO₂ value; the strip recorder prints a permanent record. The illustrations show a normal SvO₂ waveform, one from an active patient, and one that demonstrates positive end-expiratory pressure (PEEP) and fraction of inspired oxygen changes (FIO₂).

Catheter insertion follows the same technique used with any thermodilution flow-directed PA catheter. The distal lumen connects to an external PA pressure monitoring system; the proximal or central venous pressure (CVP) lumen connects to another monitoring system or to a continuous flow administration unit; and the optical module connects to the co-oximeter unit.

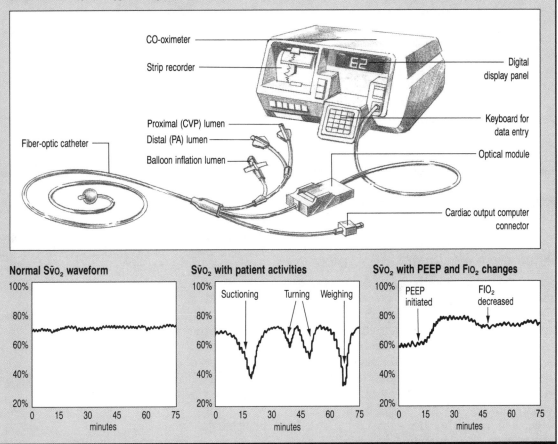

Thromboembolism also can occur if a thrombus breaks off and lodges in the circulatory system. Monitor the patient for signs and symptoms of infection—such as redness or drainage—at the catheter site.

### Documentation

Record the SvO₂ value on a flowchart and attach a tracing, as ordered. At the same time, note any significant changes in the patient's status and the results of any medical or nursing interventions. For comparison, note the SvO₂ as measured

## How oximetry works

The pulse oximeter allows noninvasive monitoring of a patient's arterial oxygen saturation ($SaO_2$) levels by measuring the absorption (amplitude) of light waves as they pass through areas of the body that are highly perfused by arterial blood. Oximetry also monitors pulse rate and amplitude.

Light-emitting diodes in a transducer (photodetector) attached to the patient's body (shown here on the index finger) send red and infrared light beams through tissue. The photodetector records the relative amounts of each color absorbed by arterial blood and transmits the data to a monitor, which displays the information with each heartbeat. If the $SaO_2$ level or pulse rate varies from preset limits, the monitor triggers visual and audible alarms.

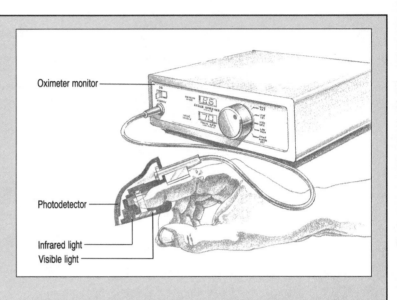

by the fiber-optic catheter whenever a blood sample is obtained for laboratory analysis of $S\bar{v}O_2$.

## Pulse and ear oximetry monitoring

Performed intermittently or continuously, oximetry is a relatively simple procedure used to monitor $SaO_2$. Pulse oximetry uses two diodes to send red and infrared light through a pulsating arterial vascular bed, like the one in the fingertip. A photodetector, which is slipped over the finger, measures the transmitted light as it passes through the vascular bed, detects the relative amount of color absorbed by arterial blood, and calculates the exact $SaO_2$ without interference from surrounding venous blood, skin, connective tissue, or bone. Ear oximetry works by monitoring the transmission of light waves through the vascular bed of a patient's earlobe. However, results will be inaccurate if the patient's earlobe is poorly perfused, as occurs with a low cardiac output. (See *How oximetry works.*)

If the patient has significantly reduced peripheral vascular pulsations, or if he is taking a vasoactive drug, oximetry may be performed through a nasal probe, which detects the pulsations of the septal anterior ethmoidal artery.

### Equipment
Oximeter ▪ finger or ear probe ▪ alcohol sponges ▪ nail polish remover, if necessary.

### Preparation of equipment
Review the manufacturer's instructions for assembly of the oximeter.

### Implementation
• Explain the procedure to the patient.

### *Performing pulse oximetry*
• Select a finger for the test. Although the index finger is commonly used, a smaller finger may be selected if the patient's fingers are too large for the equipment. Make sure the patient isn't

wearing false fingernails, and remove any nail polish from the test finger.

• Place the transducer (photodetector) probe over the patient's finger so that light beams and sensors oppose each other. If the patient has long fingernails, position the probe perpendicular to the finger if possible, or clip the fingernail.

• If you're testing a neonate or a small infant, wrap the probe around the foot so that light beams and detectors oppose each other. For a large infant, use a probe that fits on the great toe and secure it to the foot.

• Turn on the power switch. If the device is working properly, a beep will sound, a display will light momentarily, and the pulse searchlight will flash. The $SaO_2$ and pulse rate displays will show stationary zeros. After four to six heartbeats, the $SaO_2$ and pulse rate displays will supply information with each beat, and the pulse amplitude indicator will begin tracking the pulse.

### Performing ear oximetry

• Using an alcohol sponge, massage the patient's earlobe for 10 to 20 seconds. Mild erythema indicates adequate vascularization.

• Following the manufacturer's instructions, attach the ear probe to the patient's earlobe or pinna. Use the ear probe stabilizer for prolonged or exercise testing. Be sure to establish good contact on the ear; *an unstable probe may set off the low-perfusion alarm.*

• After the probe has been attached for a few seconds, an $SaO_2$ reading and pulse waveform will appear on the oximeter's screen. Leave the ear probe in place for 3 or more minutes until readings stabilize at the highest point, or take three separate readings and average them. Make sure you revascularize the patient's earlobe each time.

• After the procedure, remove the probe, turn off and unplug the unit, and clean the probe by gently rubbing it with an alcohol sponge.

### Special considerations

If oximetry has been performed properly, readings are typically accurate. However, certain factors may interfere with accuracy. For example, an elevated bilirubin level may falsely lower $SaO_2$ readings, while elevated carboxyhemoglobin or methemoglobin levels (such as occur in heavy smokers or urban dwellers) can cause a falsely elevated $SaO_2$ reading.

Certain intravascular substances — such as lipid emulsions and dyes — can also prevent accurate readings. Other factors that may interfere with accurate results include excessive light (such as from phototherapy, surgical lamps, direct sunlight, and excessive ambient lighting), excessive patient movement, excessive ear pigment, edema, hypothermia, hypotension, anemia, and vasoconstriction.

If light is a problem, cover the probes; if patient movement is a problem, move the probe or select a different probe; if ear pigment is a problem, reposition the probe, revascularize the site, or use a finger probe; and if low perfusion in the patient's finger is a problem, use a nasal sensor or place a reflective sensor on the patient's forehead. (See *What affects pulse oximetry readings,* page 78.)

Normal $SaO_2$ levels for ear and pulse oximetry are 95% to 100% for adults, and 93.8% to 100% by 1 hour after birth for healthy, full-term neonates. Lower levels may indicate hypoxemia that warrants intervention. For such patients, follow hospital policy or the doctor's orders, which may include increasing oxygen therapy. If $SaO_2$ levels decrease suddenly, you may need to resuscitate the patient immediately. Notify the doctor of any significant change in the patient's condition.

### Documentation

Document the procedure, including the date and time, the procedure type, the oximetric measurement, and any action taken. Record reading on appropriate flowcharts if indicated.

## What affects pulse oximetry readings?

If your patient is being monitored by pulse oximetry, be sure to maintain a continuous display of the oxygen saturation ($SpO_2$) value. (Arterial oxygen saturation [$SaO_2$] obtained by pulse oximetry is abbreviated $SpO_2$.) Here are some factors that commonly affect pulse oximetry readings – and measures you can take to prevent or correct false readings.

**Poor skin contact**
To prevent this problem, apply an adhesive sensor with fresh adhesive.

**Movement**
If the patient is moving the finger or toe to which the sensor is attached, the pulse oximeter may identify the motion as arterial pulsations, causing an inaccurate $SpO_2$ value. To minimize motion artifact, use an adhesive sensor or stabilize the sensor by immobilizing the monitor site.

You can also try connecting the oximeter to an electrocardiograph (ECG). The ECG will tell the sensor to work only when blood pulsation results from heart contractions (called ECG synchronization).

**Low perfusion**
Only small amounts of blood may flow through the finger's arterial bed if the patient has poor perfusion (such as from peripheral vascular disease or vasoconstrictive drugs). That

means the oximeter won't identify the arterial pulse and may not display an $SpO_2$ value. To prevent this problem, use a nasal sensor or place a reflectance sensor on the patient's forehead.

**Venous pulsation**
Normally nonpulsatile, venous blood may pulsate from right ventricular heart failure, a tight sensor, or any tourniquet-like effect. Because the oximeter looks for pulsating blood, it will detect both pulsating venous blood and pulsating arterial blood, producing a false $SpO_2$ value. Usually, you can avoid this problem simply by making sure the sensor isn't too tight.

**Outside light**
The $SpO_2$ value may be inaccurate if the photodetector senses large amounts of outside light (such as direct sunlight, procedure lamps, or bilirubin lights in the nursery). You can easily correct this by covering the sensor with a sheet or towel.

**Anemia**
Always double-check the patient's hemoglobin level. Even if he's anemic with a hemoglobin value of 5 g/dl, his $SpO_2$ value may seem normal because the hemoglobin that's available to carry oxygen is fully saturated. Yet he may have insufficient oxygen to meet his metabolic needs. To correct this problem, be prepared to administer red blood cells or whole blood.

# $ETCO_2$ monitoring

$ETCO_2$ monitoring determines the carbon dioxide concentration in exhaled gas. In this technique, a photodetector measures the amount of infrared light absorbed by airway gas during inspiration and expiration. (Light absorption increases along with the carbon dioxide concentration.) A monitor converts this data to a carbon dioxide value and a corresponding waveform, or capnogram, if capnography is used. (See *Understanding capnography*.)

$ETCO_2$ monitoring provides information about the patient's pulmonary, cardiac, and metabolic status that aids patient management and helps prevent clinical compromise. This technique has become a standard care measure during anesthesia administration and mechanical ventilation. For a patient with a stable acid-base

balance, it may be used to aid weaning from mechanical ventilation. It also reduces the need for frequent ABG measurements, especially when combined with pulse oximetry. (See *How $ETCO_2$ monitoring works*, page 80.)

Other uses for $ETCO_2$ monitoring include assessing resuscitation efforts and identifying the return of spontaneous circulation. Because no carbon dioxide is exhaled when breathing stops, this technique also detects apnea.

When used during endotracheal intubation, $ETCO_2$ monitoring can avert neurologic injury and even death by confirming correct endotracheal tube placement and detecting accidental esophageal intubation, since carbon dioxide isn't normally produced by the stomach. Ongoing $ETCO_2$ monitoring throughout intubation also can prove valuable because an endotracheal tube

## Understanding capnography

Capnographs monitor carbon dioxide ($CO_2$) levels, usually by measuring the partial pressure of end-tidal carbon dioxide ($ETCO_2$) in expired air. Most capnographs use infrared absorption spectroscopy to analyze gas samples. Of the common gases in exhaled air, only carbon dioxide and water vapor absorb infrared light. The capnograph evaporates water vapor by dehumidifying the gas sample, leaving only carbon dioxide to be measured.

Capnographs display carbon dioxide values in one of three ways: as a percentage, in millimeters of mercury (mm Hg), or in kilopascals. The monitor also displays carbon dioxide values graphically as a continuous waveform (capnograph).

Capnography allows you to measure ventilation, perfusion, and metabolism noninvasively. First used in the operating room by anesthesiologists, capnography may also be used for patients being mechanically ventilated, weaned from a mech-anical ventilator, or resuscitated by cardiopulmonary resuscitation in the intensive care unit or emergency department.

### Setting up the capnograph

Begin by calibrating the capnograph according to the manufacturer's instructions. Then attach the power cord to the receptacle on the monitor. After making sure the sample tube assembly is in good condition, connect one end to the sample inlet connector. You'll connect the other end when you're ready to use the monitor.

The capnograph has audible and visual alarms to alert you to a carbon dioxide value above or below the limits you set. The monitor also has alarms to warn of monitor failure and apnea. Be sure to set these controls as ordered, following the manufacturer's instructions.

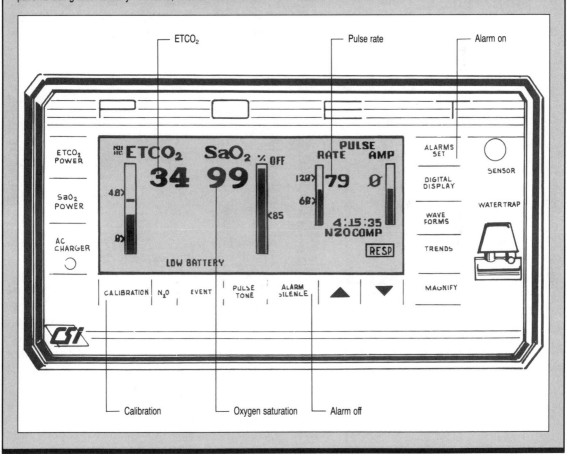

## How ETCO₂ monitoring works

The optical portion of an end-tidal carbon dioxide (ETCO₂) monitor contains an infrared light source, a sample chamber, a special carbon dioxide (CO₂) filter, and a photodetector. The infrared light passes through the sample chamber and is absorbed in varying amounts, depending on the amount of carbon dioxide the patient has just exhaled. The photodetector measures the carbon dioxide content and then relays this information to the microprocessor in the monitor, which displays the carbon dioxide value and waveform.

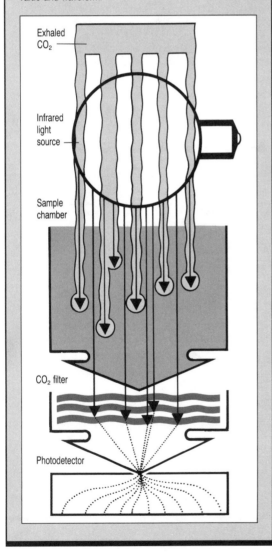

Exhaled CO₂

Infrared light source

Sample chamber

CO₂ filter

Photodetector

may become dislodged during manipulation or patient movement or transport.

Some carbon dioxide detection devices provide semiquantitative indications of carbon dioxide concentrations, supplying an approximate range rather than a specific value for ETCO₂. Other devices simply indicate whether carbon dioxide is present during exhalation. ETCO₂ monitoring has no contraindications.

### Equipment

Mainstream or sidestream ETCO₂ monitor ▪ ETCO₂ sensor ▪ airway adapter in a size appropriate for the patient, as recommended by the manufacturer. (For example, a neonatal adapter may have a much smaller dead space, making it appropriate for a smaller patient. For additional information on available equipment, see *Colorimetric ETCO₂ detection.*)

### Preparation of equipment

If the monitor you're using isn't self-calibrating, calibrate it as the manufacturer directs. If you're using a sidestream ETCO₂ monitor, be sure to replace the water trap between patients, if directed. *(The trap allows humidity from exhaled gases to be condensed into an attached container.)* Newer sidestream models don't require water traps.

### Implementation

• Wash your hands and don clean gloves.
• If the patient doesn't require intubation or is already intubated and alert, explain the purpose and expected duration of monitoring. Tell an intubated patient that the monitor will painlessly measure the amount of carbon dioxide exhaled. Inform a nonintubated patient that the monitor will track his carbon dioxide concentration *to make sure his breathing is effective.*
• Position the airway adapter and sensor as the manufacturer directs. For an intubated patient, position the adapter directly on the endotracheal tube. For a nonintubated patient, place the adapter at or near the patient's airway. (An ox-

ygen-delivery cannula may have a sample port through which gas can be aspirated for monitoring.)

The sensor, which contains an infrared light source and a photodetector, may be positioned at one of two sites in the monitoring setup. With a mainstream monitor, it's positioned directly at the patient's airway with an airway adapter, between the endotracheal tube and the breathing circuit tubing. With a sidestream monitor, the airway adapter is positioned at the airway (whether or not the patient is intubated) *to allow aspiration of gas from the patient's airway back to the sensor, which lies either within or close to the monitor.*

• Turn on all alarms and adjust alarm settings as appropriate for your patient. Make sure the alarm volume is loud enough to hear.

• Document the initial ETCO₂ value and all ventilator settings. Describe the waveform, if one appears on your monitor. If the monitor has a printer, you may want to print out a sample waveform and include it in the patient's medical record.

### Special considerations

The normal range for ETCO₂ values is from 35 to 45 mm Hg. They're usually 2 to 5 mm Hg less than a $PaCO_2$ value obtained by ABG measurement. This differential between arterial and ETCO₂ values is called the a-ADCO₂ value. This normal variance assumes that your patient has a normal ventilation-perfusion ratio and that you're sampling the gas correctly.

With adequate alveolar ventilation and blood flow to the lungs, normal ETCO₂ values should approximate $PaCO_2$ values. However, with significantly reduced pulmonary blood flow (as from cardiac arrest), ETCO₂ will drop below $PaCO_2$ — or may even measure zero.

If your patient's ETCO₂ values and $PaCO_2$ values differ, assess him for factors that can influence ETCO₂ — especially when the a-ADCO₂ value is above normal.

### Colorimetric ETCO₂ detection

A recent innovation in end-tidal carbon dioxide (ETCO₂) monitoring, colorimetric ETCO₂ detection uses a disposable device that changes color to signal the presence of carbon dioxide in the airway. On exhalation, a color change from purple to yellow or tan reveals the approximate ETCO₂ concentration. Color changes may occur for up to 2 hours of monitoring.

Colorimetric ETCO₂ detectors are commonly available in code carts, intubation kits, and emergency transport vehicles. They can be used for any intubated patient, especially if electronic ETCO₂ monitoring is unavailable.

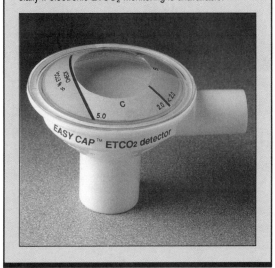

Interpreting the a-ADCO₂ value correctly will provide useful information about your patient's status. For example, an increased a-ADCO₂ value may mean your patient has worsening dead-space disease — especially if his Vᴛ remains constant.

Remember that ETCO₂ monitoring doesn't replace ABG measurements because it doesn't assess oxygenation or blood pH. Supplementing ETCO₂ monitoring with pulse oximetry may provide more complete information.

If the carbon dioxide waveform is available, assess it for height, frequency, rhythm, baseline, and shape to help evaluate gas exchange. Be sure you know how to recognize a normal waveform and can identify abnormal waveforms and

## Carbon dioxide waveform

The carbon dioxide ($CO_2$) waveform, or capnogram, produced in end-tidal carbon dioxide ($ETCO_2$) monitoring reflects the course of $CO_2$ elimination during exhalation. A normal capnogram (shown below) consists of several segments, which reflect the various stages of exhalation and inhalation.

Normally, any gas eliminated from the airway during *early exhalation* is dead-space gas, which hasn't undergone exchange at the alveolocapillary membrane. Measurements taken during this period contain no $CO_2$.

As exhalation continues, $CO_2$ *concentration rises* sharply and rapidly. The sensor now detects gas that has under-

gone exchange, producing measurable quantities of $CO_2$.

The final stages of alveolar emptying occur during late exhalation. During the *alveolar plateau* phase, $CO_2$ concentration rises more gradually because alveolar emptying is more constant.

The point at which the $ETCO_2$ value is derived is the *end of exhalation*, when $CO_2$ concentration peaks. Unless an alveolar plateau is present, this value doesn't accurately estimate alveolar $CO_2$. During inhalation, the $CO_2$ *concentration declines* sharply to zero.

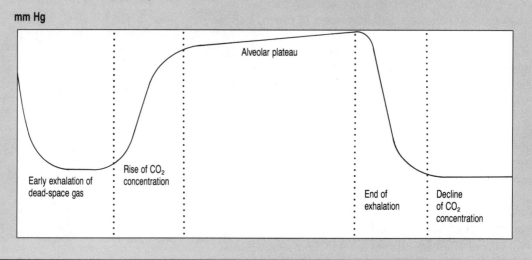

mm Hg

Alveolar plateau

Early exhalation of dead-space gas

Rise of $CO_2$ concentration

End of exhalation

Decline of $CO_2$ concentration

their possible causes. If a printer is available, record and document any abnormal waveforms in the patient's medical record. (See *Carbon dioxide waveform.*)

In a nonintubated patient, use $ETCO_2$ values to establish trends. Be aware that in this patient, exhaled gas is more likely to mix with ambient air and exhaled carbon dioxide may be diluted by fresh gas flow from the nasal cannula.

Wear gloves when handling the airway adapter to prevent cross-contamination. Make sure the adapter is changed with every breathing circuit and endotracheal tube change.

Place the adapter as close to the endotracheal tube as possible to avoid contaminating exhaled

gases with fresh gas flow from the ventilator. If you're using a heat and moisture exchanger, you may be able to position the airway adapter between the exchanger and breathing circuit.

$ETCO_2$ monitoring commonly is discontinued when the patient has been weaned effectively from mechanical ventilation or when he's no longer at risk for respiratory compromise. Carefully assess your patient's tolerance for weaning. After extubation, continuous $ETCO_2$ monitoring may detect the need for reintubation.

## Documentation

Document ETCO$_2$ values at least as often as vital signs, whenever significant changes in waveform or patient status occur, and before and after weaning, respiratory, and other interventions. Periodically obtain samples for ABG analysis as the patient's condition dictates, and document the corresponding ETCO$_2$ value.

# TcPO$_2$ and TcPCO$_2$ monitoring

Used primarily in neonates, TcPO$_2$ and TcPCO$_2$ monitoring evaluate the adequacy of gas exchange. These two noninvasive techniques may be done alone or in combination. An electrode or a sensor containing a transducer system, heating device, and temperature probe is applied to the skin with an adhesive ring. Partial pressure sensing devices measure oxygen and carbon dioxide diffusion through the skin from capillaries directly beneath the surface. This procedure supplements the established methods of observing skin color and obtaining periodic ABG values to detect hypoxemia and hyperoxemia. However, obtaining periodic ABG values is the most accurate method of evaluating gas exchange.

In TcPO$_2$ monitoring, the electrode is heated to a constant temperature above skin temperature—usually 109° to 111° F (43° to 44° C). Normally, partial pressure of oxygen (PO$_2$) of skin is near zero, although it may be higher in premature infants. Heating the electrode causes the lipid matrix of the stratum corneum epidermidis, the skin's outermost layer, to melt, enhancing capillary blood flow and promoting oxygen diffusion through the tissue under the electrode or sensor. Chemically reduced, diffused oxygen provides a current proportional to the PO$_2$ level at the oxygen-permeable membrane on the sensor surface. Because skin heating increases metabolism, this method may slightly underestimate PO$_2$. (See *How transcutaneous monitoring works,* page 84.)

Typically, carbon dioxide in unheated skin is approximately equal to carbon dioxide in venous blood. In TcPCO$_2$ monitoring, the heated sensor causes carbon dioxide to diffuse from capillaries across a carbon dioxide-permeable membrane on the sensor. Carbon dioxide then reacts with an electrolyte solution, allowing TcPCO$_2$ measurement. Because heating increases metabolism, TcPCO$_2$ values may somewhat overestimate PaCO$_2$.

## Equipment

TcPO$_2$ monitor, TcPCO$_2$ monitor, or a combination TcPO$_2$-TcPCO$_2$ monitor ▪ electrode or sensor ▪ contact medium or water ▪ alcohol sponge ▪ adhesive ring.

If the sensor requires maintenance, you may need additional equipment, as specified by the manufacturer.

## Preparation of equipment

Set up the monitor and calibrate it as required, following the manufacturer's instructions.

## Implementation

• Explain the monitoring procedure to the patient. If you're caring for an infant, explain the procedure to the parents. Provide emotional support to the parents, as needed, and answer any questions.

• Choose a site for electrode placement. The transcutaneous electrode can be placed on any flat site—preferably one with good capillary blood flow, few fatty deposits, and no bony prominences. In a neonate, the upper chest, abdomen, and inner thigh are common monitoring sites; you should avoid the extremities and costophrenic margin. If you're caring for a neonate or an infant with patent ductus arteriosus, choose a TcPO$_2$ sensor site carefully because right-to-left blood shunting may occur. A sensor placed on the right upper chest will reflect the higher, preductal PaO$_2$, whereas a sensor placed on the abdomen or thigh usually will reflect the lower, postductal PaO$_2$. In some cases, you may place

## How transcutaneous monitoring works

In transcutaneous oxygen and carbon dioxide monitoring, a heated electrode is placed on the skin, where it melts the lipid matrix of the stratum corneum epidermidis. This dramatically enhances capillary blood flow and increases oxygen and carbon dioxide diffusion through the tissue beneath the electrode. The monitor measures the amount of diffused oxygen or carbon dioxide.

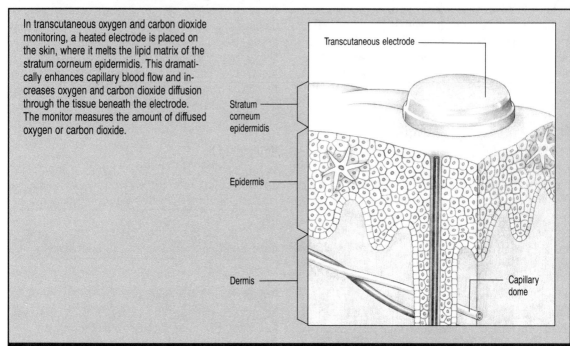

two $TcPO_2$ sensors on the infant with right-to-left shunting to monitor both preductal and postductal values, which can provide valuable data about intracardiac shunting.

• Wash your hands. Using an alcohol sponge, clean the electrode or sensor application site to remove skin oils and ensure good contact. Let the skin air-dry.

• Attach the double-sided adhesive ring to the electrode or sensor. As the manufacturer directs, moisten the site with a drop of water or a special gel to enhance contact.

• Place the electrode or sensor on the skin site, making sure the adhesive ring is tight and free from air gaps.

• Set the alarm switches and electrode or sensor temperature according to the manufacturer's instructions or hospital policy.

• Carefully monitor and rotate the sensor site every 2 to 4 hours to prevent skin irritation or burns. (An extremely premature infant may require more frequent site changes.) Ensure appropriate temperature limits.

### Special considerations

After you apply a $TcPO_2$ sensor, the patient's $TcPO_2$ value should fall rapidly because ambient air has a higher oxygen concentration than the skin surface. Once vessels at the sensor site dilate from heat (roughly 10 to 20 minutes), the value should rise accordingly. Normal $TcPO_2$ values range from 50 to 90 mm Hg.

After you apply a $TcPCO_2$ sensor, the patient's $TcPCO_2$ value should rise because ambient air has a lower carbon dioxide concentration than the skin surface. After 10 to 20 minutes, the value may drop slightly. Normal $TcPCO_2$ values range from 35 to 45 mm Hg.

Although $TcPO_2$ values estimate $PaO_2$ fairly accurately, they're most accurate with $PaO_2$ values below 80 mm Hg. This is one reason why TcPO$_2$ monitoring is generally recommended only for neonates.

With adequate blood flow to the sensor site and maximal diffusion across the skin, TcPO$_2$ values help establish the PaO$_2$ trend. However, if circumstances aren't ideal, TcPO$_2$ values may underestimate PaO$_2$ values. For example, poor perfusion (such as from hypotension, hypovolemia, or hypothermia) may decrease blood flow to the sensor even with adequate sensor temperature. Vasoconstrictive drugs and extensive edema may also impair blood flow. Variations in skin thickness may contribute to altered oxygen diffusion from the capillaries, possibly affecting the TcPO$_2$ value. Generally, the thicker the skin, the wider the variance between TcPO$_2$ and PaO$_2$ values — another reason why this form of monitoring is preferred for neonates and older people, who have thinner skin.

Falling TcPO$_2$ values that vary widely from PaO$_2$ values call for further investigation. For example, TcPO$_2$ may decrease from ineffective respiration, poor circulation, or a combination of the two. To ensure proper assessment and intervention, you should assess the patient closely for signs and symptoms of circulatory and respiratory impairment.

Because carbon dioxide diffuses more easily than oxygen, TcPCO$_2$ values correlate more closely with PaCO$_2$ values. Typically, TcPCO$_2$ values are less sensitive to changes in blood flow to the skin. Also, gestational age (in neonates and infants), body temperature, decreased blood flow, and vasoactive drugs are less likely to cause inaccurate or unreliable TcPCO$_2$ values.

Stay alert for burns and blisters from the electrode and skin reactions to the adhesive ring. Frequently assess the patient's skin integrity and tolerance for monitoring.

Although slight erythema may occur at the sensor site, it should subside shortly after sensor removal. If erythema does occur, explain the cause to the patient or his parents and reassure them that the redness probably will disappear within a few hours.

Make sure the sensor isn't occluded or covered by any source, because pressure on the sensor may interfere with blood flow to the sensor site and cause pressure necrosis and burns.

Once the sensor reaches equilibrium, expect a delayed response time (30 to 80 seconds) before the monitor responds to PaO$_2$ or PaCO$_2$ changes. Keep this in mind if you're sampling blood for ABG analysis, because monitor values may differ from ABG values if respiratory changes or activity occurs during this interval. Always note the transcutaneous value when drawing a blood sample for ABG analysis to determine how closely the values are tracking one another.

A sudden change in transcutaneous values unrelated to a change in patient status may mean the sensor has become partially or fully detached from the skin. If this happens, recalibrate the monitor and reapply the sensor as instructed by the manufacturer.

Be aware that TcPO$_2$ and TcPCO$_2$ values may change with nursing interventions. Carefully assess your patient's tolerance for care procedures, such as suctioning and chest physiotherapy, and modify these interventions as needed to prevent or minimize respiratory compromise.

Expect transcutaneous values to vary with patient oxygenation changes caused by activity, such as crying, feeding, and exercise. Be prepared to obtain a blood sample for ABG analysis and to start resuscitation if you suspect a change in transcutaneous values that may reflect patient compromise.

Be sure to obtain periodic ABG values, because transcutaneous monitoring doesn't assess pH and may not always reflect actual PaO$_2$ and PaCO$_2$ values.

Usually, transcutaneous monitoring ends when the patient regains a stable cardiopulmonary status and no longer needs mechanical ventilation and oxygen therapy. After monitoring ends, assess your patient's respirations for comfort and regularity. Consider resuming monitoring if cardiorespiratory compromise recurs.

## Documentation

Document $TcPO_2$ and $TcPCO_2$ values — at least as often as vital signs and before and after respiratory interventions — and all sensor site changes. Also document and report any changes in skin integrity, and intervene appropriately.

# Apnea monitoring in adults

Commonly used at the bedside, apnea monitoring provides an early warning of impending apneic episodes, documents the incidence and degree of apnea, and assesses the effectiveness of interventions.

In adults, apnea is defined as an absence of breathing lasting 10 seconds or longer. Apnea occurs as two distinct types: central and obstructive. Mixed apnea — a combination of central and obstructive apnea — also may occur.

In *central apnea*, the patient has no central respiratory output and therefore no respiratory effort. Central apnea is related to abnormal CNS functions that aren't fully understood.

In *obstructive apnea*, central respiratory output occurs, but pharyngeal closure prevents airflow. Obstructive apnea may result from collapse of the compliant pharyngeal muscles, altered airway configuration caused by positioning, failure of smaller airways to remain patent, anatomic airway narrowing from fat or tissue edema, chronic inflammation caused by snoring, or increased upper airway resistance secondary to swelling or obstruction.

Many people normally experience brief periods of apnea during sleep. In *sleep apnea syndrome (SAS)*, multiple episodes of obstructive or mixed apnea occur, accompanied by loud, repetitive snoring and daytime somnolence. Although definitions of SAS vary, the term usually refers to 30 or more periods of apnea per 7 hours of sleep or more than 5 such episodes per hour. SAS may cause problems ranging from mild to serious, including insomnia, daytime hypersomnolence, personality changes, cognitive dysfunction, arrhythmias, and laboratory test abnormalities (such as polycythemia, hypercapnia, and hypoxemia).

Apnea monitors may also be used for vulnerable neonates, such as those born prematurely or those with neurologic disorders, neonatal respiratory distress syndrome, seizure disorders, congenital heart disease with congestive heart failure, a tracheostomy, a personal history of sleep-induced apnea, a family history of sudden infant death syndrome, or acute drug withdrawal. (For more information on the use of apnea monitors in neonates, see Chapter 7.)

### Equipment

Thoracic impedance monitor unit ▪ chest electrodes ▪ leadwires.

The thoracic impedance monitor detects changes in thoracic impedance, which increases during inspiration and decreases during expiration. A respiratory amplifier displays the respiratory rate. Some monitors also display a respiratory waveform, whose amplitude reflects respiratory depth.

### Preparation of equipment

Plug the power cable into a grounded electrical outlet.

### Implementation

• Explain the monitoring procedure to the patient and his family. Tell them you'll be using a device to monitor the patient's breathing. Explain how the device is applied and describe the information the monitor will display. Warn them never to change the alarm settings or turn off the monitor.

• Wash your hands. Next, clean the patient's chest and abdomen with soap and warm water at the sites where electrodes will be placed. Dry the skin thoroughly.

• Place electrodes on the chest and abdomen, as the manufacturer directs. Attach the leadwires to the electrodes. Be sure to target areas where chest wall movement is greatest to help detect an adequate signal.

• Turn on the monitor. Set the high and low respiratory rate alarms and adjust the apnea time period. Make sure the alarm volume is audible and the printer (if available) is loaded with paper.

• Observe the respiratory rate, waveform, and heart rate displayed on the monitor.

## Special considerations

Normally, respirations are regular and rhythmic, without prolonged interruption. Therefore, consider frequent apnea a significant finding, especially when accompanied by other symptoms. The patient may need additional evaluation, including complete polysomnography assessment.

Apnea duration and frequency may relate to such treatments as drug therapy, continuous positive airway pressure, or surgery. As interventions change, note any improvement or deterioration in the patient's respiratory rate and pattern.

When an apnea alarm sounds, first assess the patient, checking for bradycardia and other arrhythmias, cyanosis, and airway obstruction. Be prepared to ventilate and oxygenate the patient if he remains unresponsive to stimulation. Carefully assess airway adequacy and intervene as necessary to maintain patency.

After correcting apnea, evaluate the patient for the underlying cause by thoroughly assessing his respiratory, neurologic, and metabolic status. If you suspect sepsis, obtain cultures and administer antibiotics, as ordered. Specific therapy aims to treat the underlying cause of apnea.

If your patient has obstructive apnea, stay alert for airway obstruction during apnea monitoring. The chest wall may continue to move even though the airway is obstructed. Because the apnea monitor can't distinguish between effective and ineffective ventilation, a patient with unstable respiratory status may require addi-

tional monitoring, such as pulse oximetry and capnography.

If interference or poor signal quality triggers the apnea alarm, reassess the position and integrity of chest electrodes. If necessary, reposition or replace electrodes to enhance signal quality. Also replace any loose electrodes. Remove electrodes carefully, particularly if the patient has an actual or potential skin integrity impairment.

If ordered, use airway thermistors and $ETCO_2$ monitoring devices to detect apnea. Airway thermistors produce varied electrical resistance in response to normal temperature changes that occur during inspiration and expiration (the air is cooler on inspiration than expiration). $ETCO_2$ monitoring devices detect apnea by measuring airway carbon dioxide levels, which are absent when breathing ceases.

Before discharge, teach the patient and his family how to use an apnea monitor at home, if indicated.

Apnea monitoring usually is discontinued after testing has been completed or when apneic episodes decrease in frequency and duration to a clinically acceptable level. It also may be discontinued if the doctor orders an alternative form of respiratory monitoring, such as $ETCO_2$ monitoring.

### Documentation

Document and report to the doctor the presence and degree of any apneic episodes, including their time, frequency, and duration. Also document any associated bradycardia or other findings along with any medical or nursing interventions.

# Ventilator monitoring

A mechanical ventilator moves air in and out of a patient's lungs. However, although the equipment serves to ventilate a patient, it doesn't ensure adequate gas exchange. Mechanical ventilators may use either positive or negative pressure to ventilate patients.

## High-frequency jet ventilation

This technique was developed for use when high peak-airway pressures or large intrapleural air leaks preclude conventional mechanical ventilation. The high-frequency jet ventilation (HFJV) system employs a narrow injector cannula to deliver short, rapid bursts of oxygen to the airways under low pressure.

This combination of high rate, low tidal volumes, and low pressure enhances alveolar gas exchange without elevating peak inspiratory pressures and compromising cardiac output—the major drawback of conventional high-volume, high-pressure mechanical ventilation. Thus, HFJV is valuable for patients with hemodynamic instability and those at high risk for pulmonary barotrauma, such as young children. It's also useful for ventilating patients during bronchoscopy, laryngoscopy, and laryngeal surgery because its narrow cannula doesn't obstruct the operating field.

A potential new use of HFJV is in emergency respiratory situations. Because the cannula can be inserted directly into the trachea through a cricothyrotomy, HFJV may be used when upper airway trauma or obstruction precludes intubation. Use of HFJV in cardiopulmonary resuscitation allows continuous ventilation during chest compression. And its use in patients with chest trauma decreases chest wall movement and improves stability, enhancing ventilation.

Positive pressure ventilators exert a positive pressure on the airway, which causes inspiration and, at the same time, increases the patient's $V_T$. The inspiratory cycles of these ventilators may vary according to volume, pressure, or time. For example, a volume-cycled ventilator—the type used most commonly—delivers a preset volume of air to the patient each time, regardless of the amount of resistance exerted by the patient's lungs. A pressure-cycled ventilator generates flow until the machine reaches a preset pressure, regardless of the volume delivered or the time required to achieve the pressure. A time-cycled ventilator generates flow for a preset amount of time.

High-frequency jet ventilation is the newest type of positive-pressure ventilation. This technique prevents fluctuation of pressure within the lungs and doesn't cause the detrimental effects on the cardiovascular system that other positive-pressure ventilators do. (See *High-frequency jet ventilation.*)

Negative pressure ventilators act by creating negative pressure, which pulls the patient's thorax outward and allows air to flow into the patient's lungs. Examples of negative pressure ventilators are the iron lung, the cuirass (chest shell), and the body wrap. Negative pressure ventilators are used primarily to treat patients with neuromuscular disorders, such as Guillain-Barré syndrome, myasthenia gravis, and poliomyelitis.

Other indications for ventilator use include central nervous system disorders, such as cerebral hemorrhage and spinal cord transsection, ARDS, pulmonary edema, COPD, flail chest, and acute hypoventilation.

### Equipment

Oxygen source ■ air source that can supply 50 psi ■ mechanical ventilator ■ humidifier ■ ventilator circuit tubing, connectors, and adapters ■ condensation collection trap ■ spirometer, respirometer, or electronic device to measure flow and volume ■ in-line thermometer ■ probe for gas sampling and measuring airway pressure ■ bacterial filter ■ gloves ■ hand-held resuscitation bag with reservoir ■ suction equipment ■ sterile distilled water ■ equipment for ABG analysis ■ soft restraints, if indicated ■ optional: co-oximeter.

### Preparation of equipment

In most hospitals, respiratory therapists assume responsibility for setting up the ventilator. If necessary, check the manufacturer's instructions for setting it up. In most cases, you'll need to add sterile distilled water to the humidifier and connect the ventilator to the appropriate gas source.

## Mechanical ventilation glossary

Although a respiratory therapist usually monitors ventilator settings based on the doctor's order, you should understand each of the following terms.

**Assist-control mode:** The ventilator delivers a preset tidal volume (VT) at a preset rate; however, the patient can initiate additional breaths, which trigger the ventilator to deliver the preset VT at positive pressure.

**Continuous positive airway pressure (CPAP):** This setting prompts the ventilator to deliver positive pressure to the airway throughout the respiratory cycle. It works only on patients who can breathe spontaneously.

**Control mode:** The ventilator delivers a preset VT at a fixed rate, regardless of whether the patient is breathing spontaneously or not.

**Fraction of inspired oxygen (FIO₂):** The amount of oxygen delivered to the patient by the ventilator. The dial on the ventilator that sets this percentage is labelled by the term oxygen concentration or oxygen percentage.

**I:E ratio:** This ratio compares the duration of inspiration to the duration of expiration. The I:E ratio of normal, spontaneous breathing is 1:2, meaning that expiration is twice as long as inspiration.

**Inspiratory flow rate (IFR):** The IFR denotes the VT delivered within a certain time. Its value can range from 20 to 120 liters/minute.

**Minute ventilation or minute volume (MV):** This measurement results from multiplying respiratory rate and VT.

**Peak inspiratory pressure (PIP):** Measured by the pressure manometer on the ventilator, PIP reflects the amount of pressure required to deliver a preset VT.

**Positive end-expiratory pressure (PEEP):** In this mode, the ventilator is triggered to apply positive pressure at the end of each expiration to increase the area for oxygen exchange by helping to inflate and keep open collapsed alveoli.

**Pressure support ventilation (PSV):** This mode allows the ventilator to apply a preset amount of positive pressure when the patient inspires spontaneously. PSV increases VT while decreasing the patient's breathing workload.

**Respiratory rate:** Also called frequency, this is the number of breaths per minute delivered by the ventilator.

**Sensitivity setting:** This setting determines the amount of effort the patient must exert to trigger the inspiratory cycle.

**Sigh volume:** This ventilator-delivered breath is 1½ times as large as the patient's VT.

**Synchronized intermittent mandatory ventilation (SIMV):** The ventilator delivers a preset number of breaths at a specific VT. The patient may supplement these mechanical ventilations with his own breaths, in which case the VT and rate are determined by his own inspiratory ability.

**VT:** VT refers to the volume of air delivered to the patient with each cycle, usually 12 to 15 cc/kg of body weight.

## Implementation

• Verify the doctor's order for ventilator support. If the patient is not already intubated, prepare him for intubation.

• When possible, explain the procedure to the patient and his family *to help reduce anxiety and fear.* Assure the patient and his family that staff members are nearby to provide care.

• Perform a complete physical assessment and draw blood for ABG analysis *to establish a baseline.*

• Don sterile gloves and protective gear, and suction the patient if necessary.

• Plug the ventilator into the electrical outlet and turn it on. Adjust the settings on the ventilator as ordered. (See *Mechanical ventilation glossary.*) Make sure that the ventilator's alarms are set,

as ordered, and that the humidifier is filled with sterile distilled water.

• Connect the endotracheal tube to the ventilator. Observe for chest expansion and auscultate for bilateral breath sounds *to verify that the patient is being ventilated.*

• Monitor the patient's ABG values after the initial ventilator setup (usually 20 to 30 minutes), after any changes in ventilator settings, and as the patient's clinical condition indicates *to determine whether the patient is being adequately ventilated and to avoid oxygen toxicity.* Be prepared to adjust ventilator settings depending on ABG analysis.

• Check the ventilator tubing frequently for condensation, *which can cause resistance to airflow and which may also be aspirated by the patient.* As

## Weaning the patient from the ventilator

Successful weaning depends on the patient's ability to breathe on his own. That means he must have a spontaneous respiratory effort that can keep him ventilated, a stable cardiovascular system, and sufficient respiratory muscle strength and level of consciousness to sustain spontaneous breathing. He also should meet some or all of the following criteria.

### Criteria
• Partial pressure of arterial oxygen ($PaO_2$) of 60 mm Hg (50 mm Hg or the ability to maintain baseline levels if he has chronic lung disease) or a fraction of inspired oxygen ($FIO_2$) at or below 0.4
• Partial pressure of arterial carbon dioxide ($PaCO_2$) of less than 40 mm Hg (or normal for the patient), or an $FIO_2$ of 0.4 or less if his $PaCO_2$ is 60 mm Hg or more
• Vital capacity of more than 10 ml/kg of body weight
• Maximum inspiratory pressure over $-20$ cm $H_2O$
• Minute ventilation (MV) under 10 liters/minute with a respiratory frequency of less than 28 to 30 breaths/minute
• Forced expiratory volume in the first second of more than 10 ml/kg of body weight
• Ability to double his spontaneous resting MV
• Adequate natural airway or a functioning tracheostomy
• Ability to cough and mobilize secretions
• Successful withdrawal of any neuromuscular blocker, such as pancuronium
• Clear or clearing chest X-ray
• Absence of infection, acid-base or electrolyte imbalance, hyperglycemia, arrhythmias, renal failure, anemia, fever, or excessive fatigue

### Short-term ventilation
If the patient has received mechanical ventilation for a short time, weaning may be accomplished by progressively decreasing the frequency and tidal volume of the ventilated breaths. Then the patient's endotracheal tube can be converted to a T tube to assess whether his spontaneous respirations are adequate before extubation. If the patient has been mechanically ventilated with 5 cm $H_2O$ or less of positive end-expiratory pressure, the adequacy of his spontaneous breathing can be assessed by using a trial of continuous positive airway pressure on the ventilator.

### Long-term ventilation
If the patient has received mechanical ventilation for a long time, weaning is usually accomplished by switching the ventilator to pressure support ventilation (PSV), with or without intermittent mandatory ventilation (IMV). This way, each of the patient's spontaneous breaths is augmented by the ventilator. As the patient's own respirations improve, the IMV and the PSV can be decreased.

If the patient doesn't progress satisfactorily using one of these methods, an alternative method of weaning is to disconnect the patient from the ventilator and place him on a T tube or tracheostomy collar for the ordered amount of time before reconnecting him to the ventilator. The patient then alternates between being on and off the ventilator, with the time off the ventilator increasing with each trial. Eventually, the patient will be able to breathe on his own all day. But, even then, he should be reconnected to the ventilator for a few nights so that he can obtain adequate rest and conserve the energy required to breathe on his own the next day.

---

needed, drain the condensate into a collection trap or briefly disconnect the patient from the ventilator (ventilating him with a hand-held resuscitation bag if necessary), and empty the water into a receptacle. Do not drain the condensate into the humidifier *because the condensation may be contaminated with the patient's secretions.*
• Check the in-line thermometer to make sure that the temperature of the air delivered to the patient is close to body temperature.
• When monitoring the patient's vital signs, count spontaneous breaths as well as ventilator-delivered breaths.

• Change, clean, or dispose of the ventilator tubing and equipment in accordance with hospital policy *to reduce the risk of bacterial contamination.* Typically, ventilator tubing should be changed every 24 to 48 hours, sometimes more often.
• When ordered, begin to wean the patient from the ventilator. (See *Weaning the patient from the ventilator.*)

### Special considerations
Make sure that the ventilator alarms are on at all times. *These alarms alert the nursing staff to potentially hazardous conditions and changes in patient status.* If an alarm sounds and the prob-

## Responding to ventilator alarms

| SIGNAL | POSSIBLE CAUSE | INTERVENTIONS |
|---|---|---|
| Low-pressure alarm | • Tube disconnected from ventilator<br>• Endotracheal tube displaced above vocal cords or tracheostomy tube extubated | • Reconnect the tube to the ventilator.<br>• Check tube placement and reposition if needed. If extubation or displacement has occurred, ventilate the patient manually and call the doctor immediately. |
| | • Leaking tidal volume from low cuff pressure (from an underinflated or ruptured cuff or a leak in the cuff or one-way valve) | • Listen for a whooshing sound around the tube, indicating an air leak. If you hear one, check cuff pressure. If you can't maintain pressure, call the doctor; he may need to insert a new tube. |
| | • Ventilator malfunction | • Disconnect the patient from the ventilator and ventilate him manually if necessary. Obtain another ventilator. |
| | • Leak in ventilator circuitry (from loose connection or hole in tubing, loss of temperature-sensitive device, or cracked humidification jar) | • Make sure all connections are intact. Check for holes or leaks in the tubing and replace if necessary. Check the humidification jar and replace if cracked. |
| High-pressure alarm | • Increased airway pressure or decreased lung compliance caused by worsening disease | • Auscultate the lungs for evidence of increasing lung consolidation, barotrauma, or wheezing. Call the doctor if indicated. |
| | • Patient is biting on oral endotracheal tube<br>• Secretions in airway | • Insert a bite block if needed.<br>• Look for secretions in the airway. To remove them, suction the patient or have him cough. |
| | • Condensate in large-bore tubing<br>• Intubation of right mainstem bronchus | • Check tubing for condensate and remove any fluid.<br>• Check tube position. If it has slipped, call the doctor; he may need to reposition it. |
| | • Patient coughing, gagging, or attempting to talk | • If the patient fights the ventilator, the doctor may order a sedative or neuromuscular blocking agent. |
| | • Chest wall resistance | • Reposition the patient if it improves chest expansion. If repositioning doesn't help, administer the prescribed analgesic. |
| | • Failure of high-pressure relief valve<br>• Bronchospasm | • Have the faulty equipment replaced.<br>• Assess the patient for the cause. Report to the doctor and treat as ordered. |

lem can't be identified easily, disconnect the patient from the ventilator and use a hand-held resuscitation bag to ventilate him. (See *Responding to ventilator alarms*.)

Provide emotional support to the patient during all phases of mechanical ventilation *to reduce anxiety and promote successful treatment*. Even if the patient is unresponsive, continue to explain all procedures and treatments to him.

Unless contraindicated, turn the patient from side to side every 1 to 2 hours *to facilitate lung expansion and removal of secretions*. Monitor breath sounds regularly and suction as needed. Perform active or passive range-of-motion exercises for all extremities *to reduce the hazards of immobility*. If the patient's condition permits, position him upright at regular intervals *to increase lung expansion*. When moving the patient or the ventilator tubing, be careful to prevent condensation in the tubing from flowing into the lungs *because aspiration of this contaminated moisture can cause infection.* Provide care for the patient's artificial airway as needed. Also provide adequate mouth care.

Assess the patient's peripheral circulation, and monitor his urine output for signs of decreased cardiac output. Watch for signs and symptoms of fluid volume excess or dehydration.

Place the call light within the patient's reach, and establish a method of communication, such as a communication board, *because intubation and mechanical ventilation impair the patient's ability to speak.* An artificial airway may help the patient to speak *by allowing air to pass through his vocal cords.*

Administer a sedative or neuromuscular blocking agent, as ordered, *to relax the patient or eliminate spontaneous breathing efforts that can interfere with the ventilator's action.* Remember that the patient receiving a neuromuscular blocking drug requires close observation *because of his inability to breathe or communicate.*

If the patient is receiving a neuromuscular blocking agent, make sure that he also receives a sedative. *Neuromuscular blocking agents cause paralysis without altering the patient's level of consciousness.* Reassure the patient and his family that the paralysis is temporary. Also make sure that emergency equipment is readily available in case the ventilator malfunctions or the patient is extubated accidentally. Continue to explain all procedures to the patient, and take extra steps to ensure his safety, such as raising the side rails during turning and covering and lubricating his eyes.

Ensure that the patient gets adequate rest and sleep *because fatigue can delay weaning from the ventilator.* Provide subdued lighting, safely muffle equipment noises, and restrict staff access to the area *to promote quiet during rest periods.*

When weaning the patient, continue to observe for signs of hypoxia. Schedule weaning to fit comfortably and realistically with the pa-

tient's daily regimen. Avoid scheduling sessions after meals, baths, or lengthy therapeutic or diagnostic procedures. Have the patient help you set up the schedule *to give him some sense of control over a frightening procedure.* As the patient's tolerance for weaning increases, help him sit up out of bed *to improve his breathing and sense of well-being.* Suggest diversionary activities *to take his mind off breathing.*

### Home care
If the patient will be discharged on a ventilator, evaluate the family's or the caregiver's ability and motivation to provide such care. Well before discharge, develop a teaching plan that will address the patient's needs. For example, teaching should include information about ventilator care and settings, artificial airway care, suctioning, respiratory therapy, communication, nutrition, therapeutic exercise, the signs and symptoms of infection, and ways to troubleshoot minor equipment malfunctions.

Also evaluate the patient's need for adaptive equipment, such as a hospital bed, wheelchair or walker with a ventilator tray, patient lift, and bedside commode. Determine whether the patient needs to travel; if so, select appropriate portable and backup equipment.

Before discharge, have the patient's caregiver demonstrate his ability to use the equipment. At discharge, contact a medical equipment vendor and a home health nurse to follow up with the patient. Also refer the patient to community resources, if available.

### Complications
Mechanical ventilation can cause tension pneumothorax, decreased cardiac output, oxygen toxicity, infection, fluid volume excess caused by humidification, and such GI complications as distention or bleeding from stress ulcers.

### Documentation
Document the date and time of initiation of mechanical ventilation. Name the type of ventilator

used for the patient, and note its settings. Describe the patient's subjective and objective response to mechanical ventilation (including vital signs, breath sounds, use of accessory muscles, intake and output, and weight). List any complications and nursing actions taken. Record all pertinent laboratory data, including ABG analysis results and $SaO_2$ levels.

During weaning, record the date and time of each session; the weaning method; and the baseline and subsequent vital signs, $SaO_2$ levels, and ABG values. Again describe the patient's subjective and objective responses (including level of consciousness, respiratory effort, arrhythmias, skin color, and need for suctioning).

List all complications and nursing actions taken. If the patient was receiving pressure support ventilation or using a T tube or tracheostomy collar, note the duration of spontaneous breathing and the patient's ability to maintain the weaning schedule. If using intermittent mandatory ventilation, with or without pressure support ventilation, record the control breath rate, the time of each breath reduction, and the rate of spontaneous respirations.

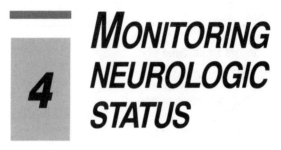

# 4 MONITORING NEUROLOGIC STATUS

## Introduction

Effective neurologic care aims to preserve and restore optimal nervous system function. Precise nursing skills, meticulously applied, are indispensable to achieving effective care. More and more, these nursing skills require mastery of sophisticated techniques and equipment.

## Neurologic assessment

Appropriate supportive care requires that you assess and document neurologic vital signs. At the same time, you also need to assess other systems for complications of neurologic dysfunction.

Be sure to assess neurologic vital signs—especially the patient's orientation level. Many patients experience changes in perception—ranging from confusion to psychosis—from neurologic dysfunction. Unaddressed, this disorientation further impairs the patient's ability to participate in his recovery. Recognizing this will help you intervene appropriately.

To record and track assessment findings, use special neurologic assessment forms or flow-charts. In common use at most hospitals, these charts separate and grade components of a neurologic assessment, assisting you and other care-givers to quickly recognize changes in neurologic status and to plan subsequent care.

Respiratory assessment constitutes an important part of an overall neurologic assessment. That's because patients with neurologic damage—especially those with traumatic brain or spinal cord injuries—are at considerable risk for respiratory complications. These injuries may depress the respiratory control center and paralyze the muscles used for breathing. As a result, brain tissue, which is especially sensitive to blood oxygen levels, can quickly be damaged by inadequate oxygenation.

Thorough respiratory care goes hand in hand with neurologic care. Frequent position changes, chest physiotherapy, and tracheal suctioning are typical interventions. Additional techniques for preventing complications and promoting comfort include pain management and therapeutic touch.

## Rehabilitation

Neurologic rehabilitation begins on admission and touches all aspects of daily care. Because neurologic impairment can alter every area of function, the patient's identity may disintegrate. Consequent rehabilitation procedures must address the psychosocial and physiologic changes associated with the patient's condition—a task that requires enormous time and patience.

# Anatomy and physiology review

The nervous system consists of the central nervous system (CNS), the peripheral nervous system, and the autonomic nervous system. Through complex and coordinated interactions, these three components integrate all physical, intellectual, and emotional activities.

## Central nervous system

The CNS includes the brain and the spinal cord. These two structures are responsible for collecting and interpreting voluntary and involuntary sensory and motor signals.

### Brain

As the highest functioning center of the nervous system, the brain collects, integrates, and interprets all stimuli. It also initiates and monitors voluntary and involuntary motor activity. The brain has three distinct regions: the cerebrum, brain stem, and cerebellum.

Encased by the skull and enclosed by three membrane layers called the meninges, the cerebrum is divided into right and left hemispheres. Each hemisphere has four lobes: parietal, occipital, temporal, and frontal. The right cerebral hemisphere controls activities on the left side of the body, and the left hemisphere controls activities on the right side of the body.

The diencephalon, a division of the cerebrum, contains the thalamus, epithalamus, subthalamus, and hypothalamus. The thalamus and hypothalamus are particularly important: The thalamus serves as a relay station for sensory impulses, and the hypothalamus has many regulatory functions, including control of temperature and pituitary hormone production and regulation of water balance.

Made up of the midbrain, pons, and medulla, the brain stem lies inferior to the diencephalon. The brain stem contains the nuclei of cranial nerves III through XII and is a major sensory and motor pathway for impulses running to and from the cerebrum. It also regulates basic body functions such as respiration, auditory and visual reflexes, swallowing, and coughing.

The cerebellum, the most posterior portion of the brain, contains the major motor and sensory pathways. It facilitates smooth, coordinated muscle movements and helps to maintain equilibrium.

### Spinal cord
The spinal cord is the primary pathway for messages traveling between the peripheral areas of the body and the brain. It also mediates the reflex arc — the natural pathway used in reflex action. An elongated mass of neural tissue, the spinal cord extends from the upper border of the first cervical vertebra to the lower border of the first lumbar vertebra. It's enclosed by the three meninges and protected by the bony vertebrae of the spine.

A cross section of the spinal cord reveals a central H-shaped mass of gray matter, surrounded by a circle of white matter. The dorsal section of gray matter contains cell bodies of sensory (afferent) nerves, and the ventral section contains cell bodies of motor (efferent) neurons. The dorsal white matter contains the ascending sensory tracts that carry impulses up the spinal cord to the higher sensory centers. The ventral white matter contains the descending motor tracts that transmit motor impulses down from the higher motor centers to the spinal cord.

### Peripheral nervous system
The peripheral nervous system includes the peripheral and cranial nerves. Peripheral sensory nerves transmit stimuli to the dorsal horn of the spinal cord from sensory receptors located in the skin, muscles, sensory organs, and viscera. The upper motor neurons of the brain and the lower motor neurons of the cell bodies in the ventral horn of the spinal cord carry impulses that affect movement.

The 12 pairs of cranial nerves are the primary motor and sensory pathways between the brain and the head and neck. (See *Cranial nerves.*)

### Autonomic nervous system
Consisting entirely of motor neurons, the autonomic nervous system regulates the activities of the visceral organs by its effect on smooth muscle, cardiac muscle, and the glands. Its two divisions — sympathetic and parasympathetic — maintain internal homeostasis.

The sympathetic (or adrenergic) nervous system controls the body's fight-or-flight reaction to stress. The parasympathetic (or cholinergic) nervous system maintains baseline body functions.

## Neurologic vital sign monitoring
Neurologic vital signs supplement the routine measurement of temperature, pulse rate, and respirations by evaluating the patient's level of consciousness (LOC), pupillary activity, and level of orientation to place, time, date, situation, and person. They provide a simple, indispensable tool for quickly checking the patient's neurologic status.

*LOC* — the degree of response to stimuli — reflects brain stem function and usually provides the first sign of CNS deterioration. Changes in *pupillary activity* — pupil size, shape, equality, and response to light — may signal a brain injury or increased intracranial pressure (ICP). *Level of orientation* evaluates higher cerebral functions and processing abilities.

Evaluating muscle strength and tone, reflexes, and posture also may help identify nervous system damage. Finally, ongoing assessment of routine vital signs helps detect neurologic changes or trends. In particular, respira-

# Cranial nerves

This illustration shows the origin of each cranial nerve (CN) and describes its type (motor, sensory, or both) and function.

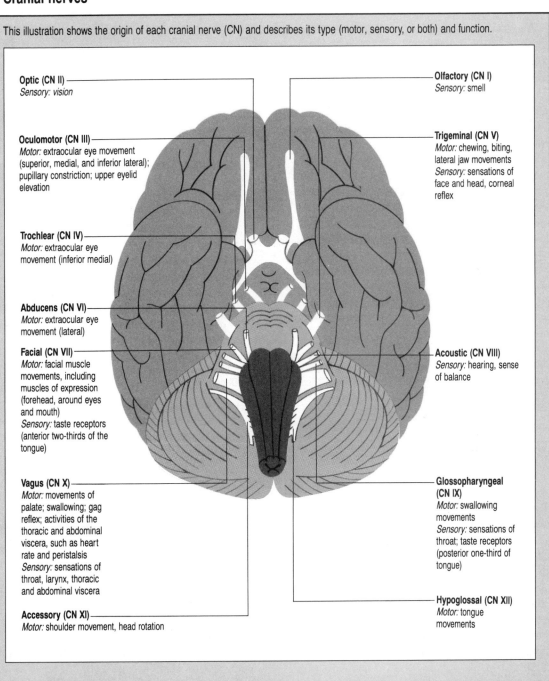

**Optic (CN II)**
*Sensory:* vision

**Oculomotor (CN III)**
*Motor:* extraocular eye movement
(superior, medial, and inferior lateral);
pupillary constriction; upper eyelid
elevation

**Trochlear (CN IV)**
*Motor:* extraocular eye
movement (inferior medial)

**Abducens (CN VI)**
*Motor:* extraocular eye
movement (lateral)

**Facial (CN VII)**
*Motor:* facial muscle
movements, including
muscles of expression
(forehead, around eyes
and mouth)
*Sensory:* taste receptors
(anterior two-thirds of the
tongue)

**Vagus (CN X)**
*Motor:* movements of
palate; swallowing; gag
reflex; activities of the
thoracic and abdominal
viscera, such as heart
rate and peristalsis
*Sensory:* sensations of
throat, larynx, thoracic
and abdominal viscera

**Accessory (CN XI)**
*Motor:* shoulder movement, head rotation

**Olfactory (CN I)**
*Sensory:* smell

**Trigeminal (CN V)**
*Motor:* chewing, biting,
lateral jaw movements
*Sensory:* sensations of
face and head, corneal
reflex

**Acoustic (CN VIII)**
*Sensory:* hearing, sense
of balance

**Glossopharyngeal
(CN IX)**
*Motor:* swallowing
movements
*Sensory:* sensations of
throat; taste receptors
(posterior one-third of
tongue)

**Hypoglossal (CN XII)**
*Motor:* tongue
movements

## Using the Glasgow coma scale

The Glasgow coma scale provides a standard reference for assessing or monitoring a patient with suspected or confirmed brain injury. You measure three responses to stimuli—eye opening, motor response, and verbal response—and assign a number to each of the possible responses within these categories. A score of 3 is the lowest and 15 is the highest. A score of 7 or less indicates coma. This scale is commonly used in the emergency department, at the scene of an accident, and for periodic evaluation of the hospitalized patient.

| CHARACTERISTIC | RESPONSE | SCORE |
|---|---|---|
| Eye opening | • Spontaneous | 4 |
| | • To verbal command | 3 |
| | • To pain | 2 |
| | • No response | 1 |
| Best motor response | • Obeys commands | 6 |
| | • To painful stimuli | |
| | Localizes pain; pushes stimulus away | 5 |
| | Flexes and withdraws | 4 |
| | Abnormal flexion | 3 |
| | Extension | 2 |
| | No response | 1 |
| Best verbal response (Arouse patient with painful stimuli, if necessary.) | • Oriented and converses | 5 |
| | • Disoriented and converses | 4 |
| | • Uses inappropriate words | 3 |
| | • Makes incomprehensible sounds | 2 |
| | • No response | 1 |
| | Total: | 3 to 15 |

tory rate and pattern can help locate brain lesions and determine their size.

### Equipment

Penlight ▪ thermometer ▪ sterile cotton ball or cotton-tipped applicator ▪ stethoscope ▪ sphygmomanometer ▪ pupil size chart ▪ optional: pencil or pen.

### Implementation

• Explain the procedure to the patient, even if he's unresponsive. Then wash your hands and provide privacy.

### *Assessing LOC and orientation*

• Assess the patient's LOC by evaluating his responses. Use standard guidelines, such as the Glasgow coma scale. (See *Using the Glasgow coma scale.*) Begin by measuring the patient's response to verbal, light tactile (touch), or painful (nail bed pressure) stimuli. First, ask the patient his full name. If he responds appropriately, assess his orientation to place, time, date, and situation. Ask the patient where he is and then what day, season, and year it is. (Expect disorientation to affect the sense of date first, then time, place, caregivers, and finally self.) When the patient responds verbally, assess the quality of replies. For example, garbled words indicate difficulty with the motor nerves that govern speech muscles. Rambling responses indicate difficulty with thought processing and organization.

• Assess the patient's ability to understand and follow one-step commands that require a motor response. For example, ask him to open and close his eyes or stick out his tongue. Note whether the patient can maintain his LOC. If you must gently shake the patient to keep him focused on your verbal commands, he may sustain neurologic compromise.

• If the patient doesn't respond to commands, apply a painful stimulus. With moderate pressure, squeeze the nail beds on fingers and toes, and note his response. Check motor responses bilaterally *to rule out monoplegia (paralysis of a single area) and hemiplegia (paralysis of one side of the body).*

### Examining pupils and eye movement

• Ask the patient to open his eyes. If he doesn't respond, gently lift his upper eyelids. Inspect each pupil for size and shape, and compare the two for equality. *To evaluate pupil size more precisely,* use a chart showing the various pupil sizes (in increments of 1 mm, with the normal diameter ranging from 2 to 6 mm). Remember, pupil size varies considerably, and some patients have normally unequal pupils (anisocoria). Also see if the pupils are positioned in, or deviated from, the midline.

• Test the patient's direct light response. First, darken the room. Then hold each eyelid open in turn, keeping the other eye covered. Swing the penlight from the patient's ear toward the midline of the face. Shine the light directly into the eye. Normally, the pupil constricts immediately. When you remove the penlight, the pupil should dilate immediately. Wait about 20 seconds before testing the other pupil *to allow it to recover from reflex stimulation.*

• Now test consensual light response. Hold both eyelids open, but shine the light into one eye only. Watch for constriction in the other pupil, *which indicates proper nerve function at the optic chiasm.*

• Brighten the room and have the conscious patient open his eyes. Observe the eyelids for ptosis or drooping. Then check extraocular movements. Hold up one finger and ask the patient to follow it with his eyes alone. As you move the finger up, down, laterally, and obliquely, see if the patient's eyes track together to follow your finger (conjugate gaze). Watch for involuntary jerking or oscillating eye movements (nystagmus).

• Check accommodation. Hold up one finger midline to the patient's face and several feet away. Have the patient focus on your finger. Then gradually move your finger toward his nose while he still focuses on your finger. This should cause his eyes to converge and both pupils to constrict equally.

• Test the corneal reflex by rapidly moving the palm of your hand toward the patient's open eyes. *This forces a cushion of air against the corneas, which normally causes an immediate blink reflex.* Repeat for the other eye.

• If the patient is unconscious, test the oculocephalic (doll's eye) reflex. Hold the patient's eyelids open. Then quickly, but gently, turn the patient's head to one side, then the other. If the patient's eyes move in the opposite direction from the side to which you turn the head—eyes move right when the head moves left—the reflex is intact.

***Nursing alert:*** Never test the doll's eye reflex if you know or suspect that the patient has a cervical spine injury.

## Identifying warning postures

Decorticate and decerebrate posturing are ominous signs of central nervous system deterioration.

### Decorticate (abnormal flexion)
In decorticate posturing, the patient's arms are adducted and flexed, with the wrists and fingers flexed on the chest. The legs may be stiffly extended and internally rotated, with plantar flexion of the feet.

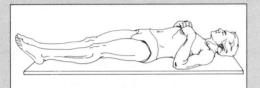

The decorticate posture may indicate a lesion of the frontal lobe, internal capsule, or cerebral peduncles.

### Decerebrate (extension)
In decerebrate posturing, the patient's arms are adducted and extended with the wrists pronated and the fingers flexed. One or both of the legs may be stiffly extended, with plantar flexion of the feet.

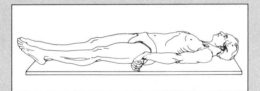

The decerebrate posture may indicate lesions of the upper brain stem.

### *Evaluating motor function*
• If the patient is conscious, test his grip strength in both hands at the same time. Extend your hands, ask the patient to squeeze your fingers as hard as he can, and compare the strength of each hand. Grip strength is usually slightly stronger in the dominant hand.
• Test arm strength by having the patient close his eyes and hold his arms straight out in front of him with the palms up. See if either arm drifts downward or pronates, *which indicates muscle weakness.*
• Test leg strength by having the patient raise his legs, one at a time, against gentle downward pressure from your hand. Gently push down on each leg at the midpoint of the thigh *to evaluate muscle strength.*
• If the patient is unconscious, estimate the strength of spontaneous and reflex movements. Apply a painful stimulus to elicit movement. Exert pressure on each fingernail bed with a pencil or pen. If the patient withdraws from this stimulus, compare the strength of each limb.
   ***Nursing alert:*** If decorticate or decerebrate posturing develops in response to painful stimuli, notify the doctor immediately. (See *Identifying warning postures.*)
• Flex and extend the extremities on both sides *to evaluate muscle tone.*
• Test the plantar reflex in all patients. Stroke the lateral aspect of the sole of the patient's foot with your thumbnail or another moderately sharp or blunt, pointed object. Normally, this elicits flexion of all toes. Watch for a positive Babinski's sign—dorsiflexion of the great toe with fanning of the other toes—*which indicates an upper motor neuron lesion.*
• Test for Brudzinski's and Kernig's signs in patients suspected of having meningitis. In Brudzinski's sign, the patient's knee flexes involuntarily when you flex his neck. In Kernig's sign, the patient can easily extend his leg when lying supine; however, when sitting up or lying with his thigh flexed upon his abdomen, he can't extend his leg completely. (See also *Assessing the sensory system.*)

### *Completing the neurologic examination*
• Take the patient's temperature, pulse rate, respiration rate, and blood pressure. Especially note his pulse pressure—the difference between systolic pressure and diastolic pressure—*because widening pulse pressure can indicate increasing ICP.*

## Assessing the sensory system

Further evaluate the patient's sensory function by assessing for two-point discrimination, temperature sensation, sense of position (proprioception), and point localization. Also assess number identification, superficial pain, response to vibration, extinction, and the patient's ability to recognize objects by the sense of touch (stereognosis). Perform all sensory testing with the patient's eyes closed.

### Two-point discrimination
Alternately touch one or two sharp objects to the patient's skin. First assess whether he can feel one or two points; then assess the smallest distance between the two points at which he can still discriminate the presence of two points. Acuity varies in different body areas. On the finger pads, an area rich in tactile sensory receptors, the average distance necessary for two-point discrimination is less than 5 mm. On the back, however, two-point discrimination requires a much wider distance.

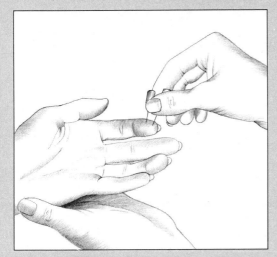

### Temperature sensation
First fill two test tubes with water, one hot and the other cold. Alternately touch the patient's skin with the hot and cold tubes, and ask him to differentiate between them. Test and compare distal and proximal portions of all extremities.

### Sense of position
Grasp the sides of the patient's great toe between your thumb and forefinger. Move the toe upward or downward, asking the patient to describe the position. Repeat on the other foot, as shown, and then perform the same technique on the patient's fingers.

If the patient exhibits an impaired sense of position, proceed to the next joint on the extremity and repeat the procedure. On the leg, progress from the ankle to the knee; on the arm, from the wrist to the elbow.

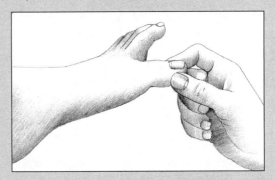

### Point localization
Have the patient close both eyes while you briefly touch a point on his skin. Ask him to open his eyes and point to the place just touched. He should be able to identify the spot.

### Number identification
Trace a number on the patient's palm with an object, such as the blunt end of a pencil. He should be able to identify the number.

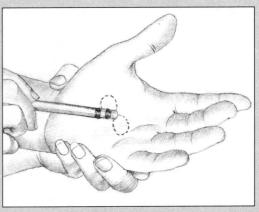

*(continued)*

### Assessing the sensory system *(continued)*

#### Superficial pain
Lightly touch – but don't puncture – the patient's skin using a sharp object, such as a sterile needle. Occasionally alternate sharp and blunt ends. (Remember to discard the sharp object safely after use, and never use the same object on another patient.)

Ask the patient to identify the sensation as sharp or dull. Test and compare the distal and proximal portions of all extremities. If he displays abnormal pain sensation, test for temperature sensation.

#### Response to vibration
Tap a low-pitched tuning fork (preferably 128 cycles/second) on the heel of your hand, then place the base of the tuning fork firmly on an interphalangeal joint (any of the patient's fingers or his great toe).

Ask the patient to describe the sensation, differentiating between pressure and vibration, and then to state when the feeling stops. Proceed from distal to proximal areas.

If the patient has intact distal vibration sensation, further testing is unnecessary. However, if he suffers from an absence of distal vibration sensation, test the next most proximal bony prominence. When assessing the leg, progress from the medial malleolus to the patella, to the anterior superior iliac spine, to the spinous process of the vertebra. For the arm, progress from the wrist to the elbow to the shoulder.

#### Extinction
Touch two corresponding parts on the patient (such as the forearms just above the wrist) simultaneously. Ask him to describe the location of the touch. He should sense the touch in both locations.

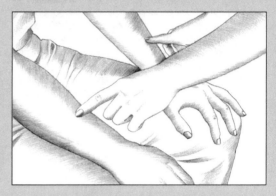

#### Stereognosis
Place a familiar object, such as a key, pencil, or paper clip, in the patient's hand and ask him to identify the object by feel – which he should be able to do. A particularly sensitive test of stereognosis involves having the patient identify the "heads" and "tails" sides of a coin.

## Special considerations
If the previously stable patient suddenly develops a change in neurologic or routine vital signs, further assess his condition, and notify the doctor immediately.

## Documentation
Baseline data require detailed documentation; subsequent notes can be brief unless the patient's condition changes. Record the patient's LOC and orientation, pupillary activity, motor function, and routine vital signs, as hospital policy directs. To save time while keeping complete records, the hospital may let you use abbreviations. Use only commonly understood abbreviations and terms to avoid misinterpretation of the patient's status. Examples include the following:

• A + O × 4 – alert and oriented to person, place, time, and date
• PERRLA – pupils equal, round, reactive to light and accommodation
• PERL – pupils equal, reactive to light
• EOM – extraocular movements

Also describe the patient's behavior – difficult to arouse by gentle shaking, sleepy, unresponsive to painful stimuli.

## ICP monitoring
This procedure measures pressure exerted by the brain, blood, and cerebrospinal fluid (CSF) against the inside of the skull. Indications for monitoring ICP include head trauma with bleeding or edema, overproduction or insufficient ab-

sorption of CSF, cerebral hemorrhage, neurologic surgery, and space-occupying brain lesions. ICP monitoring can detect elevated ICP early, before clinical danger signs develop. Prompt intervention can then help avert or diminish neurologic damage caused by cerebral hypoxia and shifts of brain mass.

The four basic ICP monitoring systems include ventricular catheter, subarachnoid bolt, epidural sensor, and intraparenchymal pressure monitoring. (See *Understanding ICP monitoring*, pages 104 and 105.) Regardless of the system used, the procedure is always performed by a neurosurgeon in the operating room, emergency department, or critical care unit. Inserting an ICP monitoring device requires sterile technique to reduce the risk of CNS infection. Setting up equipment for the monitoring systems also requires strict asepsis.

## Equipment

Monitoring unit and transducers, as ordered ▪ 16 to 20 sterile 4″ × 4″ gauze pads ▪ linen-saver pads ▪ shaving preparation tray or hair scissors ▪ sterile drapes ▪ povidone-iodine solution ▪ sterile gown ▪ surgical mask ▪ two pairs of sterile gloves ▪ povidone-iodine ointment ▪ head dressing supplies (two rolls of 4″ elastic gauze dressing, one roll of 4″ roller gauze, adhesive tape) ▪ optional: suction apparatus, a yardstick.

## Preparation of equipment

Monitoring units and setup protocols are varied and complex and differ among hospitals. Check your hospital's guidelines for your particular unit and its preparation.

Various models of preassembled ICP monitoring units are available, each with its own setup protocols. These units are designed to reduce the risk of infection by eliminating the need for multiple stopcocks, manometers, and transducer dome assemblies. Some hospitals use units that have miniaturized transducers rather than transducer domes.

## Implementation

• Explain the procedure to the patient or his family. Make sure the patient or a responsible family member has signed a consent form. Determine if the patient is allergic to iodine preparations.

• Provide privacy if the procedure is being done in an open emergency department or intensive care unit.

• Obtain baseline routine and neurologic vital signs *to aid in prompt detection of decompensation during the procedure.*

• Place the patient in the supine position and elevate the head of the bed 30 degrees, or as ordered. Document the number of bed crank rotations, or hang a yardstick on an I.V. pole and mark the exact elevation.

• Place linen-saver pads under the patient's head. Shave or clip his hair at the insertion site, as indicated by the doctor, *to decrease the risk of infection.* Carefully fold and remove the linen-saver pads *to avoid spilling loose hair onto the bed.*

• Wash hands and don sterile gloves and a mask. Drape the patient with sterile drapes. Scrub the insertion site for 2 minutes with povidone-iodine solution.

• The doctor puts on the sterile gown, mask, and sterile gloves. He then opens the interior wrap of the sterile supply tray and proceeds with insertion of the catheter or bolt.

• *To facilitate placement of the device,* hold the patient's head in your hands. Alternatively, run a strip of tape across the patient's forehead and attach it to either side of the bed, or attach a long strip of 4″ roller gauze to one side rail and bring it across the patient's forehead to the opposite rail. Reassure the conscious patient *to help ease his anxiety.* Talk to him frequently *to assess his LOC and detect signs of deterioration.* Watch for cardiac arrhythmias and abnormal respiratory patterns.

• After insertion, apply povidone-iodine ointment (if in accordance with hospital policy) and a sterile dressing to the site. The doctor will then

## Understanding ICP monitoring

Intracranial pressure (ICP) can be monitored using one of four systems.

### Intraventricular catheter monitoring

In this procedure, which monitors ICP directly, the doctor inserts a small polyethylene or silicone rubber catheter into the lateral ventricle through a burr hole.

Although this method measures ICP most accurately, it carries the greatest risk of infection. This is the only type of ICP monitoring that allows evaluation of brain compliance and drainage of significant amounts of cerebrospinal fluid (CSF).

Contraindications usually include stenotic cerebral ventricles, cerebral aneurysms in the path of catheter placement, and suspected vascular lesions.

### Subarachnoid bolt monitoring

This procedure involves insertion of a special bolt into the subarachnoid space through a twist-drill burr hole that's positioned in the front of the skull behind the hairline.

Placing the bolt is easier than placing an intraventricular catheter, especially if a computerized tomography (CT) scan reveals that the cerebrum has shifted or the ventricles have collapsed. This type of ICP monitoring also carries less risk of infection and parenchymal damage because the bolt doesn't penetrate the cerebrum.

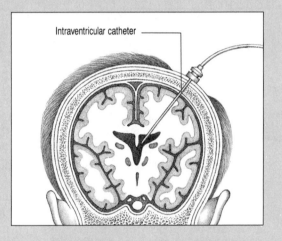

Intraventricular catheter

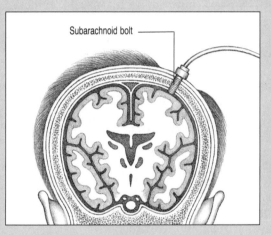

Subarachnoid bolt

connect the catheter to the appropriate monitoring device, depending on the system used.

• If the doctor has set up a drainage system, attach the drip chamber to the headboard or the bedside I.V. pole, as ordered.

*Nursing alert:* Position the chamber in accordance with the degree of bed elevation. Be aware that positioning the drip chamber too high may raise ICP; positioning it too low may cause excessive CSF drainage.

• Inspect the insertion site at least every 24 hours or according to hospital policy for redness, swelling, and drainage. Clean the site, reapply povidone-iodine, and apply a fresh sterile dress-

ing. (Some institutions recommend that the doctor change the catheter dressings.)

• Hourly, or as ordered, assess the patient's clinical status, and take routine and neurologic vital signs. Make sure you have obtained orders for waveforms and pressure parameters from the doctor.

• Observe digital ICP readings and waves. Remember, the pattern of readings is more significant than any single reading. (See *Interpreting ICP waveforms,* page 106.) If you observe continually elevated ICP readings, note how long they're sustained. If they last several minutes,

### Epidural sensor monitoring

The least invasive with the lowest incidence of infection, this method uses a tiny fiber-optic sensor inserted into the epidural space through a burr hole.

Unlike an intraventricular catheter or a subarachnoid bolt, the sensor can't become occluded with blood or brain tissue. Accuracy is questionable, however, because the epidural sensor doesn't measure ICP directly from a CSF-filled space. Several types of sensors are available; some can be recalibrated repeatedly. Fiber-optic sensors must be calibrated before they're inserted.

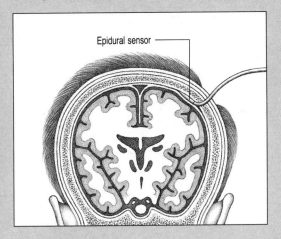

### Intraparenchymal monitoring

In this procedure, the doctor inserts a catheter through a small subarachnoid bolt and, after puncturing the dura, advances the catheter a few centimeters into the brain's white matter. There's no need to balance or calibrate the equipment after insertion.

Although this method doesn't provide direct access to CSF, measurements are accurate because brain tissue pressures correlate well with ventricular pressures. Intraparenchymal monitoring may be used to obtain ICP measurements in patients with compressed or dislocated ventricles.

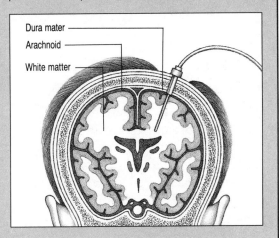

notify the doctor immediately. Finally, record and describe any CSF drainage.

### Special considerations

In infants, ICP monitoring can be performed without penetrating the scalp. In this external method, a photoelectric transducer with a pressure-sensitive membrane is taped to the anterior fontanel. The transducer responds to pressure at the site and transmits readings to a bedside monitor and recording system. The external method is restricted to infants *because pressure readings can be obtained only at fontanels, the incompletely ossified areas of the skull.*

Osmotic diuretic agents, such as mannitol, reduce cerebral edema by shrinking intracranial contents. Given by I.V. drip or bolus, mannitol draws water from tissues into plasma; it does not cross the blood-brain barrier. Monitor serum electrolyte levels and osmolality readings closely *because the patient may become dehydrated very quickly.* Be aware that a rebound increase in ICP may occur. (See *Nursing management of increased ICP,* page 107.) If your patient has congestive heart failure or severe renal dysfunction, monitor for problems in adapting to the increased intravascular volumes. Fluid restriction, usually

## Interpreting ICP waveforms

Three waveforms, A, B, and C, are used to monitor intracranial pressure (ICP). *A waves* are an ominous sign of intracranial decompensation and poor compliance. *B waves* correlate with changes in respiration, and *C waves* with changes in arterial pressure.

A normal ICP waveform typically shows a steep upward systolic slope followed by a downward diastolic slope with a dicrotic notch. In most cases, this waveform occurs continuously and indicates an ICP between 0 and 15 mm Hg – normal pressure.

### Normal waveform

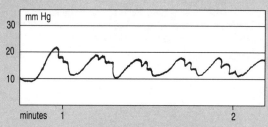

The most clinically significant ICP waveforms are A waves (shown below), which may reach elevations ranging from 50 to 100 mm Hg, persist for 5 to 20 minutes, then drop sharply – signaling exhaustion of the brain's compliance mechanisms. A waves may come and go, spiking from temporary rises in thoracic pressure or from any condition that increases ICP beyond the brain's compliance limits. Activities such as sustained coughing or straining with bowel movements can cause temporary elevations in thoracic pressure.

### A waves

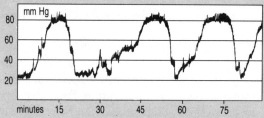

B waves, which appear sharp and rhythmic, with a sawtooth pattern, occur every 1½ to 2 minutes and may reach elevations of 50 mm Hg. The clinical significance of B waves isn't clear, but they correlate with respiratory changes and may oc-

cur more frequently with decreasing compensation. *Because B waves sometimes precede A waves,* notify the doctor if B waves occur frequently.

### B waves

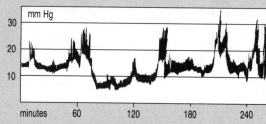

Like B waves, C waves are rapid and rhythmic, but not as sharp. Clinically insignificant, they may fluctuate with respirations or systemic blood pressure changes.

### C waves

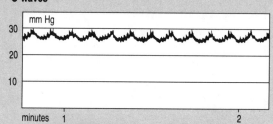

A waveform that looks like the one shown below signals a problem with the transducer or monitor. Check for line obstruction, and determine if the transducer needs rebalancing.

### Waveform showing equipment problem

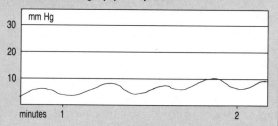

## Nursing management of increased ICP

By performing nursing care gently, slowly, and cautiously, you can best help to manage increased intracranial pressure (ICP) rather than possibly compound it. You may even be able to reduce it significantly. If possible, urge your patient to participate in his own care. Here are some steps you can take to manage increased ICP.

• Plan your care to include rest periods between activities. *This allows the patient's ICP to return to baseline, thus avoiding lengthy and cumulative pressure elevations.*

• Try to speak to the patient before attempting any procedures, even if he appears comatose. Touch him on an arm or leg first before touching him in a more personal area, such as the face or chest. This is especially important if the patient doesn't know you, or if he's confused or sedated.

• Suction the patient only when needed *to remove secretions and maintain airway patency.* Avoid depriving him of oxygen for long periods while suctioning; always hyperventilate the patient with oxygen after the procedure. Monitor his heart rate while suctioning. If multiple catheter passes are needed to clear secretions, hyperventilate the patient between them *to bring ICP as close to baseline as possible.*

• Promote venous drainage. Keep the patient's head in the midline position, even when he's positioned on his side. Avoid neck flexion or hip flexion greater than 90 degrees, and keep the head of the bed elevated 30 to 45 degrees.

• *To avoid increasing intrathoracic pressure, which raises ICP,* discourage Valsalva's maneuver and isometric muscle contractions. To avoid isometric contractions, distract the patient when giving him painful injections (by asking him to wiggle his toes and by massaging the area before injection to relax the muscle) and have him concentrate on breathing through difficult procedures such as bed-to-stretcher transfers. Tell the patient to relax as much as possible during position changes, *to keep him from holding his breath when moving around in bed.* If necessary, administer a stool softener *to help prevent constipation and unnecessary straining at stool.*

• If the patient is heavily sedated, monitor respiratory rate and blood gas levels. *Depressed respirations will compromise ventilations and oxygen exchange. Maintaining adequate respiratory rate and volume helps reduce ICP.*

• If you're in a specialty unit, you may be able to routinely hyperventilate the patient to counter sustained ICP elevations. This procedure is one of the best ways to reduce high ICP at bedside for short periods. Consult your hospital's policy before using this technique.

1,200 to 1,500 ml per day, decreases the incidence of increased cerebral edema.

Although steroid therapy is controversial, steroids may be used to lower elevated ICP by reducing sodium and water concentration in the brain. *Because they may also produce peptic ulcers,* they're usually given with antacids and cimetidine or ranitidine. Observe for possible GI bleeding. Also monitor urine glucose and acetone levels *because steroids may cause glycosuria in patients with borderline diabetes.*

Barbiturate-induced coma depresses the reticular activating system and reduces the brain's metabolic demand. Reduced demand for oxygen and energy reduces cerebral blood flow (CBF), thereby lowering ICP.

Hyperventilation with oxygen from a hand-held resuscitation bag or respirator helps rid the patient of excess carbon dioxide, thereby constricting cerebral vessels and reducing cerebral blood volume and ICP. However, only normal brain tissues respond, because blood vessels in damaged areas have reduced vasoconstrictive ability.

Before tracheal suctioning, hyperventilate the patient with 100% oxygen, as ordered. Apply suction for a maximum of 15 seconds. Avoid inducing hypoxia *because it greatly increases CBF.*

*Because fever raises brain metabolism, which increases CBF,* fever-reduction (achieved by administering acetaminophen, alcohol sponge baths, and a hypothermia blanket) also helps to reduce ICP. However, rebound increases in ICP and brain edema may occur if rapid rewarming takes place after hypothermia or if cooling measures induce shivering.

Withdrawal of CSF through the drainage system reduces CSF volume, and thus reduces ICP. Although less commonly used, surgical removal of a skull-bone flap provides room for the swollen brain to expand. If this procedure is performed, keep the site clean and dry *to prevent infection* and maintain sterile technique when changing the dressing.

## Complications

CNS infection, the most common hazard of ICP monitoring, can result from contamination of the equipment setup or of the insertion site.

*Nursing alert:* Excessive loss of CSF can result from faulty stopcock placement or a drip chamber that's positioned too low. Such loss can rapidly decompress the cranial contents and damage bridging cortical veins, leading to hematoma formation. Decompression can also lead to rupture of existing hematomas or aneurysms, causing hemorrhage.

Watch for signs of impending or overt decompensation: papilledema; pupillary dilation (unilateral or bilateral); decreased pupillary response to light; decreasing LOC; rising systolic blood pressure and widening pulse pressure; bradycardia; and slowed, irregular respirations. In late decompensation, be alert for decerebrate posturing.

## Documentation

Record the time and the date of the insertion procedure and the patient's response. Note the insertion site and the type of monitoring system used. Record ICP digital readings and waveforms hourly in your notes, on a flowchart, or directly on readout strips, depending on the hospital's policy. Document any factors that may affect ICP—for example, drug therapy, stressful procedures, or sleep.

Record routine and neurologic vital signs hourly, and describe the patient's clinical status. Note the amount, character, and frequency of any CSF drainage (for example, "between 6 p.m. and 7 p.m., 15 ml of blood-tinged CSF").

# CBF monitoring

Traditionally, caregivers have estimated CBF in neurologically compromised patients by calculating cerebral perfusion pressure. However, modern technology permits continuous regional blood flow monitoring at the bedside. A sensor placed on the cerebral cortex calculates CBF in the capillary bed by thermal diffusion. Thermistors within the sensor sense the temperature differential between two metallic plates—one heated, one neutral. This differential relates inversely to CBF: As the differential decreases, CBF increases—and vice versa. This monitoring technique yields important information about the effects of interventions on CBF. It also yields continuous real-time values for CBF, which are essential in conditions where compromised blood flow may put the patient at risk, such as ischemia and infarction.

CBF monitoring is indicated whenever CBF alterations are anticipated. It's used most commonly in patients with subarachnoid hemorrhage (in which a vasospasm may restrict blood flow), trauma associated with high ICP, or vascular tumors. Use of this new technology is likely to grow as practitioners become more familiar with the information it provides. (See *Why monitor CBF?*)

As with ICP monitoring, CBF monitoring may lead to infection. To help prevent this complication, the doctor may order prophylactic antibiotics. You can help prevent infection by correctly administering any ordered antibiotics and by maintaining a sterile dressing around the insertion site. To prevent CSF leakage, another potential complication, the surgeon usually places an additional suture at the sensor insertion site.

## Equipment

Computer data system or analog monitor ∎ sensor ∎ povidone-iodine solution. (See *CBF monitoring systems,* page 110.)

### For monitor removal

Suture removal set ∎ mask ∎ sterile gloves ∎ sutures ∎ sterile 4″ × 4″ gauze pads ∎ adhesive tape.

## Why monitor CBF?

Cerebral blood flow (CBF) monitoring yields important information about the effects of interventions on CBF. By carefully correlating CBF with other assessment findings, you can detect complications and intervene promptly, improving the patient's chances of avoiding multiple deficits caused by reduced oxygen flow to the brain. Take, for example, the case of Edna Thompson, age 52.

**Initial treatment**
Ms. Thompson underwent a craniotomy to remove an aneurysm of the right middle cerebral artery and is still at risk for vasospasm. Anesthesia was not reversed at the completion of surgery. Postoperatively, she was admitted to your unit after a ventriculostomy and with a CBF monitor in place.

**Care on your unit**
When first assessing Ms. Thompson, you measure her pupils at 3 mm and note that they're reactive to light. But there are no other significant assessment findings. You also find that her intracranial pressure (ICP), measured by an intraventricular catheter, ranges from 12 to 15 mm Hg. CBF ranges from 40 to 65 ml/100 g/minute.

Eight hours after the patient arrived on your unit, you note that Ms. Thompson has begun to localize to painful stimulus — but more quickly with her right side than her left side. Her pu-

pils continue to appear small and reactive to light. CBF values remain stable at 45 to 58 ml/100 g/minute, and ICP remains unchanged.

At the end of the first 24 hours of postoperative care, Ms. Thompson's CBF consistently measures 75 to 80 ml/100 g/minute. On assessment, you find that she can follow commands intermittently, her right and left extremities move equally, and her pupils are equal and react briskly to light.

During the second day of postoperative care, Ms. Thompson's CBF drops to 40 to 45 ml/100 g/minute, and her right extremities become weaker than her left. All other assessment findings remain unchanged. Other hemodynamic parameters show a normal fluid volume status.

You report these findings to the doctor, who then orders an albumin infusion. Over the next 3 hours, Ms. Thompson's CBF rises, remaining at 75 to 85 ml/100 g/minute, and she regains some strength in her left side.

**Conclusion**
By correlating the patient's reduced CBF with her extremity weakness and normal fluid volume status, you were able to intervene promptly. As a result, all parameters returned to baseline, demonstrating that the faster a health care team can respond to CBF decreases, the better the patient's prognosis.

## Preparation of equipment
You won't have to set up special equipment for CBF monitoring. Depending on the type of system you're using, you may need to verify that a battery has been inserted in the monitor to allow CBF monitoring during patient transport to the ICU.

## Implementation
• Make sure that the patient or a family member is fully informed about the procedures involved in CBF monitoring, and that the appropriate person has signed an informed consent form. If the patient will need CBF monitoring after surgery, inform him that a sensor will be in place for about 3 days postoperatively to measure CBF. Tell him that the insertion site will be covered

with a dry sterile dressing. Mention that the sensor may be removed at the bedside.
• The surgeon typically inserts the sensor in the operating room, during or at completion of a craniotomy. (Occasionally, he may place it through a burr hole.) He implants the sensor far from major blood vessels and verifies that the metallic plates have good contact with the brain surface. (See *Placing a CBF sensor,* page 111.)
• If ordered, attach the distal end of the sensor to the monitor. Once the sensor is in place, turn the monitor on. Turn the RUN/CAL switch to CAL, and adjust the ZERO ADJUST knob until the digital readout is 0.00. This calibrates the system. Then adjust the knob to the lock position, and turn the RUN/CAL switch to RUN. (Or, if the monitor is different from the one illustrated, follow the manufacturer's instructions.)

## CBF monitoring systems

To monitor cerebral blood flow (CBF) at the patient's bedside, you may use a monitor such as the one shown below. This monitor has a digital display; some also display waveforms. The CBF sensor, placed in the cerebral cortex, continuously measures cortical blood flow.

**Bedside CBF monitor**

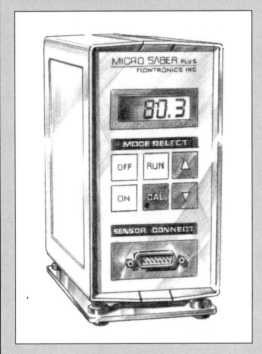

**CBF sensor**

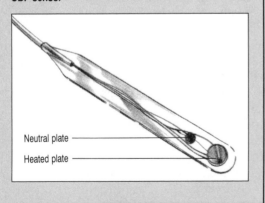

Neutral plate
Heated plate

• Document the baseline CBF value and then obtain values hourly.

### Removing the monitor

• The surgeon typically removes the monitor 72 hours after insertion. To do so, he removes the anchoring suture and then gently removes the sensor from the insertion site. He closes the wound with a stitch.

### Special considerations

CBF fluctuates with the brain's metabolic demands. The normal range for CBF is from 60 to 90 ml/100 g/minute. However, the patient's neurologic condition dictates the acceptable range. For instance, in a patient in a coma, CBF may be half the normal value; in a patient in a barbiturate-induced coma with burst suppression on the electroencephalogram, CBF may be as low as 10 ml/100 g/minute. Vasospasm secondary to subarachnoid hemorrhage may result in CBF below 40 ml/100 g/minute. In an awake patient, CBF above 90 ml/100 g/minute may indicate hyperemia.

Be aware that stimulation or activity may cause a 10% increase or decrease in CBF. If you note a 20% increase or decrease, suspect poor contact between the sensor and the cerebral cortex. To correct this, turn the patient toward the side of the sensor and then, after prepping the exit point of the catheter with a povidone-iodine solution, gently move the catheter back and forth (using a sterile-gloved hand). To determine if these maneuvers have improved contact between the sensor and the cortex, observe the CBF value on the monitor as you perform them.

If your patient has low CBF but no neurologic symptoms that indicate ischemia, suspect a fluid layer (a small hematoma) between the sensor and the cortex.

To reduce the risk of infection, change the dressing at the insertion site daily. After cleaning the site with a povidone-iodine solution (if ordered), apply a new dry sterile dressing. Be sure to use sterile technique during dressing

## Placing a CBF sensor

Typically, the surgeon inserts a cerebral blood flow (CBF) sensor during a craniotomy. He tunnels the sensor toward the craniotomy site and then carefully inserts the metallic plates of the thermistor to make sure that they continuously contact the surface of the cerebral cortex. After closing the dura and replacing the bone flap, he closes the scalp.

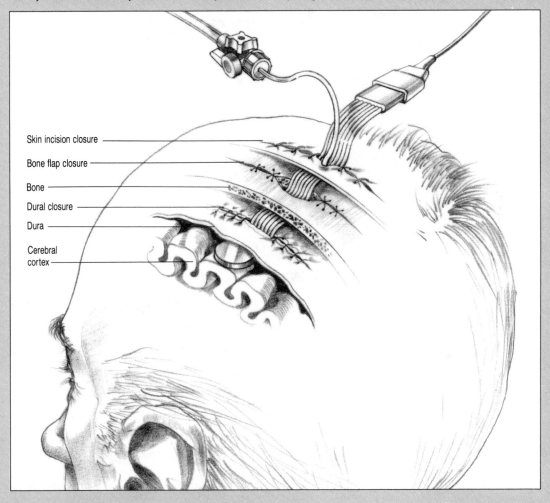

Skin incision closure

Bone flap closure

Bone

Dural closure

Dura

Cerebral cortex

changes. If ordered, administer prophylactic antibiotics. Observe the site for CSF leakage, which increases the risk of infection. (The surgeon may place an additional suture to prevent or stop any such leakage.)

**Documentation**

Record hourly CBF values. Be sure to check for trends and correlate values with the patient's clinical status. Also document the condition of the site and leakage, if any.

# MONITORING FLUID AND ELECTROLYTE STATUS

**5**

## Introduction

Whether you work in a hospital, an extended care facility, or some other health care setting, maintaining fluid and electrolyte balance in your patient is a primary goal. To accomplish this goal, you must know how to monitor for both actual and potential fluid and electrolyte disturbances.

Many problems—illness, injury, surgery, and even some treatments, for instance—can disrupt a patient's fluid and electrolyte balance. Yet the changes that herald such disruptions may be quite subtle. To identify these changes before serious problems occur, you need keen observational skills and expertise in measuring and recording intake and output. You must also know which laboratory studies to monitor—and what abnormal results could mean.

This chapter begins by describing the physiology of fluids and electrolytes, including the body's fluid compartments and the mechanisms that regulate fluid and electrolyte balance. It then explains how to ensure your patient's fluid and electrolyte balance by monitoring intake and output, I.V. fluid therapy, and blood and urine studies. The chapter also explains how to use the vascular intermittent access system to evaluate a patient's electrolyte status and how to monitor intra-abdominal pressure to help assess fluid balance.

## Physiology review

Water, the essential component of body fluid, accounts for approximately 60% of total body weight in the normal adult. Body water transports gases and nutrients, helps regulate temperature, transports wastes to excretion sites, and helps maintain cell shape.

Solutes include electrolytes and various nonionized substances. Electrolytes, such as sodium, potassium, calcium, and chloride, are essential to maintaining the body's fluid and acid-base balance. They also conduct the electrical current needed to maintain homeostasis.

Nonionized substances include glucose, creatinine, and urea.

### Fluid compartments

Two-thirds of body water is *intracellular*, remaining within cells. The other third is *extracellular*, remaining outside cells. Intracellular fluid (ICF) totals about 25 liters and accounts for 40% of total body weight. Extracellular fluid (ECF) totals roughly 15 liters and accounts for 20% of total body weight.

ECF is subdivided into interstitial, intravascular, and transcellular fluid. *Interstitial fluid,* which surrounds cells, makes up 80% of the total ECF. *Intravascular fluid* consists of plasma, the liquid component of blood. It accounts for about 20% of the total ECF. *Transcellular fluid,* found in such spaces as the cerebrospinal column, GI tract, and peritoneal cavity, makes up only a minute portion of the total ECF. Consisting of epithelial cell secretions, transcellular fluid differs from interstitial and intravascular fluid in ionic composition.

Body composition affects total body water. Unlike skeletal tissue, adipose (fat) tissue contains little water. Consequently, the typical woman, with more fat cells than the typical man, has a somewhat lower percentage of total body fluid. Elderly people have less total body fluid because body fluid diminishes with age while the number of fat cells increases. These differences have important nursing implications: Fluid and electrolyte replacement dosages that are appropriate for a lean man may be excessive for an obese, female, or elderly patient. (See also *Fluid gains and losses,* page 114.)

### Electrolytes

These chemical compounds dissociate in solution into electrically charged particles called ions. *Cations* form a positive charge, whereas *anions* form a negative charge. The electrical charge conducts the electrical current required for normal cell function.

## Fluid gains and losses

Each day the body gains—and loses—roughly 2,600 ml of fluid. This illustration shows the various sources of fluid gain and loss.

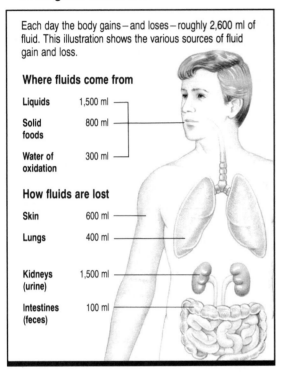

**Where fluids come from**

| | |
|---|---|
| Liquids | 1,500 ml |
| Solid foods | 800 ml |
| Water of oxidation | 300 ml |

**How fluids are lost**

| | |
|---|---|
| Skin | 600 ml |
| Lungs | 400 ml |
| Kidneys (urine) | 1,500 ml |
| Intestines (feces) | 100 ml |

Electrolytes exist within both ECF and ICF. Although the various electrolytes differ in concentration, their totals balance to achieve a neutral electrical charge. (*Concentration* refers to the number of dissolved particles or solutes in a liter of fluid.)

Most electrolytes help maintain acid-base balance by interacting with hydrogen ions. The acid-base balance—the amount of bicarbonate (base) in relation to carbonic acid—is normally 20:1. A body pH of 7.35 to 7.45 reflects a normal ratio of bicarbonate to carbonic acid. The major electrolytes also have specialized functions that contribute to metabolism and fluid and electrolyte balance. An explanation of their special functions follows.

**Sodium.** The main ECF cation, sodium ($Na^+$) is crucial in maintaining normal ECF osmolality.

(*Osmolality* refers to the total number of osmotically active particles in a volume of solution.) A sodium concentration change causes an ECF volume change as the kidneys, influenced by antidiuretic hormone, adjust water reabsorption to maintain normal osmolality.

Besides influencing ECF osmolality, sodium plays at least two other major roles: It contributes to acid-base balance (in association with bicarbonate ions) and activates nerve and muscle cells.

**Chloride.** Like sodium, chloride ($Cl^-$), the major ECF anion, also helps maintain normal ECF osmolarity. Chloride and sodium levels usually rise and fall together because most bodily chloride exists in combination with sodium. Chloride also affects pH by playing a vital role in acid-base balance and producing hydrochloric acid (HCl).

**Potassium.** The major ICF cation, potassium ($K^+$) helps control ICF osmolarity and energy metabolism. However, its main role is to regulate cell excitability. All excitable cells have an electric charge difference across the cell membrane, called the *resting membrane potential;* negativity inside the cell exceeds negativity outside the cell. Because potassium ions permeate cell membranes while most other ions can't, potassium movement greatly affects the cell's electric state as well as ICF concentration and composition.

**Phosphate.** The major ICF anion, phosphate ($HPO_4^{-2}$) proves essential to many cell processes, including energy storage and carbohydrate, protein, and fat metabolism. It also serves as hydrogen's major intracellular buffer, helping to maintain acid-base balance. When paired with calcium, it forms an essential bone and tooth component.

**Calcium.** Crucial to many physiologic functions, calcium ($Ca^{++}$) exists in blood as a physiologically active ionized form as well as in an albumin-bound form. In cell membranes, calcium helps cells adhere to one another and maintain their shape. An enzyme activator within cells, it must exist in muscle cell cytoplasm for contraction to occur. As a cofactor, it's involved in several steps leading to blood coagulation. And, along with phosphate, it hardens and strengthens bones and teeth.

Calcium also profoundly affects excitable cells' membrane permeability and firing level. It's largely responsible for the membrane's relative impermeability to sodium, which accounts for nerve and skeletal muscle cells' resting membrane potential. An above-normal calcium level makes cell stimulation more difficult — the membrane becomes less permeable to sodium while the firing level (threshold) increases. A below-normal calcium level makes the membrane more permeable to sodium, facilitating stimulation. Muscle cells, for example, respond with increasing tension until they reach tetany, a prolonged contraction state.

**Magnesium.** A major ICF cation, magnesium ($Mg^{++}$) serves as a cofactor in many enzymatic and metabolic processes, particularly protein synthesis. Within nerve cells, it affects synaptic acetylcholine release, thus modifying nerve impulse transmission and subsequent skeletal muscle response. As with calcium, an increase or decrease in the magnesium level can severely depress neuromuscular activity or cause marked neuromuscular irritability.

Electrolytes contribute to homeostasis through these various functions, both specifically and in relation to other electrolytes. An imbalance of one electrolyte commonly affects several others. Electrolytes are also affected by fluid intake and output, acid-base balance, hormone secretion, and normal cell functioning.

### Fluid and solute movement

Fluid and solutes constantly move between fluid compartments by passing through the semipermeable cell membrane. Movement occurs through one of four mechanisms: diffusion, osmosis, capillary filtration, or active transport.

Most solutes move by *diffusion*. In this passive process, the solute moves from an area of high concentration to one of lower concentration. Eventually, such movement leads to equal solute distribution in fluid.

*Osmosis* occurs when two areas with different concentrations are separated by a membrane that allows water but not solutes to pass. Water moves passively across such a membrane, from an area of low solute concentration to one of higher solute concentration, until solute concentrations on both sides are equal. Volume on one side of the membrane increases as more water enters to dilute the concentration; volume on the other side decreases.

Water moves by osmosis between ECF and ICF according to the osmolarity of these compartments. (*Osmolarity* refers to the concentration of a solute in a volume of solution.) Normally, ECF and ICF have equal osmotic pressures. If ECF osmolarity increases, water shifts by osmosis from ICF to ECF. Conversely, if ICF osmolarity increases, water shifts from ECF to ICF.

*Filtration* occurs when water and dissolved substances move through a semipermeable membrane from an area of high pressure to one of lower pressure. In body fluids, hydrostatic (capillary) pressure resulting from the heart's pumping action aids filtration. When blood pressure inside the capillary exceeds pressure outside the capillary, water and solutes are forced out through pores in capillary walls and into the interstitial fluid.

In *active transport*, physiologic pumps move substances against a concentration gradient — a process that requires adenosine triphosphate for energy. The sodium-potassium pump, for instance, moves sodium ions from ICF, an area of greater concentration, to ECF, where concentration is lower. The reverse occurs with potassium, so greater amounts of potassium remain in ICF. Active transport of sodium, potassium, chloride, sugars, and amino acids also requires a carrier substance, which provides specific attachment sites for the solute.

# Intake and output monitoring

The cornerstone of assessing fluid and electrolyte balance, intake and output monitoring is indicated for any patient with an actual or potential fluid or electrolyte imbalance. Accurate intake and output records are mandatory for patients with burns, renal failure, dehydration, an electrolyte imbalance, congestive heart failure (CHF), or severe vomiting or diarrhea; for those who've had surgery recently; and for those receiving diuretics or corticosteroids. They're also important for patients with nasogastric (NG) tubes or drainage collection devices, for those on ventilators, and for those receiving I.V. therapy.

## Implementation

• Explain to the patient that you will be measuring his intake and output. Enlist the patient's help, if possible, *to ensure the most accurate records.*
• When recording intake, include all fluids entering the body, including beverages, fluids contained in solid foods taken by mouth, and foods that are liquid at room temperature, such as flavored gelatin, custard, and ice cream. Intake also should include GI instillations, bladder irrigations, and I.V. fluids.
• When recording output, include all fluid that leaves the patient's body, including urine, loose stools, vomitus, aspirated fluids, and drainage from surgical drains, NG tubes, and chest tubes. Also estimate and record output from other sources, such as insensible losses from the lungs and skin.
• If required, record 8-hour summaries with 24-hour totals. Depending on the patient's condition, you may also need to document hourly intake and output.

## Special considerations

Normally, the patient's intake and output record should show a balance between the amount of fluid he takes in and the amount he loses. Suspect a fluid volume deficit (hypovolemia) if his output exceeds his intake; suspect a fluid volume excess (hypervolemia) if his intake exceeds his output. However, if he's receiving fluid replacement therapy to treat hypovolemia, his intake should exceed his output.

Make sure not to overlook any source of fluid gain or loss when recording your patient's intake and output. *Such an error could delay detection and treatment of a fluid imbalance.* (See *Avoiding common mistakes in intake and output monitoring.*)

Whenever possible, measure — don't estimate — intake and output. For a small child, weigh diapers, if appropriate.

Review intake and output during each shift, and notify the doctor if amounts differ significantly over a 24-hour period. *To identify trends,* review daily totals for several consecutive days.

## Documentation

On the patient's intake and output record, note the date and time you initiated monitoring, and document appropriate patient information. Record all fluid gained or lost as separate entries on the intake and output record. Record amounts in milliliters. Also describe any fluid restrictions and the patient's compliance with them.

# Monitoring I.V. fluids

Patients receive I.V. fluids to meet daily nutritional needs, replace abnormal fluid losses, or correct electrolyte imbalances. The I.V. route also allows rapid, effective drug administration. Patients receiving I.V. fluids require careful monitoring for fluid imbalances. (See *Recognizing fluid volume deficits and excess,* page 119.)

Balanced I.V. solutions, used to treat and correct specific electrolyte imbalances, resemble plasma in fluid and electrolyte content. After adequate renal function has been established,

## Avoiding common mistakes in intake and output monitoring

Measuring fluid intake and output accurately can pose a challenge unless you're aware of potential sources of error – and take steps to prevent them. This chart lists common mistakes caregivers make when measuring and recording intake and output and describes measures you can take to prevent them.

| MISTAKE | PREVENTIVE MEASURES |
|---|---|
| Discarding body fluids without measuring them | • Make sure all staff members know which patients require intake and output measurement. For instance, verify that the card file contains a list of these patients' names, and post a list of the names in a convenient area for quick reference.<br>• Supply an adequate patient report to all personnel.<br>• Attach a "Measure intake and output" sign to the patient's bed. |
| Failing to elicit the patient's cooperation | • Make sure the patient and his family understand the importance of monitoring intake and output.<br>• Teach the patient and his family how to help caregivers maintain an accurate record of intake and output. |
| Incorrectly measuring small amounts of oral fluids | • Use an appropriate device to measure small amounts of oral fluids.<br>• Keep small, calibrated paper cups at the patient's bedside to more easily measure oral fluids. |
| Ascribing inconsistent volumes to fluid containers | • Designate a specific volume for each container used to measure fluids, and make sure all staff members record the same volume consistently.<br>• Keep a bedside record that lists the designated volumes for each container. |
| Overestimating fluid intake from iced beverages | • Be aware that iced beverages have a lower fluid volume than uniced beverages (from fluid displacement by ice).<br>• Record intake from ice chips as roughly half the volume of the ice chips; an ounce of ice chips equals roughly 15 ml of water.<br>• Keep ice in beverages to a minimum to promote more accurate intake measurement. |
| Inaccurately estimating fluids ingested from meal trays | • Don't assume the patient drank the entire contents of an empty fluid container. Instead, ask him if he drank all the fluid himself or gave some to another person. |
| Underestimating fluid intake from parenteral fluid | • Keep in mind that parenteral fluid bottles are overfilled. A 1,000-ml bottle may contain 1,100 ml of fluid; a 100-ml bottle, 150 ml.<br>• Run excess fluid through tubing during setup, or record actual volume infused. |
| Failing to estimate fluid lost through perspiration | • Record the amount of clothing and bed linens saturated with perspiration. Be aware that each necessary bed change represents at least 1 liter of fluid lost.<br>• If required, estimate perspiration as 1, 2, 3, or 4 (with 1 representing barely visible sweating and 4 representing profuse sweating). |
| Failing to record vomitus | • Don't record uncaught vomitus as a lost specimen. Instead, estimate and document the amount of fluid lost in vomitus. |

*(continued)*

**Avoiding common mistakes in intake and output monitoring** *(continued)*

| MISTAKE | PREVENTIVE MEASURES |
|---|---|
| Failing to record fluid lost in liquid stools | • Encourage the patient to use a bedpan, or place a measuring device over the toilet to allow direct measurement.<br>• Estimate the amount of fluid lost in liquid stools through fecal incontinence. |
| Failing to estimate fluid lost in wound exudate | • Measure and document the amount of drainage on a dressing by measuring the width of the stained area and determining dressing thickness.<br>• If necessary, weigh the dressing before applying and after removing it to estimate fluid loss.<br>• If the patient has a fistula, apply a stoma bag to catch and measure drainage. |
| Failing to assess urinary catheter patency if urine drainage decreases | • Don't assume that decreased drainage from an indwelling urinary catheter results from reduced urine formation. If drainage decreases, first determine if the catheter is patent. |
| Inaccurately measuring small amounts of urine | • Obtain an appropriate measuring device for frequent checks of urine output. (An error as small as 10 ml could have important consequences when dealing with small amounts of urine.)<br>• Use a collecting device calibrated to measure small amounts of urine. |
| Failing to record intake and output from irrigation | • Add the amount of irrigating solution infused to the intake column, and add the amount of fluid withdrawn during irrigation to the output column.<br>  Alternatively, you may compare the amount of irrigating solution to the amount of fluid withdrawn during irrigation. If the amount added exceeds the amount removed, record the excess in the intake column. If the amount removed exceeds the amount added, record the excess in the output column. |

the patient may receive Ringer's or lactated Ringer's solution. The latter is especially useful in treating mild acidosis.

Therapeutic solutions, usually infused through a subclavian catheter, are indicated when oral intake is contraindicated for a prolonged period. Hypertonic solutions, used in parenteral nutrition, contain 20% to 50% glucose in 500 ml of water (depending on the patient's needs) or 5% to 8% amino acids in 500 ml of water. These solutions, which supply roughly 440 calories and 4 g of nitrogen/liter, replace lost GI fluids and electrolytes, volume for volume.

Colloids draw fluid into the bloodstream by increasing intravascular osmotic pressure. They remain in the vascular space for several days, provided that the capillary endothelium is normal. (Colloids are not considered true I.V. fluid solutions because they contain undissolved proteins or starch molecules that are uniformly distributed.) Colloids include albumin, plasma protein fraction, dextran, and hetastarch. (See *Guide to colloids,* pages 120 and 121.)

Selection of an I.V. delivery method depends upon the therapy's purpose and duration; the patient's diagnosis, age, and health history; and the condition of his veins. For example, in peripheral I.V. therapy, you'll administer I.V. solutions through a vein in the arm, the hand or, less frequently, the leg or foot. Typically, this method is used for short-term or intermittent therapy.

# Recognizing fluid volume deficits and excess

Too much or too little fluid volume can have serious consequences. To ensure prompt detection and correction of an imbalance, make sure you're familiar with common assessment findings and the appropriate interventions.

## Fluid volume deficit

Fluid volume deficit reflects loss of water and electrolytes from the extracellular fluid (ECF) compartment. Three types of fluid volume deficits exist. A *hypertonic deficit* occurs when the ECF loses proportionately more water than sodium or when its sodium content increases. In contrast, a *hypotonic deficit* occurs when the ECF loses proportionately more sodium than water. An *isotonic deficit* reflects a proportionate loss of sodium and water from the ECF.

### Assessment findings

The patient with a fluid volume deficit may complain of thirst, fatigue, and urine output changes. He may experience vomiting or diarrhea, abdominal pain, and difficulty concentrating. Physical findings include a systolic blood pressure decrease of 10 mm Hg or more when the patient moves from a supine to a standing position. You may also note a subnormal temperature, elevated pulse and respiratory rates, and a weak pulse.

Other findings include dry mucous membranes, poor skin turgor, sunken eyes, pinched facial expression, flat neck veins when supine, slow hand-vein filling, cold extremities, and increased tongue furrows (wrinkles). With a severe fluid volume deficit, stupor or coma may occur. A weight loss of 2% suggests a mild fluid volume deficit; 5%, a moderate deficit; 8% or more, a severe deficit.

### Interventions

• Assess the patient's vital signs and level of consciousness (LOC) at least every 4 hours or as necessary.
• Check for signs and symptoms of dehydration: decreased skin turgor, dry oral mucous membranes, and thirst.
• Monitor serum electrolyte levels and check urine specific gravity every 8 hours.
• Weigh the patient daily at the same time, on the same scale, while he's wearing the same type of clothing.
• Maintain accurate intake and output records. Record intake and output every 8 hours, and report and correct an imbalance.
• Encourage adequate fluid intake. To promote compliance with increased intake, determine the patient's fluid likes and dislikes.

• If the patient experiences diarrhea, notify the doctor.
• If indicated, initiate parenteral fluid administration.
• Teach the patient how to recognize fluid volume deficit.

## Fluid volume excess

Fluid volume excess reflects an increased accumulation of water and electrolytes in the ECF.

### Assessment findings

The patient with fluid volume excess may complain of lethargy, shortness of breath, acute weight gain, and a bloated sensation. He may be experiencing ankle and eyelid edema, anorexia, nausea, vomiting, or abdominal cramps. Suspect fluid volume excess if the patient has seizures and you detect an altered LOC.

During the physical examination, check for edema, distended neck veins, ascites, pleural effusion, and crackles. Other findings may include engorged peripheral veins; slow hand-vein emptying; a full, bounding pulse; an increase in blood pressure; and polyuria.

Note whether the patient is receiving corticosteroids, chlorpropamide, vasopressin, phenylbutazone, or guanethidine. All of these drugs can cause a fluid volume excess.

A weight gain of 2% indicates a mild fluid volume excess; 5%, a moderate excess; 8% or more, a severe excess.

### Interventions

• Assess the patient's vital signs and LOC at least every 4 hours or as necessary.
• Check for ankle or sacral edema.
• Monitor serum electrolyte levels and check urine specific gravity every 8 hours.
• Weigh the patient daily at the same time, on the same scale, while he's wearing the same type of clothing.
• Maintain accurate intake and output records. Record intake and output every 8 hours, and notify the doctor if an imbalance occurs.
• Maintain dietary sodium restrictions, if indicated. Teach the patient about his prescribed diet, advising him of the sodium content of various foods.
• Maintain fluid restrictions, as indicated. Teach the patient about fluid restrictions and the signs and symptoms of fluid retention.
• Evaluate the effectiveness of diuretics and watch for any adverse reactions.

## Guide to colloids

You may need to administer colloids to a patient with a fluid volume deficit. This chart provides essential information about major colloids.

| COLLOID | CONTENTS | USES | NURSING IMPLICATIONS |
|---|---|---|---|
| Albumin (normal human serum albumin): albumin protein from human plasma. Supplied in two strengths: 5% albumin (which is osmotically equal to plasma) and 25% albumin (which draws about four times its volume in interstitial fluid into the circulation within 15 minutes of administration). | *5% albumin*<br>• Albumin (50 g/liter)<br>• Sodium (130 mEq/liter)<br>• Potassium (1 mEq/liter)<br>• pH 6.4 to 7.4<br>*25% albumin*<br>• Albumin (240 g/liter)<br>• Globulins (10 g/liter)<br>• Sodium (130 mEq/liter)<br>• pH 6.4 to 7.4 | Volume replacement in hypovolemic shock, hemorrhagic shock, cerebral edema, exchange transfusion, and hypoproteinemia | • Albumin is heat treated to reduce the risk of hepatitis transmission.<br>• It can be given without typing or crossmatching.<br>• Although 25% albumin was once called salt-poor, the term is a misnomer; it contains 130 to 160 mEq/liter of sodium.<br>• Infusion rate depends on the patient's condition and response. For patients in hypovolemic shock, infuse as rapidly as possible to restore vascular volume. For patients with normal vascular volume, infuse 5% solution at 2 to 4 ml/minute, 25% solution at 1 ml/minute.<br>• Monitor the patient for signs and symptoms of allergic reaction: fever, rash, chills.<br>• Don't administer more than 250 g in 48 hours.<br>• Use opened containers immediately; albumin solutions have no preservatives. |
| Dextran (Gentran): Large polysaccharide glucose polymer (combination of simpler molecules) that's water-soluble. Supplied in two strengths: low-molecular-weight dextran (LMD) and high-molecular-weight dextran (HMD). LMD expands vascular volume one to two times more than amount of LMD infused. With HMD, plasma expansion slightly exceeds the volume infused. | *LMD*<br>• 500-ml solution containing 10% dextran (molecular weight 40,000) in 0.9% sodium chloride solution or dextrose 5% in water ($D_5W$)<br>*HMD*<br>• 500-ml solution containing 6% dextran (molecular weight 70,000) in 0.9% sodium chloride solution or $D_5W$ | Volume replacement in hypovolemic shock, hemorrhagic shock, and thromboembolism prophylaxis (LMD only) | • Dextran solutions may prolong bleeding time. (LMD decreases red blood cell adhesiveness. HMD increases platelet adhesiveness and blood viscosity.) Use cautiously in patients with hemorrhagic or coagulation disorders.<br>• Dextran infusion may interfere with blood typing and crossmatching, so draw blood samples before starting the infusion.<br>• Dextran increases urine specific gravity and osmolality (50% to 70% is excreted unchanged in urine).<br>• Dextran is less expensive than Plasmanate.<br>• Infuse only clear solution. If you see dextran flakes in a stored, unopened I.V. bag, put the bag in warm water until flakes dissolve.<br>• Stop the infusion if the patient develops signs of renal failure – for example, oliguria and increasing levels of blood urea nitrogen or creatinine.<br>• Monitor the patient for an anaphylactic reaction. |
| Hetastarch (Hespan): synthetic starch similar to human glycogen with a side range of molecular weights mixed in 0.9% sodium chloride solution | *In 500 ml*<br>• Sodium (154 mEq/liter)<br>• Chloride (154 mEq/liter)<br>• 6% hetastarch | Volume replacement in hemorrhagic and hypovolemic shock | • Expansion of plasma volume slightly exceeds the amount of hetastarch given.<br>• About 40% of hetastarch dose is excreted in 24 hours.<br>• Use opened containers immediately; hetastarch contains no preservatives. |

*(continued)*

## Guide to colloids *(continued)*

| COLLOID | CONTENTS | USES | NURSING IMPLICATIONS |
|---------|----------|------|----------------------|
| Hetastarch (Hespan) *(continued)* | | | • Monitor the patient for an anaphylactic reaction.<br>• Monitor hematology and coagulation results for prolonged prothrombin, plasma thrombin, and clotting times. |
| Plasma protein fraction (Plasmanate): 5% solution of human plasma proteins mixed in 0.9% sodium chloride solution | • Albumin (44 g/liter)<br>• Alpha and beta globulin (6 g/liter)<br>• Sodium (145 mEq/liter)<br>• Chloride (85 mEq/liter)<br>• Potassium (2 mEq/liter)<br>• pH 6.7 to 7.3 | Volume replacement in hypovolemic shock, hemorrhagic shock, and hypoproteinemia | • Solution is heat treated to reduce the risk of hepatitis transmission.<br>• It doesn't require crossmatching.<br>• Adverse reactions are unusual. However, patients with heart failure may develop circulatory overload or pulmonary edema. At infusion rates above 10 ml/minute, peripheral vasodilation and hypotension may occur.<br>• Solution doesn't replace lost clotting factors.<br>• Because solution is osmotically equal to plasma, plasma expansion equals the amount of solution infused.<br>• Don't administer cloudy or sedimented solutions. |

In central venous (CV) therapy, you'll administer I.V. solutions through a central vein, such as the right or left subclavian or the internal or external jugular. This method is typically used for patients who need a large volume of fluid or a hypertonic solution, caustic drug, or high-calorie parenteral nutrition solution. Implanted vascular access devices provide a variation on CV infusion. The infused solution enters a central vein through an access device surgically implanted in a subcutaneous pocket or attached to a catheter in the chest wall or abdomen. A percutaneous central line may also be used for this purpose. This catheter is inserted through the brachial artery and threaded up to the vena cava or right atrium. These methods of delivery are ordered for patients needing long-term (months to years) I.V. therapy.

## Implementation

• Administer the correct solutions at the prescribed rate and volume using the appropriate delivery system.

• Consider the patient's normal electrolyte requirements when providing I.V. fluids. The sodium requirement is 1 to 2 mEq/kg of body weight per day; potassium, 0.5 to 1 mEq/kg of body weight per day; and chloride, 1 to 2 mEq/kg of body weight per day, for instance. Are the solutions being infused providing these electrolytes? Also consider how long the patient has been receiving I.V. fluids and whether his electrolyte requirements are being supplemented by oral intake. Be aware that elderly patients and those with cardiovascular disorders are especially prone to fluid overload.

• If you're caring for a patient receiving parenteral nutrition, be alert for changes in fluid and electrolyte status and in glucose, amino acid, mineral, and vitamin levels. Make sure the patient is receiving adequate calories for his age, height, weight, and medical condition. Monitor the patient's response to the nutrient solution and watch for early signs of complications.

• Carefully assess the I.V. insertion site for signs of infiltration, phlebitis, local infection, and catheter occlusion. *These complications may alter the rate and volume of fluid administration, leading to fluid imbalance.*

## Special considerations
Make sure you know how the prescribed I.V. fluid therapy will affect the patient's fluid and electrolyte balance.

## Documentation
Record on an I.V. flow sheet or in the nurses' notes the date and time of administration, the signature of the person giving the therapy, the infusion starting date and time, the solution name, the device and needle gauge inserted in the vein, the insertion site, the administration rate, and any additives, including their dosages.

Also record the number of attempts required to start the I.V. line, including reasons for any change of site, such as extravasation, phlebitis, occlusion, patient removal of cannula, or routine change according to hospital policy. Include details of any problems with I.V. flow or site condition.

When administering I.V. medications, record the drug given on the medication record, including the date and your signature. If the drug wasn't given, circle the indicated time, note the reason the drug was not given, and sign your name.

Also chart on an input and output record all large-volume parenteral solutions, including those containing drug admixtures.

## Monitoring electrolytes through venipuncture

Monitoring a patient's electrolytes often requires obtaining blood samples for laboratory analysis. The blood samples are typically obtained through venipuncture, a technique which involves piercing a vein with a needle and collecting blood in a syringe or evacuated tube. Typically, venipuncture is performed using the antecubital fossa. If necessary, however, it can be performed on a vein in the wrist, the dorsum of the hand or foot, or another accessible location. Usually, laboratory personnel carry out the procedure in the hospital setting; however, a nurse may perform it occasionally.

## Equipment
Tourniquet ▪ gloves ▪ syringe or evacuated tubes and needle holder ▪ 70% ethyl alcohol or povidone-iodine sponges ▪ 20G or 21G needle for the forearm or 25G for the wrist, hand, ankle, or for children ▪ color-coded tubes containing appropriate additives ▪ labels ▪ laboratory request form ▪ 2″ × 2″ gauze pads ▪ adhesive bandage.

## Preparation of equipment
If you're using evacuated tubes, open the needle packet, attach the needle to its holder, and select the appropriate tubes. If you're using a syringe, attach the appropriate needle to it. Be sure to choose a syringe large enough to hold all the blood required for the test. Label all collection tubes clearly with the patient's name and room number, the doctor's name, and the date and time of collection.

## Implementation
• Wash your hands thoroughly and don gloves *to prevent cross-contamination.*
• Tell the patient that you're about to take a blood sample, and explain the procedure *to ease his anxiety and encourage his cooperation.* Ask him if he's ever felt faint, sweaty, or nauseated when having blood drawn.
• If the patient is on bed rest, ask him to lie supine, with his head slightly elevated and his arms at his sides. Ask the ambulatory patient to sit in a chair and support his arm securely on an armrest or table.
• Assess the patient's veins *to determine the best puncture site.* (See *Possible venipuncture sites.*) Observe the skin for the vein's blue color, or palpate the vein for a firm rebound sensation.

• Tie a tourniquet 2″ (5 cm) proximal to the area chosen. *By impeding venous return to the heart while still allowing arterial flow,* a tourniquet produces venous dilation. If arterial perfusion remains adequate, you'll be able to feel the radial pulse. (If the tourniquet fails to dilate the vein, have the patient open and close his fist repeatedly. Then ask him to close his fist as you insert the needle and to open it again when the needle is in place.)

• Clean the venipuncture site with a povidone-iodine sponge or with an alcohol sponge. Don't wipe off the povidone-iodine with alcohol *because alcohol cancels the effect of povidone-iodine.* Wipe in a circular motion, spiraling outward from the site *to avoid introducing potentially infectious skin flora into the vessel during the procedure.* If you use alcohol, apply it with friction for 30 seconds, or until the final sponge comes away clean. Allow the skin to dry before performing venipuncture.

• Immobilize the vein by pressing just below the venipuncture site with your thumb and drawing the skin taut.

• Position the needle holder or syringe with the needle bevel up and the shaft parallel to the path of the vein and at a 30-degree angle to the arm. Insert the needle into the vein. If you're using a syringe, venous blood will appear in the hub; withdraw the blood slowly, pulling the plunger of the syringe gently *to create steady suction* until you obtain the required sample. *Pulling the plunger too forcibly* may collapse the vein. If you're using a needle holder and evacuated tube, a drop of blood will appear just inside the needle holder. Grasp the holder securely to stabilize it in the vein, and push down on the collection tube until the needle punctures the rubber stopper. Blood will flow into the tube automatically.

• Remove the tourniquet as soon as blood flows adequately *to prevent stasis and hemoconcentration, which can impair test results.* If the flow is sluggish, leave the tourniquet in place longer, but always remove it before withdrawing the needle.

## Possible venipuncture sites

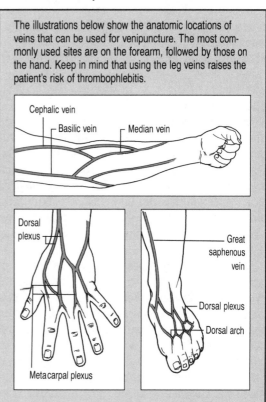

The illustrations below show the anatomic locations of veins that can be used for venipuncture. The most commonly used sites are on the forearm, followed by those on the hand. Keep in mind that using the leg veins raises the patient's risk of thrombophlebitis.

Cephalic vein

Basilic vein

Median vein

Dorsal plexus

Metacarpal plexus

Great saphenous vein

Dorsal plexus

Dorsal arch

• After you've drawn the sample, place a gauze pad over the puncture site, and slowly and gently remove the needle from the vein. When using an evacuated tube, remove it from the needle holder *to release the vacuum before withdrawing the needle from the vein.*

• Apply gentle pressure to the puncture site for 2 or 3 minutes or until bleeding stops. *This prevents extravasation into the surrounding tissue,* which causes hematoma.

• After bleeding stops, apply an adhesive bandage.

• If you've used a syringe, transfer the sample to a collection tube. Detach the needle from the syringe, open the collection tube, and gently

empty the sample into the tube, being careful to avoid foaming, *which may cause hemolysis.*
• Finally, check the venipuncture site *to make sure a hematoma hasn't developed.* If it has, apply warm soaks.
• Discard used gloves in the appropriate container.

### Special considerations
Never draw a venous sample from an arm or leg already being used for I.V. therapy or blood administration *because this may affect test results.* Don't draw a venous sample from an infection site *because this risks introduction of pathogens into the vascular system.* Likewise, avoid drawing blood from edematous areas, arteriovenous shunts, or sites of previous hematoma or vascular injury.

If you use a blood pressure cuff as a tourniquet, inflate it to a level between the patient's systolic and diastolic pressures *to allow for venous distention without constricting arterial flow.* If the patient has large, distended, highly visible veins, perform venipuncture without a tourniquet *to minimize the risk of hematoma.*

If the patient has a clotting disorder or is receiving anticoagulant therapy, maintain firm pressure on the venipuncture site for at least 5 minutes after withdrawing the needle *to prevent possible formation of a hematoma.* Perform venipuncture cautiously in patients who have clotting disorders or who are receiving anticoagulant therapy.

Avoid using veins in the patient's legs for venipuncture, if possible, *because this increases the risk of thrombophlebitis.*

### Complications
Hematoma at the needle insertion site is the most common complication of venipuncture. Infection may result from poor technique.

### Documentation
Record the date, time, and site of venipuncture; the name of the test; the time the sample was sent to the laboratory; and any adverse effects the patient experiences, such as a hematoma or anxiety.

# Monitoring electrolytes with a vascular intermittent access system

The vascular intermittent access system measures electrolyte levels automatically in patients who have an indwelling arterial or venous line. In just 1 minute, it obtains such critical indices as potassium, calcium, sodium, glucose, hematocrit, and arterial blood gas levels. Then it reinfuses the blood sample into the patient.

By monitoring electrolyte levels repeatedly, this system allows you to respond quickly to any abnormalities. The arterial or venous line can be accessed as often as every 3 minutes. This avoids the need to draw blood manually for laboratory samples and eliminates problems that an indwelling sensor sometimes causes. Easily transported with the patient from one area to another, the system can be used in the operating room, intensive care unit, emergency department, and other special care units.

### Equipment
Monitor and a sensor array ▪ isotonic I.V. solution with tubing (lactated Ringer's solution).

The I.V. solution serves to keep the I.V. line patent. With the appropriate calibrant additives, the solution calibrates the sensors before each measurement. A printer provides a hard copy of test results, and an automatic timer automatically initiates the process at predetermined intervals. (See *Vascular intermittent access system.*)

## Vascular intermittent access system

Used to measure electrolyte levels automatically, the vascular intermittent access system includes a sensor array, an I.V. administration set, an I.V. solution with additives for sensor calibrations, and a monitor that processes signals from the sensors. A pumping mechanism infuses the solution and withdraws blood samples.

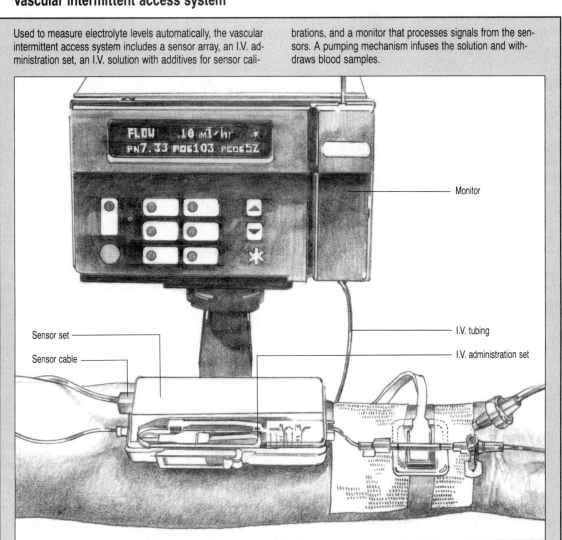

### Preparation of equipment

Set up the vascular intermittent access system, following the manufacturer's directions. Place the sensor array at the distal end of the I.V. administration set.

### Implementation

Perform blood chemistry testing as often as desired by simply pressing the sampling key on the monitor. This triggers a series of automatic steps. First, the sensors are calibrated against known reference values in the I.V. solution. Next, the system reverses its usual pumping action and withdraws a small amount of blood (0.6 ml), which then contacts the sensors. Roughly 30 seconds later, test results appear on the monitor screen. Finally, the system flushes the blood back into the patient along with the I.V. solution.

### Special considerations
Abnormal electrolyte values measured by this system indicate electrolyte imbalances, which can disrupt various body systems and cause serious health problems. Make sure you know normal and abnormal laboratory values as well as the implications of abnormal results. (See *Laboratory tests used to monitor fluid and electrolyte balance.*)

Be aware that the vascular intermittent access system doesn't require long-term compatibility between the sensors and the patient's blood. Except for the few seconds during which the measurement is being made, the sensors are exposed only to the I.V. solution, not the blood.

Because the system is closed, blood handling by caregivers is avoided and blood loss in the patient is prevented.

### Documentation
Document the date and time of the automatic blood sampling, the arterial or venous line accessed, and the name of the test. If the access system is set at predetermined times, document the intervals. If available, attach a duplicate of the hard copy to patient's chart.

# Urine specific gravity monitoring
The kidneys maintain homeostasis by varying urine output and its concentration of dissolved salts. Urine specific gravity measures the concentration of urine solutes, which reflects the kidneys' capacity to concentrate urine. The capacity to concentrate urine is among the first functions lost when renal tubular damage occurs.

Urine specific gravity is determined by comparing the weight of a urine specimen with that of an equivalent volume of distilled water, which is 1.000. Because urine contains dissolved salts and other substances, it's heavier than 1.000. Urine specific gravity ranges from 1.003 (very dilute) to 1.035 (highly concentrated); normal values range from 1.010 to 1.025. Specific gravity is commonly measured with a urinometer (a specially calibrated hydrometer designed to float in a cylinder of urine.) The more concentrated the urine, the higher the urinometer floats — and the higher the specific gravity. It may also be measured by a refractometer, which measures the refraction of light as it passes through a urine sample, or by a reagent strip test.

Elevated specific gravity reflects an increased concentration of urine solutes, which occurs in conditions causing renal hypoperfusion, and may indicate CHF, dehydration, hepatic disorders, or nephrosis. Low specific gravity reflects failure to reabsorb water and concentrate urine; it may indicate hypercalcemia, hypokalemia, alkalosis, acute renal failure, pyelonephritis, glomerulonephritis, or diabetes insipidus.

Although urine specific gravity is commonly measured with a random urine specimen, more accurate measurement is possible with a controlled specimen collected after fluids are withheld for 12 to 24 hours.

### Equipment
Calibrated urinometer and cylinder, refractometer, or reagent strips (Multistix) ▪ gloves ▪ graduated specimen container.

### Implementation
• Explain the procedure to the patient, and tell him when you will need the specimen. Explain why you're withholding fluids and for how long *to ensure his cooperation.*

#### Measuring with a urinometer
• Don gloves and collect a random urine specimen. Allow it to come to room temperature (71.6° F [22° C]) before testing *because this is the temperature at which most urinometers are calibrated.*

*(Text continues on page 130.)*

## Laboratory tests used to monitor fluid and electrolyte balance

Monitoring certain laboratory tests can help you evaluate your patient's fluid and electrolyte status. This chart presents normal values for relevant blood and urine tests, along with related nursing considerations.

| TEST | NORMAL RANGE | NURSING CONSIDERATIONS |
|---|---|---|
| **BLOOD TESTS** | | |
| Fasting blood glucose | 65 to 110 mg/dl (3.58 to 6.05 mmol/liter) | • Marked serum glucose elevations cause osmotic diuresis, resulting in hypovolemia.<br>• Expect increased levels in patients receiving parenteral glucose therapy. |
| Serum albumin | 3.5 to 4.8 g/dl (35 to 48 g/liter) | • When the albumin level drops, colloidal osmotic pull in the intravascular space decreases; fluid then shifts to the interstitial space, causing edema.<br>• Be sure to consider your patient's albumin level when evaluating total calcium values. |
| Serum calcium | *Total calcium*<br>8.9 to 10.3 mg/dl (2.23 to 2.57 mmol/liter) | • Total serum calcium represents the sum of ionized (47%) and nonionized (53%) calcium components. Of the nonionized portion, albumin-bound calcium makes up 40%, and the portion chelated to anions (such as phosphate and citrate) accounts for 13%.<br>• Total calcium is the most commonly performed serum calcium test.<br>• To determine the serum calcium level from the serum albumin, first obtain the serum albumin level, then correct total serum calcium for variations in albumin by assuming that each serum albumin change of 1 g/dl (10 g/liter) will alter the total serum calcium level by 0.8 mg/dl (0.2 mmol/liter).<br>    However, don't calculate serum calcium this way if your patient has a condition that affects the degree of calcium-albumin binding or the blood pH (which alters the percentage of ionized calcium). Calcium-albumin binding rises with alkalosis and increased free fatty acid levels (common in stressed patients). Increased levels of lactate, bicarbonate, citrate, phosphate, and some substances in radiographic contrast media also may reduce the ionized calcium level. |
| | *Ionized calcium*<br>4.6 to 5.1 mg/dl (1.15 to 1.27 mmol/liter) | • Direct ionized calcium measurement is especially valuable in critically ill patients because ionized calcium is physiologically active.<br>• Be aware that the sampling technique may affect test results. For instance, prolonged tourniquet application or an inappropriate amount of heparin in the collecting syringe may cause misleading results. |
| Serum chloride | 97 to 110 mEq/liter (97 to 110 mmol/liter) | • Below-normal level indicates hypochloremia, as from metabolic alkalosis or hypokalemia.<br>• Above-normal level signifies hyperchloremia, as from excessive administration of isotonic sodium chloride solution. |
| Serum magnesium | 1.3 to 2.1 mEq/liter (0.65 to 1.05 mmol/liter) | • Hemolysis of the sample causes release of magnesium from red blood cells (RBCs) into serum, invalidating test results. |
| Serum phosphate | 2.5 to 4.5 mg/dl (0.81 to 1.45 mmol/liter) | • Evaluate the value in conjunction with serum calcium levels. Keep in mind that phosphate and calcium relate inversely; if the phosphate level increases, the calcium level drops. |

*(continued)*

## Laboratory tests used to monitor fluid and electrolyte balance *(continued)*

| TEST | NORMAL RANGE | NURSING CONSIDERATIONS |
|---|---|---|
| **BLOOD TESTS** *(continued)* | | |
| Serum phosphate *(continued)* | | • Expect a higher serum phosphate level in a child than in an adult.<br>• Infusing I.V. glucose before or during sample collection will cause a decreased value (from carbohydrate metabolism).<br>• Insulin aids entry of extracellular phosphate into cells.<br>• Hemolysis of the sample causes phosphate release from RBCs into serum, invalidating test results. |
| Serum potassium | 3.5 to 5 mEq/liter (3.5 to 5 mmol/liter) | • Increased value may indicate acidosis, which causes potassium to shift out of cells into blood.<br>• Decreased value may indicate alkalosis, which causes potassium to shift from blood into cells.<br>• Insulin triggers entry of extracellular potassium into cells, causing a transient drop in the serum potassium level.<br>• Serum potassium level may be raised an additional 2.7 mEq/liter by a tight tourniquet around an exercising extremity (as when a patient opens and closes his hand).<br>• Hemolysis of the sample causes movement of potassium from RBCs into serum, invalidating test results. |
| Serum sodium | 135 to 145 mEq/liter (135 to 145 mmol/liter) | • Value relates closely to body water. For adults, each 3-mEq/liter elevation of serum sodium above the normal range represents a deficit of roughly 1 liter of body water.<br>• Expect the value to drop as the serum glucose level rises (from movement of water from cells to extracellular fluid). Every 62-mg/dl increase in the serum glucose level draws enough water from cells to dilute serum sodium concentration by 1 mEq/liter. Thus, if the patient's serum glucose level is 1,000 mg/dl (930 mg/dl above normal), the serum sodium level should decrease 15 mEq/liter. |
| Blood urea nitrogen (BUN) | 8 to 25 mg/dl (2.9 to 8.9 mmol/liter) | • Increased value may result from decreased renal blood flow secondary to fluid volume deficit (which reduces urea clearance).<br>• Conditions that enhance urea production, including excessive protein intake and increased catabolism (as from starvation, trauma, bleeding into the intestines, or catabolic drugs), may elevate BUN levels.<br>• Below-normal value may result from overhydration or low protein intake. |
| Serum creatinine | 0.6 to 1.6 mg/dl (53 to 133 μmol/liter) | • This test evaluates renal disease more sensitively and specifically than BUN because few nonrenal causes of creatinine elevation exist.<br>• Value increases when at least half of the renal nephrons are nonfunctional.<br>• Slight elevations may occur with severe fluid volume depletion (from a reduced glomerular filtration rate [GFR]). |

## Laboratory tests used to monitor fluid and electrolyte balance *(continued)*

| TEST | NORMAL RANGE | NURSING CONSIDERATIONS |
|---|---|---|
| **BLOOD TESTS** *(continued)* | | |
| BUN-creatinine ratio | 10:1 | • This test helps evaluate hydration status. A ratio above 10:1 suggests hypovolemia, low perfusion pressure to the kidney, or increased protein metabolism. A ratio below 10:1 suggests hepatic insufficiency or low protein intake.<br>• When both BUN and creatinine levels rise but remain in a 10:1 ratio, suspect intrinsic renal disease. (However, this result also may occur when fluid volume depletion causes the GFR to drop.) |
| Hematocrit | Men: 44% to 52%<br>Women: 39% to 47% | • Hematocrit measures the percentage by volume of packed RBCs in plasma.<br>• An increased value suggests hypovolemia. (RBCs are contained in a relatively smaller plasma fluid volume.) A decreased value suggests hypervolemia. (RBCs are contained in a relatively larger plasma fluid volume.) However, with hemolysis or bleeding, test results don't accurately reflect fluid balance. |
| **URINE TESTS** | | |
| Urine calcium | 50 to 300 mg/24 hours (depending on dietary intake) | • Value may reach 900 mg/24 hours in patients with hypercalcemia secondary to metastatic tumors.<br>• Subnormal value may indicate hypocalcemia.<br>• Qualitative test is done on a single specimen by observing for precipitate after adding a few drops of calcium oxalate. A heavy white precipitate indicates an above-normal urine calcium level; a clear specimen, a below-normal urine calcium level. |
| Urine chloride | 110 to 250 mEq/liter/ 24 hours (110 to 250 mmol/dl/24 hours) | • Sodium intake may affect the value.<br>• Value usually approximates urine sodium value in patients with hypovolemia because sodium and chloride are reabsorbed together.<br>• This test helps differentiate the various forms of metabolic alkalosis. A decreased value indicates metabolic alkalosis secondary to vomiting, gastric suctioning, or diuretic therapy. An increased value indicates metabolic alkalosis resulting from profound potassium depletion or mineralocorticoid excess. |
| Urine potassium | 25 to 125 mEq/liter/24 hours (25 to 125 mmol/liter/ 24 hours)<br>Random specimen: usually above 40 mEq/liter | • The 24-hour test is used mainly to assess hormonal function and determine if hypokalemia has a renal or nonrenal cause.<br>• Value varies with diet and with serum aldosterone or cortisol level. (Increased amounts of these substances enhance potassium excretion.)<br>• Below-normal value may indicate acute renal failure. In the presence of hypokalemia, however, a below-normal value indicates a nonrenal cause. |
| Urine sodium | 40 to 220 mEq/liter/24 hours (40 to 220 mmol/liter/ 24 hours)<br>Random specimen: usually above 40 mEq/liter | • A decreased value indicates hypovolemia characterized by renal sodium conservation to maintain blood volume.<br>• An increased value indicates hypovolemia associated with underlying renal disease, hypoaldosteronism, osmotic diuresis, or diuretic therapy.<br>• Value varies with diet. Be sure to record dietary intake during the test period to permit correct interpretation of test result. |

*(continued)*

## Laboratory tests used to monitor fluid and electrolyte balance *(continued)*

| TEST | NORMAL RANGE | NURSING CONSIDERATIONS |
|---|---|---|
| **URINE TESTS** *(continued)* | | |
| Urine osmolality | Range:<br>50 to 1,400 mOsm/kg<br>Average:<br>500 to 800 mOsm/kg | • After an overnight fast of 14 hours, urine osmolality should be triple the serum osmolality.<br>• Value rises with hypovolemia as the kidneys conserve needed fluid, causing greater urine concentration. Value decreases with hypervolemia as the kidneys excrete unneeded fluid, causing more diluted urine.<br>• Simultaneous serum and urine osmolality tests measure renal concentrating ability more accurately than the urine specific gravity test. |
| Urine pH | 4.5 to 8.0 | • In pooled daily output, urine pH averages roughly 5.0; in most random specimens, it measures less than 6.6.<br>• Value normally fluctuates throughout the day.<br>• Urine pH reflects serum pH and helps confirm acidosis or alkalosis (except with paradoxical aciduria in hypokalemic alkalosis, or alkaline urine caused by infections or renal tubular acidosis).<br>• Value increases with use of alkalinizing agents (such as sodium bicarbonate and potassium citrate) and decreases with use of acidifying agents (such as ascorbic acid, sodium acid phosphate, and methenamine mandelate).<br>• Specimen should be examined soon after collection to avoid alkalinization from bacteria-induced splitting of urea into ammonia. |
| Urine specific gravity | 1.003 to 1.035 | • In most random specimens, specific gravity measures 1.012 to 1.025.<br>• In elderly patients, normal range may be lower because of reduced renal concentrating ability.<br>• Value reflects hydration status and varies with urine volume and the solute load to be excreted.<br>• In patients with normal renal function, increased value indicates hypovolemia (the kidneys attempt to retain needed fluid and excrete solutes in a small, concentrated urine volume).<br>• Specific gravity fixed at 1.010 indicates significant renal disease.<br>• Heavy molecules (such as glucose, albumin, and dyes) increase specific gravity disproportionately to the actual concentration. Therefore, urine osmolality is a more accurate test in patients with glycosuria or proteinuria and in those who've recently been injected with radiopaque dyes. |

• Fill the cylinder about three-fourths full of urine. Then, gently spin the urinometer and drop it into the cylinder.

• When the urinometer stops bobbing, read the specific gravity from the calibrated scale marked directly on the stem of the urinometer. Make sure the instrument floats freely and doesn't touch the sides of the cylinder. Read the scale at the lowest point of the meniscus *to ensure an accurate reading.* (For specific instructions, see *Using a urinometer.*)

• Discard the urine, and rinse the cylinder and urinometer in cool water. *Warm water coagulates proteins in urine, making them stick to the instrument.*

• Remove gloves and wash your hands thoroughly *to prevent cross-contamination.*

### Measuring with a refractometer
• Don gloves and collect a random or controlled urine specimen.
• Place a single drop of urine on the refractometer slide.
• Turn on the light and look through the eyepiece, where you will see the specific gravity indicated on a scale. (Some instruments use a digital display.)

### Measuring with a reagent strip
• Don gloves and obtain a random or controlled urine specimen.
• Dip the reagent end of the test strip into the specimen for 2 seconds.
• Tap the strip on the rim of the specimen container *to remove excess urine,* and compare the resultant color change with the color chart supplied with the kit.

### Special considerations
Test the urinometer in distilled water at room temperature *to check that its calibration is 1.000.* If necessary, correct the urinometer reading for temperature effects; add 0.001 to your observed reading for every 5.4° F (3° C) above the calibration temperature of 71.6° F (22° C); subtract 0.001 for every 5.4° F below 71.6° F.

### Documentation
Record the specific gravity, volume, color, odor, and appearance of the collected urine specimen.

# Urine pH monitoring
The pH of urine — its alkalinity or acidity — reflects the ability of the kidneys to maintain a normal hydrogen ion concentration in plasma and extracellular fluids. The normal hydrogen ion concentration in urine varies, ranging from pH 4.6 to 8.0, but it usually averages around pH 6.0.

## Using a urinometer

With the urinometer floating in a cylinder of urine, position your eye at a level even with the bottom of the meniscus and read the specific gravity from the scale printed on the urinometer.

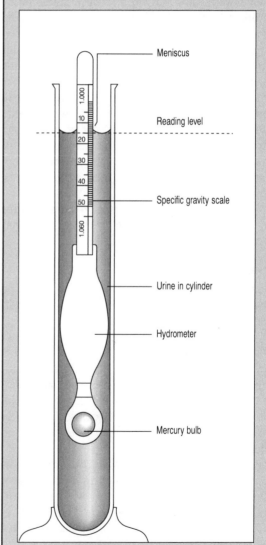

The simplest procedure for testing the pH of urine consists of dipping a reagent strip (such as a Combistix) into a fresh specimen of the patient's urine and comparing the resultant color change with a standardized color chart.

An alkaline pH (above 7.0), resulting from a diet low in meat but high in vegetables, dairy products, and citrus fruits, causes turbidity and formation of phosphate, carbonate, and amorphous crystals. Alkaline urine may also result from urinary tract infection and from metabolic or respiratory alkalosis.

An acid pH (below 7.0), resulting from a high-protein diet, also causes turbidity, with formation of oxalate, cystine, amorphous urate, and uric acid crystals. Acid urine may also result from renal tuberculosis, phenylketonuria, alkaptonuria, pyrexia, diarrhea, starvation, and all forms of acidosis.

Measuring urine pH can also help monitor some medications, such as methenamine, that are active only at certain pH levels.

### Equipment
Urine specimen container ▪ gloves ▪ reagent strips ▪ color chart. (The reagent strip has a pH indicator as part of a battery of indicators.)

### Implementation
• Wash your hands thoroughly and don gloves.
• Provide the patient with a specimen container, and instruct him to collect a clean-catch midstream specimen. Dip the reagent strip into the urine, remove it, and tap off the excess urine from the strip.
• Hold the strip horizontally *to avoid mixing reagents from adjacent test areas on the strip.* Then, compare the color on the strip with the standardized color chart on the strip package. This comparison can be made up to 60 seconds after immersing the strip.
• Discard the urine specimen. If you're monitoring the patient's intake and output, measure the amount of urine discarded.

• Discard gloves and wash your hands thoroughly *to prevent cross-contamination.*

### Special considerations
Use only a fresh urine specimen *because bacterial growth at room temperature changes urine pH.* Avoid letting a drop of urine run off the pH reagent onto adjacent reagent spots on the strip *because these other reagents will change the pH result.*

Urine collected at night is usually more acidic than urine collected during the day.

### Documentation
Record the test results, time of voiding, and amount voided.

## Timed urine collection
Because hormones, proteins, and electrolytes are excreted in small variable amounts in urine, specimens for measuring these substances must typically be collected over an extended time to yield quantities of diagnostic value.

A 24-hour specimen is used most commonly because it provides an average excretion rate for substances eliminated during this period. Timed specimens may also be collected for shorter periods, such as 2 or 12 hours, depending on the specific information needed.

A timed urine specimen may also be collected after administering a challenge dose of a chemical — inulin, for example — to detect various renal disorders.

### Equipment
Large collection bottle with a cap or stopper, or a commercial plastic container ▪ preservative, if necessary ▪ gloves ▪ bedpan or urinal, if patient does not have an indwelling catheter ▪ graduated container, if patient is on intake and output measurement ▪ gloves ▪ ice-filled container, if a refrigerator isn't available ▪ label ▪ laboratory request form ▪ four patient care reminders.

Check with the laboratory to see what preservatives may be needed in the urine specimen, or if a dark collection bottle is required.

## Implementation

• Explain the procedure to the patient and his family members, as necessary, *to enlist their co-operation and prevent accidental disposal of urine during the collection period.* Emphasize that loss of even *one* urine specimen during the collection period invalidates the test and requires that it begin again.

• Place patient-care reminders over the patient's bed, in his bathroom, on the bedpan hopper in the utility room, and on the urinal or indwelling catheter collection bag. Include the patient's name and his room number, the date, and the collection interval.

• Instruct the patient to save all urine during the collection period, to notify you after each voiding, and to avoid contaminating the urine with stool or toilet tissue. Explain any dietary or drug restrictions and be sure he understands and is willing to comply with them.

### Obtaining a 2-hour collection

• If possible, instruct the patient to drink two to four 8-oz glasses (480 to 960 ml) of water about 30 minutes before collection begins. After 30 minutes, tell him to void. Don gloves and discard this specimen *so the patient starts the collection period with an empty bladder.*

• If ordered, administer a challenge dose of medication (such as glucose solution or corticotropin), and record the time.

• If possible, offer the patient a glass of water at least every hour during the collection period *to stimulate urine production.* After each voiding, don gloves and add the specimen to the collection bottle.

• Instruct the patient to void about 15 minutes before the end of the collection period, if possible, and add this specimen to the collection bottle.

• At the end of the collection period, remove and discard gloves and send the appropriately la-

beled collection bottle to the laboratory immediately, along with a properly completed laboratory request form.

### Obtaining a 12- and a 24-hour collection

• Put on gloves and ask the patient to void. Then discard this urine *so he starts the collection period with an empty bladder.* Record the time.

• After putting on gloves and pouring the first urine specimen into the collection bottle, add the required preservative. Then refrigerate the bottle or keep it on ice until the next voiding, as appropriate.

• Collect all urine voided during the prescribed period. Just before the collection period ends, ask the patient to void again, if possible. Add this last specimen to the collection bottle, pack it in ice *to inhibit deterioration of the specimen,* and remove and discard gloves. Send the specimen to the laboratory. Include a properly completed laboratory request form.

### Special considerations

The patient should be hydrated before and during the test *to ensure adequate urine flow.*

Before collection of a timed specimen, make sure the laboratory will be open when the collection period ends *to help ensure prompt, accurate results.* Never store a specimen in a refrigerator containing food or medication *to avoid contamination.* If the patient has an indwelling catheter in place, put the collection bag in an ice-filled container at his bedside.

Instruct the patient to avoid exercise, ingestion of coffee or tea, or any drugs (unless otherwise directed by the doctor) before the test *to avoid altering test results.*

If you accidentally discard a specimen during the collection period, restart the collection. Accidentally discarding a specimen during the test period may result in an additional day of hospitalization, possibly causing the patient personal and financial hardship. Therefore, emphasize the need to save all the patient's urine during the collection period to all persons in-

## Dangers of increased intra-abdominal pressure

If your patient has increased intra-abdominal pressure, he may face potential renal, respiratory, and cardiovascular compromise.

Renal complications of increased intra-abdominal pressure ultimately may lead to renal failure. As intra-abdominal pressure rises, the mean glomerular filtration rate and renal blood flow decrease while renal vascular resistance rises. In response, urine output falls. Eventually, renal failure may occur.

Respiratory complications can be equally serious. As intra-abdominal pressure pushes the diaphragm upward, pulmonary compliance diminishes, making the lungs stiffer and harder to ventilate. As a result, peak end-inspiratory pressure rises. The bulging diaphragm also contributes to greater intrathoracic pressure, which compresses the pulmonary alveoli and blood vessels. This may lead to a ventilation-perfusion imbalance and a drop in the partial pressure of arterial oxygen. As blood flow decreases, the arterial pH falls and the lungs and, possibly, some organs may suffer ischemia.

Cardiovascular effects of increased intra-abdominal pressure include reduced cardiac output, increased systemic vascular resistance, elevated right atrial pressure (RAP), and increased pulmonary artery wedge pressure (PAWP). These problems, more common when intra-abdominal pressure exceeds 20 mm Hg, result from various factors. For example, the drop in cardiac output may stem from both rising systemic vascular resistance and reduced venous return caused by increased pressure on the vena cava. RAP and PAWP rise as increased intra-abdominal pressure is transmitted across the diaphragm to the thoracic cavity. However, these hemodynamic elevations may not be true increases but only reflect rising pleural pressures.

volved in his care, as well as to family or other visitors.

### Home care

If the patient must continue collecting urine at home, provide written instructions for the appropriate method. Tell the patient he can keep the specimens in a brown bag in his refrigerator at home, separate from other refrigerator contents.

### Documentation

In the Kardex and in your notes, record the date and the interval of collection and that the specimen was sent to the laboratory.

# Intra-abdominal pressure monitoring

In this procedure, a pressure transducer monitoring system is attached to an indwelling urinary catheter to measure intra-abdominal pressure — pressure within the abdominal cavity. When filled with fluid, the urinary bladder wall acts as a passive diaphragm, allowing transmission of the intra-abdominal pressure into the catheter tubing. The monitoring system converts the signal to a waveform and pressure value, which are displayed on the monitor.

Intra-abdominal pressure monitoring is indicated for patients with conditions that could increase this pressure, such as ascites, abdominal bleeding, intestinal obstruction, or bowel edema or ischemia. Increased intra-abdominal pressure may lead to renal, respiratory, and cardiovascular complications. (See *Dangers of increased intra-abdominal pressure.*)

### Equipment

Indwelling urinary catheter irrigation tray ■ 16G or 18G needle ■ sterile 0.9% sodium chloride solution for irrigation ■ sterile gloves ■ one or two sterile Kelly clamps ■ sterile towel ■ povidone-iodine swabs ■ bedside pressure monitor ■ carpenter's level ■ disposable, fluid-filled, pressure transducer monitoring system.

### Preparation of equipment

Attach the 16G or 18G needle to the pressure transducer tubing. Then flush the transducer tubing with the appropriate flush solution, making sure to remove all air from the tubing. Take all equipment to the patient's bedside.

## Implementation

• Explain the purpose of the procedure to the patient. Place him in the supine position, with the head of the bed flat. *(If the head remains elevated, thoracic cavity contents will push downward on the abdomen, falsely increasing intra-abdominal pressure.)* If the patient can't tolerate a flat position, document the degree of bed elevation and make sure all other staff members use the same elevation when obtaining readings. Although measurements taken with the head slightly elevated will be falsely high, you can use them to check for trends in intra-abdominal pressure as long as the elevation remains consistent.

• Next, attach the pressure transducer to the monitoring system. Level the transducer with the top of the patient's symphysis pubis by using a carpenter's level or similar device. Then zero and calibrate the transducer, following the directions supplied by the monitor manufacturer.

• Using sterile technique, open the irrigation tray and prepare the irrigation syringe.

• Create a sterile field by placing the sterile towel under the catheter where the catheter tubing connects to the catheter. Place all other sterile supplies on this field.

• Wearing sterile gloves, clamp or cross-clamp the tubing of the urinary drainage bag distal to the aspiration port, using one or two sterile Kelly clamps.

• Disconnect the catheter from the drainage bag. Place the end of the drainage bag tubing on the sterile field.

• With your gloved hand, hold the end of the catheter. Instill 50 to 100 ml of sterile 0.9% sodium chloride solution, using the syringe.

• Pinch the catheter closed to prevent fluid leakage, and remove the irrigating syringe. Reconnect the clamped drainage bag tubing to the catheter.

• Slowly release the Kelly clamp (or clamps) just enough so that air escapes and fluid fills the catheter tubing. Then reclamp the drainage bag tubing distal to the aspiration port. (Air in the tubing may cause a false reading.)

• Prepare the aspiration port with povidone-iodine swabs. Then insert the needle on the pressure tubing into this port.

• Note the intra-abdominal pressure reading on the bedside monitor and watch for the waveform, which should appear as a relatively flat line. (See also *How to monitor intra-abdominal pressure,* pages 136 and 137.)

• Remove the needle from the aspiration port.

• Unclamp the Kelly clamp (or clamps). Watch for urinary drainage flow to resume.

• Remove your gloves and discard disposable supplies.

• Document the intra-abdominal pressure reading. *Because it may vary with the phase of the respiratory cycle,* you should record the reading at end expiration, when the diaphragm rises and intrathoracic pressure has the least effect. This is especially important if the patient is on a mechanical ventilator or is receiving high levels of positive end-expiratory pressure.

• Replace the needle on the pressure tubing with a new sterile needle to prepare for the next intra-abdominal pressure measurement.

## Special consideration

Normally, mean intra-abdominal pressure is 0 mm Hg to subatmospheric. It typically increases just after abdominal surgery, possibly rising to 15 mm Hg, or if the patient is wearing a pneumatic antishock garment. At all other times, above-normal intra-abdominal pressure suggests intestinal obstruction, ascites, ruptured abdominal aortic aneurysm, or postoperative bleeding.

Make sure the transducer is leveled, zeroed, and calibrated correctly before each measurement *to avoid inaccurate readings.*

If the monitor reveals an abnormal reading, determine the need for interventions to help avert renal, respiratory, and cardiovascular complications. However, be sure to consider other assessment and diagnostic findings in conjunction

## How to monitor intra-abdominal pressure

If your patient has increased intra-abdominal pressure, you may need to monitor it to avert complications. These illustrations show essential steps for setting up the equipment and taking intra-abdominal measurements.

Level the transducer with the top of the patient's symphysis pubis.

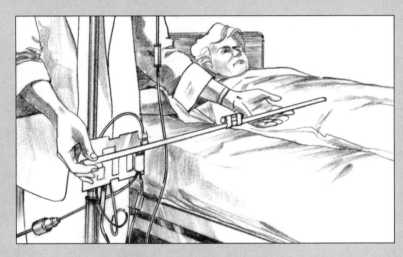

Clamp the catheter distal to the injection port.

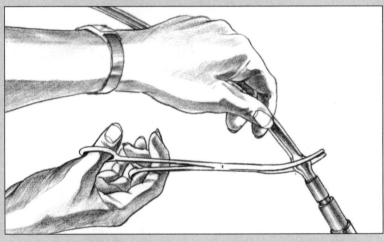

with intra-abdominal pressure values. Also, analyze successive values for trends rather than focus solely on isolated values.

Make sure you know which laboratory results and clinical findings suggest that your patient's condition is worsening. For instance, increasing blood urea nitrogen (BUN) and serum creatinine levels may indicate renal dysfunction; if urine output continues to fall, reflecting reduced renal blood flow, the patient may need I.V. fluids and vasopressor therapy.

Using strict sterile technique, instill 50 to 100 ml of 0.9% sodium chloride solution.

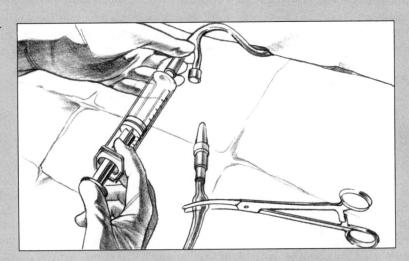

Insert the needle on the pressure tubing into the injection port. Then read the intra-abdominal pressure value on the monitor.

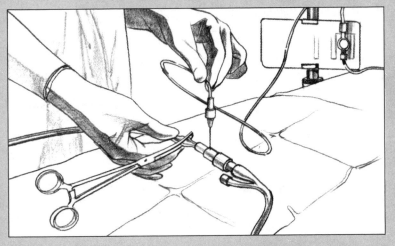

Be aware that each time you measure intra-abdominal pressure, you increase your patient's risk for urinary tract infection and sepsis by interrupting the closed urinary drainage system. *To reduce the infection risk,* use strict sterile technique and a new sterile disposable irrigation tray and sterile needle for each measurement. Assess the patient regularly for signs and symptoms of infection by monitoring his temperature and white blood cell count and noting urine color and clarity.

If the pulmonary artery catheter is in place, monitor the patient's cardiac output, pulmonary artery pressure, pulmonary artery wedge pressure, right atrial pressure, mean arterial pressure, and systemic vascular resistance (SVR). Watch for hemodynamic values indicating decreased cardiac output and increased SVR. If cardiac output starts to fall, be prepared to administer inotropic or fluid therapy *to support the patient's cardiovascular status and prevent renal failure.*

Monitor the patient's respiratory status continuously. If his intra-abdominal pressure increases, take measures to prevent respiratory complications. For instance, except when taking intra-abdominal pressure readings, always keep the head of the bed elevated (unless contraindicated) *to promote maximum lung expansion and minimize any ventilation-perfusion imbalance caused by pulmonary alveolar and blood vessel compression.* Encourage the patient to cough and deep-breathe *to prevent atelectasis,* which may worsen the ventilation-perfusion imbalance.

Discontinue intra-abdominal pressure monitoring, as ordered, when the patient's condition stabilizes. Expect to maintain the indwelling urinary catheter in place even after the monitoring ends.

Continue to assess the patient's fluid balance by monitoring intake and output, evaluating laboratory studies (especially BUN and serum creatinine levels), and assessing abdominal girth and skin turgor. Changes in abdominal girth usually occur late, after other signs and symptoms appear.

### Documentation
Document the date and the time monitoring began and the patient's tolerance of the procedure. Document the intra-abdominal pressure readings along with the degree of bed elevation and the amount of fluid inserted. Also note any complications and the results of any nursing or medical interventions.

## Monitoring for fluid gain by measuring abdominal girth

Fluid accumulation, abdominal obstruction, or post-operative complications may cause a patient to develop increasing abdominal distension. When this occurs, you should monitor the patient's status by measuring his girth on a regular basis.

### Equipment
Disposable tape measure.

### Implementation
• Explain the procedure to the patient and provide privacy. Wash your hands.
• Place the patient in a supine position with the head of the bed flat. If the patient can't tolerate a flat position, document the degree of bed elevation and make sure all other staff members use the same elevation when obtaining measurements.
• Wrap the tape measure around the patient's abdomen at the widest point—usually the umbilical area. Mark the area measured *to insure consistency with future measurements.*

### Special considerations
Obtain abdominal measurements as often as the patient's condition dictates. Be sure to monitor for trends in increasing or decreasing girth.

### Documentation
Record the measurement, the date, and the time on the patient's flow chart.

## Urine glucose and ketone monitoring

Reagent tablet and strip tests are used to monitor urine glucose and ketone levels and to screen for diabetes. *Urine ketone tests* monitor fat metabolism, help diagnose carbohydrate deprivation and diabetic ketoacidosis, and help distinguish between diabetic and nondiabetic coma. However, urine glucose tests are less accurate than blood glucose tests, and are now used less frequently because of the increasing convenience of blood self-testing.

The *copper reduction test (Clinitest)* measures the concentration of reducing substances in the urine through the reactions of these substances with a tablet composed of sodium hydroxide, cupric sulfate, and other reagents. When this tablet is added to a test tube containing drops of water and urine, the reaction generates heat. Simultaneously, reduction of cupric ions in the presence of glucose causes a color change. Comparison of this test color with a standardized color chart gives the approximate level of urine glucose. Similarly, the Acetest tablet test produces a color reaction that allows an estimate of urine ketone levels by comparison to a standardized chart.

*Glucose oxidase tests (such as Diastix, Tes-Tape, and Chemstrip UG strips)* produce color changes when patches of reagents implanted in hand-held plastic strips react with glucose in the patient's urine; *urine ketone strip tests (such as Chemstrip K and Ketostix)* are similar. All test results are read by comparing color changes against a standardized reference chart.

## Equipment

*For reagent tablet tests:* Specimen container ■ 10-ml test tube ■ medicine dropper ■ gloves ■ Clinitest or Acetest tablets ■ Clinitest or Acetest color chart.

*For reagent strip tests:* Specimen container ■ gloves ■ glucose or ketone test strips ■ reference color chart.

Wear gloves as barrier protection when performing all urine tests.

## Implementation

• Explain the test to the patient, and if he's a newly diagnosed diabetic, teach him to perform the test himself. Check his history for medications that may interfere with test results.

• Before each test, instruct the patient not to contaminate the urine specimen with stool or toilet tissue.

• Test the urine specimen immediately after the patient voids.

### Administering the Clinitest tablet test

• Ask the patient to void, and then ask him to drink a glass of water, if possible. Don gloves and collect a second-voided urine specimen 30 to 45 minutes later.

• Perform the 5-drop test: With the medicine dropper, transfer 5 drops of urine from the specimen container to the test tube. Rinse the dropper and add 10 drops of water to the test tube. Then add one Clinitest tablet to the tube.

• Hold the test tube near the top during the reaction *because the test solution will come to a boil.* Observe the color change that occurs during the reaction.

• Fifteen seconds after effervescence subsides, shake the tube gently. Observe the solution's color and compare it with the Clinitest color chart.

• Remove and discard gloves, and record the test results. Ignore any changes that develop after 15 seconds.

• If the color changes rapidly in the 5-drop test, record the result as "over 2%" glucosuria.

• Alternatively, perform the 2-drop test: Transfer 2 drops of urine from the specimen container to the test tube, and then add 10 drops of water and a Clinitest tablet. After the reaction, observe the color of the test solution, and compare it with the Clinitest color chart.

• Remove and discard your gloves, and record the test results.

• Rapid color change in the 2-drop test indicates glycosuria up to 5%.

### Administering the Acetest tablet test

• Don gloves and collect a second-voided specimen, as for the Clinitest tablet test.

• Place the Acetest tablet on a piece of white paper, and add 1 drop of urine to the tablet.

## How to use a bedside blood glucose and hemoglobin monitor

Monitoring blood glucose and hemoglobin levels at the patient's bedside is a straightforward procedure. Follow the three steps shown below to use the HemoCue system to obtain a blood sample and place it in the photometer for a reading.

After you pierce the skin, the microcuvette draws blood automatically.

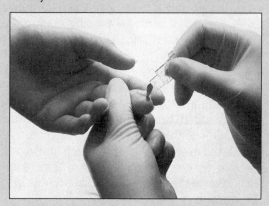

Next, place the microcuvette into the photometer.

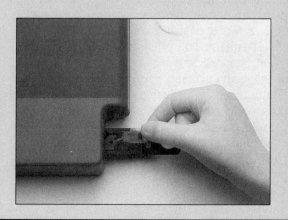

• After 30 seconds, compare the tablet's color (white, lavender, or purple) with the Acetest color chart. Remove gloves and record the test results.

### Administering glucose oxidase strip tests
• Explain the test to the patient and, if he's diagnosed as diabetic, teach him to perform it himself. Check his history for medications that may interfere with test results. Don gloves before collecting specimens for each of these tests, and remove them to record test results.
• Instruct the patient to void. Ask him to drink a glass of water, if possible, and collect a second-voided specimen after 30 to 45 minutes.
• If you're using Clinistix, dip the reagent end of the strip into the urine for 2 seconds. Remove excess urine by tapping the strip against the container's rim, wait for exactly 10 seconds, and then compare its color with the color chart on the container. Ignore color changes that occur after 10 seconds. Record the result.
• If you're using a Diastix strip, dip the reagent end of the strip into the urine for 2 seconds. Tap

off excess urine, wait for exactly 30 seconds, and then compare its color with the standardized color chart on the container. Ignore color changes that occur after 30 seconds. Record the result.
• If you're using a Tes-Tape strip, pull about 1½" (3.8 cm) of the reagent strip from the dispenser, and dip one end about ¼" (0.6 cm) into the specimen for 2 seconds. Tap off excess urine, wait exactly 60 seconds, and then compare the darkest part of the tape with the standardized color chart. If the test result exceeds 0.5%, wait an additional 60 seconds and make a final comparison. Record the result.

### Administering ketone strip tests
• Explain the procedure to the patient, and if he's diagnosed as diabetic, teach him to perform the test. Check his medication history. If he's receiving phenazopyridine or levodopa, use Acetest tablets instead *because reagent strips will give inaccurate results.*
• Don gloves and collect a second-voided midstream specimen.

Because Clinitest tablets contain caustic soda, keep the container tightly closed and in a dry place. If you must handle these tablets, keep your fingers dry *to prevent the tablet from leaving a deposit,* which could then be accidentally ingested or brought into contact with eyes, skin, mucous membranes, or clothing, causing caustic burns. Time limits for interpretation of results vary with each product. Be sure to read the manufacturer's instructions carefully before using strips or tablets.

### Documentation
In your notes, record the time, date, test results, and color changes according to the information on the charts on the reagent containers. Or, use special flowcharts designed to record this information. If you're teaching a patient how to perform these tests, keep a record of his progress.

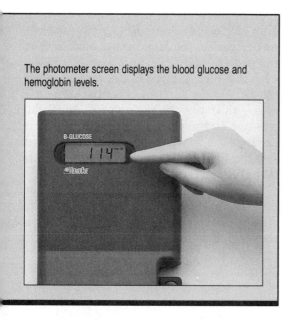

The photometer screen displays the blood glucose and hemoglobin levels.

• If you're using Ketostix, dip the reagent end of the strip into the specimen and remove it immediately. Wait exactly 15 seconds, and then compare the color of the strip with the standardized color chart on the container. Ignore color changes that occur after 15 seconds. Record the result.

• If you're using Keto-Diastix, dip the reagent end of the strip into the specimen and remove it immediately. Tap off excess urine, and hold the strip horizontally *to prevent mixing of chemicals between the two reagent squares.* Wait exactly 15 seconds, and then compare the color of the ketone part of the strip with the standardized color chart. After 30 seconds, compare the color of the glucose part of the strip with the chart. Record the results.

### Special considerations
Keep reagent strips in a cool, dry place at a temperature below 86° F (30° C), but don't refrigerate them. Keep the containers tightly closed. Don't use discolored or outdated strips.

## Blood glucose monitoring
Increasingly, nurses are monitoring blood glucose levels at the patient's bedside. The fast, accurate results obtained this way allow immediate intervention, if necessary. In contrast, with traditional monitoring methods, blood samples must be sent to the laboratory for interpretation. A blood sample that sits at room temperature for an hour may undergo glycolysis, which reduces glucose concentration by 3% to 30%, leading to inaccurate test results.

Numerous testing systems are available for bedside monitoring. Bedside systems are also convenient for the patient's home use. HemoCue, a widely used system, gives accurate results without having to dispense, pipette, or mix blood and reagents to obtain readings. Thus, it eliminates the risk of leakage, broken tubes, and splattered blood.

Rapid, easy-to-perform reagent strip tests (such as Glucostix, Chemstrip bG, or Multistix) use a drop of capillary blood obtained by fingerstick, heelstick, or earlobe puncture as a sample. These tests can detect or monitor elevated blood glucose levels in patients with diabetes, screen for diabetes mellitus and neonatal hypoglycemia, and help distinguish diabetic coma from nondiabetic coma. In these tests, a reagent patch on the tip of a hand-held plastic strip changes color in response to the amount of glucose in the blood sample. Comparing the color change with a standardized color chart provides a semiquantitative measurement of blood glucose levels; inserting the strip in a portable blood glucose meter (such as a Glucometer II, Accu-Chek II, or One Touch) provides quantitative measurements that compare in accuracy with other laboratory tests. Some meters store successive test results electronically to help determine glucose patterns.

## Equipment
Reagent strips ▪ gloves ▪ portable blood glucose meter, if available ▪ gauze pads ▪ alcohol sponges ▪ disposable lancets ▪ small adhesive bandage ▪ watch or clock with a second hand.

## Implementation
• Explain the procedure to the patient or to the infant's parents.
• Select the puncture site — usually the fingertip or earlobe for an adult or the heel or great toe for an infant.
• Wash your hands and don gloves.
• If necessary, dilate the capillaries by applying warm, moist compresses to the area for about 10 minutes.
• Wipe the puncture site with an alcohol sponge and dry it thoroughly with a gauze pad.
• To draw a sample from the patient's fingertip with a disposable lancet (smaller than 2 mm), make the puncture on the side of the fingertip and position the lancet perpendicular to the lines of the patient's fingerprints. Pierce the skin sharply and quickly *to minimize the patient's anxiety and pain, and to increase blood flow.* Alternatively, you may want to use a mechanical

bloodletting device, such as an Autolet, which uses a spring-loaded lancet.
• After puncturing the finger, wipe away the first drop of blood *to avoid diluting the sample with tissue fluid.* For the same reason, avoid squeezing the puncture site.
• Touch a drop of blood to the reagent patch on the strip; make sure you cover the entire patch.
• After collecting the blood sample, briefly apply pressure to the puncture site *to prevent painful extravasation of blood into subcutaneous tissues.* Ask the adult patient to hold a gauze pad firmly over the puncture site until bleeding stops.
• Leave the blood on the strip for exactly 60 seconds, and then quickly wash it off with a stream of water from a wash bottle. Don't hold the strip under a faucet *because a strong stream of water will wash off too much blood.* Some reagent strips require only that the blood be wiped off, without washing. Follow the manufacturer's instructions exactly *because results will influence insulin dosage.*
• Immediately after washing, compare the color change on the strip with the standardized color chart on the product container. If you're using a blood glucose meter, follow the manufacturer's instructions. Meter designs vary, but they all analyze a drop of blood placed on a reagent strip that comes with the unit, and they provide a digital display of the resulting glucose level. (See *How to use a bedside blood glucose and hemoglobin monitor,* pages 140 and 141.)
• After bleeding has stopped, you may apply a small adhesive bandage to the puncture site.

## Special considerations
Before using reagent strips, check the expiration date on the package and replace outdated strips. Also check for special instructions related to the specific reagent. The reagent area of a fresh strip should match the color on the "0" block on the color chart. Protect the strips from light, heat, and moisture.

Before using a blood glucose meter, calibrate it and run it with a control sample *to ensure*

## Oral and intravenous glucose tolerance tests

For monitoring trends in glucose metabolism, two tests may offer benefits over testing blood with reagent strips.

### Oral glucose tolerance test
The most sensitive test for detecting borderline diabetes mellitus, the oral glucose tolerance test (OGTT) measures carbohydrate metabolism after ingestion of a challenge dose of glucose. The body absorbs this dose rapidly, causing plasma glucose levels to rise and peak within 30 minutes to 1 hour. The pancreas responds by secreting insulin, causing glucose levels to return to normal within 2 to 3 hours. During this period, plasma and urine glucose levels are monitored to assess insulin secretion and the body's ability to metabolize glucose.

Although you may not collect the blood and urine specimens (usually five of each) required for this test, you will be responsible for preparing the patient for the test and monitoring his physical condition during the test.

Begin by explaining the OGTT to the patient. Then, tell him to maintain a high-carbohydrate diet for 3 days and to fast for 10 to 16 hours before the test, as ordered. The patient must not smoke, drink coffee or alcohol, or exercise strenuously for 8 hours before or during the test. Inform him that he will then receive a challenge dose of 100 g of carbohydrate (usually a sweetened carbonated beverage or gelatin).

Tell the patient who will perform the venipunctures and when, and that he may feel slight discomfort from the needle punctures and the pressure of the tourniquet. Reassure him that collecting each blood sample usually takes less than 3 minutes. As ordered, withhold drugs that may affect test results. Remind him not to discard the first voided urine specimen on waking.

During the test period, watch for signs and symptoms of hypoglycemia—weakness, restlessness, nervousness, hunger, and sweating—and report these to the doctor immediately. Encourage the patient to drink plenty of water to promote adequate urine excretion. Provide a bedpan, urinal, or specimen container when necessary.

### I.V. glucose tolerance test
This test may be chosen for patients unable to absorb an oral dose of glucose—for example, those with malabsorption disorders, short-bowel syndrome, or those who have had a gastrectomy. The I.V. glucose tolerance test measures blood glucose after an I.V. infusion of 50% glucose over 3 or 4 minutes. Blood samples are then drawn after 30 minutes, 1 hour, 2 hours, and 3 hours. After an immediate glucose peak of 300 to 400 mg/dl (accompanied by glycosuria), the normal glucose curve falls steadily, reaching fasting levels within 1 to 1¼ hours. Failure to achieve fasting glucose levels within 2 to 3 hours typically confirms diabetes.

---

*accurate test results.* Follow the manufacturer's instructions for calibration.

Avoid selecting cold, cyanotic, or swollen puncture sites *to ensure an adequate blood sample.* If you can't obtain a capillary sample, perform venipuncture and place a large drop of venous blood on the reagent strip. If you want to test blood from a refrigerated sample, allow the blood to return to room temperature before testing it.

To help detect abnormal glucose metabolism and diagnose diabetes mellitus, the doctor may order other blood glucose tests. (See *Oral and intravenous glucose tolerance tests.*)

## Home care
If the patient will be using the reagent strip system at home, teach him the proper use of the lancet or Autolet, the reagent strips and color chart, and the portable blood glucose meter, as necessary. Also provide written guidelines.

## Documentation
Record the reading from the reagent strip (using a portable blood glucose meter or a color chart) in your notes or on a special flowchart, if available. Also record the time and date of the test.

# 6 MONITORING GI AND NUTRITIONAL STATUS

## Introduction

From birth, the quality of a patient's life is affected by the quality and quantity of nutrients consumed and used. The body's nutritional status—the balance between nutrient intake and energy expenditure or need—reflects the degree to which the physiologic need for nutrients is being met. Proper nutrition promotes growth, maintains health, and helps the body resist infection and recover from disease or surgery. Malnutrition impedes these natural processes.

You may encounter patients with nutritional disorders in settings that range from pediatric clinics to schools to hospitals, and your involvement in the patient's nutritional status can vary. In some health care facilities, you may have the primary responsibility for the patient's nutritional assessment and care. In other settings, you may refer the patient to a specially trained dietitian who performs these functions. In still other facilities, you may work with members of a nutritional support team to provide complete nutritional services.

Many people assume that malnutrition occurs only in underdeveloped countries. Unfortunately, this assumption is false. Malnutrition affects about two-thirds of the world's population and occurs in people of every nationality, race, and age. In North America, certain groups—especially those with low incomes—run a particularly high risk of developing nutritional deficiencies. These groups include children, adolescents, pregnant or lactating women, and people over age 60. Malnutrition may be a primary disorder caused by insufficient nutrient intake, or a secondary disorder caused by a condition that impairs digestion, absorption, or use of nutrients or by a condition that increases nutrient requirements or excretion.

Because a functional GI system is vital for optimal nutrition, the chapter begins by reviewing the anatomy and physiology of the GI system with a focus on nutritional status. Then it describes how to monitor for bowel sounds, fecal occult blood, and altered nutritional status. The chapter also includes information about methods for promoting nutrition, such as total parenteral nutrition (TPN) and tube feedings.

## Anatomy and physiology review

The GI system comprises two major components: the alimentary canal and the accessory GI organs. The alimentary canal, or GI tract, consists essentially of a hollow muscular tube that begins in the mouth and extends to the anus. It includes the pharynx, esophagus, stomach, small intestine, and large intestine. Accessory organs aiding GI function include the salivary glands, liver, biliary duct system (gallbladder and bile ducts), and pancreas. (See *Reviewing GI structure and innervation,* pages 146 and 147.)

Together, the GI tract and accessory organs serve two major functions: digestion, the breaking down of food and fluid into simple chemicals that can be absorbed into the bloodstream and transported throughout the body, and the elimination of waste products from the body through excretion of feces.

### Ingestion, digestion, absorption, and excretion

Ingestion is the act of eating or taking food into the body; it is affected by age and cultural, psychological, socioeconomic, physiologic, and religious factors. Digestion is a series of physical and chemical changes by which ingested food undergoes hydrolysis (addition of water) and is broken down in preparation for absorption.

Absorption of some nutrients occurs in the stomach. However, most nutrients are absorbed in the duodenal and jejunal segments of the small intestine, with the remainder absorbed in the ileum.

After absorption by any of these processes, water-soluble nutrient components from carbohydrates and proteins readily dissolve in plasma and enter the portal circulation en route to the liver. Fat and fat-soluble vitamins (A, D, E, and K) are absorbed as mixed micelles, soluble complexes

*(Text continues on page 148.)*

## Reviewing GI structure and innervation

The GI tract is a hollow tube extending from the lips to the anal opening. Along its entire length are associated glands and accessory organs devoted to breaking down ingested foods into useful components and to eliminating unabsorbed residues. The GI tract's walls alternate muscle tissue with nerve tissue and blood vessels to regulate peristalsis, digestion, and absorption. The diagram below depicts the major anatomic structures of this system.

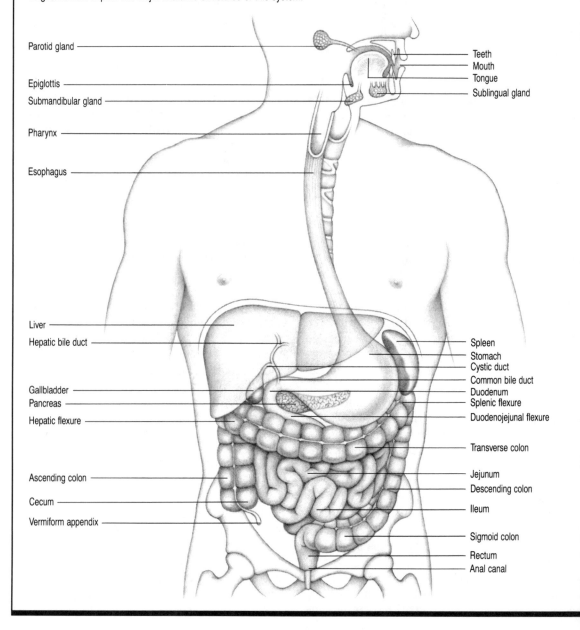

## Cellular anatomy

The GI tract wall, shown below, consists of several layers. The innermost layer (tunica mucosa, or mucosa) consists of epithelial and surface cells and loose connective tissue. In the small intestine, epithelial cells elaborate into millions of finger-like projections (villi) that vastly increase their absorptive surface area. They also secrete gastric and protective juices and absorb nutrients. Surface cells overlie connective tissue (lamina propria), supported by a thin layer of smooth muscle (muscularis mucosae).

The submucosa (tunica submucosa) encircles the mucosa. It's composed of loose connective tissue, blood and lymphatic vessels, and a nerve network (submucosal, or Meissner's, plexus). Around this layer lies the tunica muscularis, composed of skeletal muscle in the mouth, pharynx, and upper esophagus, and of longitudinal and circular smooth muscle fibers elsewhere in the tract. During peristalsis, longitudinal fibers shorten the lumen length and circular fibers reduce the lumen diameter. At points along the tract, circular fibers thicken to form sphincters. Between the two muscle layers lies another nerve network — myenteric, or Auerbach's, plexus.

The GI tract's outer covering — the tunica adventitia in the esophagus and rectum, the tunica serosa elsewhere — consists of connective tissue protected by epithelium. Also called the visceral peritoneum, this layer covers most of the abdominal organs and is contiguous with an identical layer (parietal peritoneum) lining the abdominal cavity. The visceral peritoneum becomes a double-layered fold around the blood vessels, nerves, and lymphatics supplying the small intestine and attaches the jejunum and ileum to the posterior abdominal wall to prevent twisting. A similar mesenteric fold attaches the transverse colon to the posterior abdominal wall.

## GI innervation

Distention of the submucosal or myenteric plexus stimulates neural transmission to the smooth muscle, initiating peristalsis and mixing contractions. Parasympathetic stimulation — via the vagus nerve for most of the intestines and the sacral spinal nerves for the descending colon and rectum — increases gut and sphincter tone and frequency, strength, and velocity of smooth muscle contractions. Vagal stimulation also increases motor and secretory activities. Sympathetic stimulation, via spinal nerves from levels T6 to L2, reduces peristalsis and inhibits GI activity.

### Structure of GI tract wall

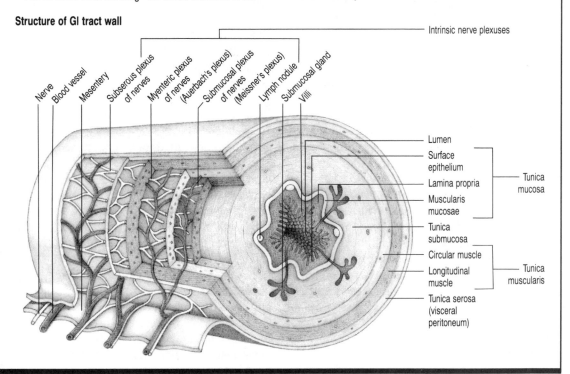

Intrinsic nerve plexuses

Nerve · Blood vessel · Mesentery · Subserous plexus of nerves · Myenteric plexus of nerves (Auerbach's plexus) · Submucosal plexus of nerves (Meissner's plexus) · Lymph nodule · Submucosal gland · Villi

Lumen
Surface epithelium
Lamina propria — Tunica mucosa
Muscularis mucosae
Tunica submucosa
Circular muscle
Longitudinal muscle — Tunica muscularis
Tunica serosa (visceral peritoneum)

formed from bile salts coating the fat globules in the small intestine. The bile salts, released after the micelles are absorbed into mucosal cells of the small intestine, reenter the intestinal lumen for reabsorption in the ileum and circulation to the liver for reuse.

The lipid components (diglycerides and monoglycerides) reform into triglycerides within the intestinal epithelial cells. They then circulate through the lymph vessels, through the systemic circulation, and into the liver.

Most of the water in the intestinal contents is absorbed in the intestines. The remaining water and related nutrients, such as minerals and vitamins, are absorbed in the colon, primarily in the proximal half. Electrolytes, principally sodium, are transported into the bloodstream from the colon. Bacteria in the colon synthesize vitamin K and some B complex vitamins, which are then absorbed from the colon.

Excretion is the process by which undigested food residue, including dietary fiber, inorganic matter such as minerals, metabolic waste products, and dietary excesses such as water-soluble vitamins (B complex and vitamin C), are eliminated through the large intestine, the kidneys and, to a lesser extent, the lungs and skin.

# Bowel sounds monitoring

Bowel sounds result when peristalsis propels air and fluid through the bowel. These high-pitched sounds may be heard by auscultating the abdomen with a stethoscope.

Monitoring bowel sounds provides information on bowel motility and the underlying vessels and organs. Evaluate your patient's bowel sounds upon his admission to the hospital (to establish a baseline). Thereafter, evaluate bowel sounds once each shift or whenever a change in GI status occurs.

## Equipment
Stethoscope.

## Preparation of equipment
Warm your hands as well as the diaphragm of the stethoscope.

## Implementation
• Explain the procedure to patient and provide privacy. Wash your hands.
• Make sure the patient has voided before the abdominal examination. Then place him in the supine position. Place a pillow behind his head and another behind his knees *to help him relax the abdominal muscles.*
• After inspecting the patient's abdomen, lightly press the stethoscope diaphragm against the patient's abdomen.
• Systematically auscultate all four quadrants, listening for the sounds of air and fluid moving through the bowel. Note the character and frequency of the sounds you hear. If you don't hear bowel sounds right away, be sure to listen for at least 2 minutes. (See *Auscultating the abdomen.*)

## Special considerations
Normally, air and fluid moving through the bowel by peristalsis create soft, bubbling sounds with no regular pattern, often with soft clicks and gurgles interspersed, every 5 to 15 seconds. A hungry patient normally may have a familiar "stomach growl," a condition of hyperperistalsis called borborygmi. Rapid, high-pitched, loud, and gurgling bowel sounds are *hyperactive*, and may occur normally in a hungry patient. Hyperactive bowel sounds may also occur as an emotional response or following the administration of certain medications. Hyperactive sounds may also occur with diarrhea, GI bleeding, or early intestinal obstruction.

Sounds occurring at a rate of one every minute or longer are *hypoactive* and normally occur after bowel surgery or when the colon is feces filled. Other causes of hypoactive bowel sounds include reduced food intake, gaseous distention, general anesthesia, and narcotic medications. If the patient has nausea, vomiting, or increasing abdom-

## Auscultating the abdomen

Before using a stethoscope to auscultate the abdomen, warm your hands and the stethoscope to prevent muscular contraction, which can alter auscultatory findings. Auscultate for bowel sounds throughout all four quadrants, using the diaphragm of the stethoscope, as shown. Then, using the bell of the stethoscope, listen for vascular sounds in the sites shown.

**Stethoscope placement for auscultation**

**Auscultation sites for vascular sounds**

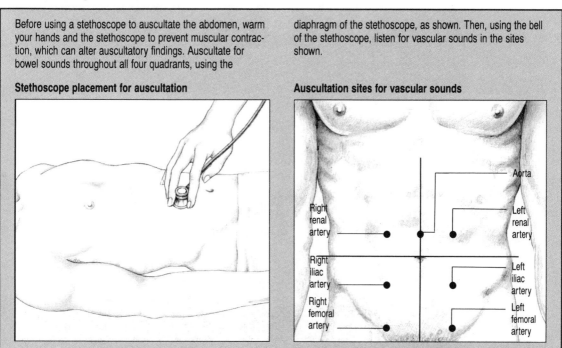

inal distention in addition to decreasing bowel sounds, notify the doctor. Together, these signs signal a worsening bowel obstruction. (See *Identifying a bowel obstruction,* page 150.)

Before reporting absent bowel sounds, make sure the patient has an empty bladder; a full bladder may obscure the sounds. Gently pressing on the abdominal surface may initiate peristalsis and audible bowel sounds, as will having the patient eat or drink something.

Realize that bowel sounds may differ in intensity throughout the four abdominal quadrants. Also, bowel sounds may be diminished in obese patients or when the abdominal cavity contains a large amount of fluid.

Always auscultate a patient's abdomen before percussing and palpating *because percussion and palpation can affect bowel activity and thus bowel sounds.* If the patient has abdominal pain, assess the painful area last.

Establish a regular sequence for ausculating bowel sounds. For instance, start in the right upper quadrant and move clockwise. By using the same sequence every time, you'll ensure a thorough assessment.

### Documentation
Document the presence of bowel sounds along with the frequency, pitch, and intensity of the sounds. If the patient has any abnormal bowel sounds, note the location of the sounds by documenting the quadrant in which they occurred. Also document any related findings, such as nausea, vomiting, or distention.

## Identifying a bowel obstruction

A bowel obstruction requires prompt medical intervention. Because a worsening bowel obstruction produces a characteristic pattern of sounds, routine auscultation of the patient's bowel sounds may help identify a bowel obstruction before it becomes complete.

In a patient with a partial bowel obstruction, bowel sounds will typically be hyperactive and produce a high-pitched, tinkling sound proximal to the obstruction. These sounds represent the presence of fluid and air in a dilated bowel. At the same time, you may see peristaltic waves moving across the patient's abdomen.

As the obstruction progresses, the tinkling sounds decrease in intensity and frequency. In addition, you may hear a "rushing" sound that mimics splashing water. The patient may also complain of abdominal cramping as the bowel attempts to move its contents past the obstruction.

Finally, if the obstruction continues, bowel sounds become absent. (Absent bowel sounds may also result from paralytic ileus, bowel perforation, peritonitis, general anesthesia, electrolyte imbalance, and spinal cord injury.) If the patient has absent bowel sounds, a rigid abdomen, guarding, or rebound tenderness, contact the patient's doctor immediately.

# Fecal occult blood monitoring

Fecal occult blood tests are valuable for determining the presence of occult blood (hidden GI bleeding) and for distinguishing between true melena and melena-like stools. Certain medications, such as iron supplements and bismuth compounds, can darken stools so that they resemble melena.

Two common occult blood screening tests are Hematest (an orthotolidin reagent tablet) and the Hemoccult slide (filter paper impregnated with guaiac). Both tests produce a blue reaction in a fecal smear if occult blood loss exceeds 5 ml in 24 hours. A newer test, Colocare, requires no fecal smear.

Occult blood tests are particularly important for early detection of colorectal cancer because 80% of patients with this disorder test positive. However, a single positive test result doesn't necessarily confirm GI bleeding or indicate co-

lorectal cancer. For a confirmed positive result, the test must be repeated at least three times while the patient follows a meatless, high-residue diet. Still, a confirmed positive test doesn't necessarily indicate colorectal cancer. It does indicate the need for further diagnostic studies; GI bleeding can result from many causes other than cancer, such as ulcers and diverticula. These tests are easily performed on collected specimens or smears from digital rectal examination.

### Equipment
Test kit ∎ glass or porcelain plate ∎ tongue blade or other wooden applicator ∎ gloves.

### Implementation
• Put on gloves and collect a stool specimen.

#### *Hematest reagent tablet test*
• Use a wooden applicator to smear a bit of the stool specimen on the filter paper supplied with the kit. Or, after performing a digital rectal examination, wipe the finger you used for examination on a square of the filter paper.
• Place the filter paper with the stool smear on a glass plate.
• Remove a reagent tablet from the bottle, and immediately replace the cap tightly. Then, place the tablet in the center of the stool smear on the filter paper.
• Add one drop of water to the tablet, and allow it to soak in for 5 to 10 seconds. Add a second drop, letting it run from the tablet onto the specimen and filter paper. If necessary, tap the plate gently to dislodge any water from the top of the tablet.
• After 2 minutes, the filter paper will turn blue if the test is positive. Don't read the color that appears on the tablet itself or develops on the filter paper after the 2-minute period.
• Note the results, and discard the filter paper.
• Remove and discard your gloves, and wash your hands thoroughly.

### *Hemoccult slide test*
• Open the flap on the slide packet, and use a wooden applicator to apply a thin smear of the stool specimen to the guaiac-impregnated filter paper exposed in box A. Or, after performing a digital rectal examination, wipe the finger you used for examination on a square of the filter paper.
• Apply a second smear from another part of the specimen to the filter paper exposed in box B *because some parts of the specimen may not contain blood.*
• Open the flap at the rear of the slide package, and place 2 drops of Hemoccult developing solution on the paper over each smear. A blue reaction will appear in 30 to 60 seconds if the test is positive.
• Record the results of the test and discard the slide package.
• Remove and discard your gloves, and wash your hands thoroughly.

### Special considerations
Make sure stool specimens aren't contaminated with urine, soap solution, or toilet tissue, and test them as soon as possible after collection.

Test samples from several different portions of the same specimen *because occult blood from the upper GI tract isn't always evenly dispersed throughout the formed stool;* likewise, blood from colorectal bleeding may occur mostly on the outer stool surface.

Check the condition of the reagent tablets and note their expiration date. Use only fresh tablets and discard outdated ones. Protect Hematest tablets from moisture, heat, and light.

If repeated testing is necessary after a positive screening test, explain the test to the patient. Instruct him to maintain a high-fiber diet and to refrain from eating red meat, poultry, fish, turnips, and horseradish for 48 to 72 hours before the test as well as throughout the collection period *because these substances may alter test results.*

As ordered, have the patient discontinue use of iron preparations, bromides, iodides, rauwolfia derivatives, indomethacin, colchicine, salicylates, potassium, phenylbutazone, oxyphenbutazone, bismuth compounds, steroids, and ascorbic acid for 48 to 72 hours before the test and during it *to ensure accurate test results and to avoid possible bleeding* that some of these compounds may cause.

### Documentation
Record the time and date of the test, the result, and any unusual characteristics of the stool tested. Report positive results to the doctor.

# Daily weight monitoring
Height and weight are routinely measured for most patients during admission to the hospital. An accurate record of the patient's height and weight is essential for calculating dosages of drugs, anesthetics, and contrast media; assessing the patient's nutritional status; and determining the height-weight ratio. Body weight provides the best overall picture of fluid status; it also may provide clues to undernutrition or to overnutrition. Although most adults state their height correctly, take a baseline measurement.

Body weight is the total weight of lean body mass (extracellular fluid, protoplasm, and bone) and fat. Comparison with standard measurements shows whether the patient's weight, height, and body frame are above or below that standard, indicating whether the patient is undernourished or overnourished.

To determine ideal body weight for an adult patient (age 18 and over), first determine body frame size. Then, based on body frame size, compare the patient's height and weight with the values on a standard height-weight chart. (See *Suggested weights for adults,* page 152.)

Some authorities believe that any patient who has had an unmonitored 10% weight loss over 6 months, or is either 20% above or 20% below the standard, risks developing a nutritional dis-

## Suggested weights for adults

This chart provides a guideline for determining healthy weights. Higher weights in each category typically apply to men, who average more muscle and bone; lower weights usually apply to women, who have less muscle and bone. Suggested weights for people age 35 and older are higher than those for younger adults because recent research shows that older people can carry somewhat more weight without impairing their health. Height is measured without shoes; weight is measured without clothes.

| HEIGHT | WEIGHT (LB) | | HEIGHT | WEIGHT (LB) | |
|---|---|---|---|---|---|
| | Ages 19 to 34 | Ages 35 and over | | Ages 19 to 34 | Ages 35 and over |
| 5'0" | 97 to 128 | 108 to 138 | 5'10" | 132 to 174 | 146 to 188 |
| 5'1" | 101 to 132 | 111 to 143 | 5'11" | 136 to 179 | 151 to 194 |
| 5'2" | 104 to 137 | 115 to 148 | 6'0" | 140 to 184 | 155 to 199 |
| 5'3" | 107 to 141 | 119 to 152 | 6'1" | 144 to 189 | 159 to 205 |
| 5'4" | 111 to 146 | 122 to 157 | 6'2" | 148 to 195 | 164 to 210 |
| 5'5" | 114 to 150 | 126 to 162 | 6'3" | 152 to 200 | 168 to 216 |
| 5'6" | 118 to 155 | 130 to 167 | 6'4" | 156 to 205 | 173 to 222 |
| 5'7" | 121 to 160 | 134 to 172 | 6'5" | 160 to 211 | 177 to 228 |
| 5'8" | 125 to 164 | 138 to 178 | 6'6" | 164 to 216 | 182 to 234 |
| 5'9" | 129 to 169 | 142 to 183 | | | |

Source: U.S. Department of Agriculture, U.S. Department of Health and Human Services. *Nutrition and Your Health: Dietary Guidelines for Americans,* 3rd ed. Washington, D.C., 1990.

order and may need referral for medical evaluation and follow-up.

Weight can be measured with a standing scale, chair scale, or bed scale; height can be measured with the measuring bar on a standing scale or with a tape measure for a supine patient.

### Equipment
Scale — standing (with measuring bar), chair, or bed ▪ wheelchair (if needed to transport patient) ▪ tape measure if needed.

### Preparation of equipment
Select the appropriate scale — usually, a standing scale for an ambulatory patient or a chair or bed scale for an acutely ill or debilitated patient. Then check scale balance. Standing scales and, to a lesser extent, bed scales may become unbalanced when transported.

### Implementation
• Explain the procedure to the patient.

### Using a standing scale

• Place a paper towel on the scale's platform.
• Tell the patient to remove his robe and slippers or shoes *to ensure accurate measurement of height and weight.* If the scale has wheels, lock them before the patient steps on. Assist the patient onto the scale *to prevent falls.* Remain close to the patient *so you can steady him if necessary.*
• If you're using an upright balance (gravity) scale, slide the lower rider to the groove representing the largest increment below the patient's estimated weight. Grooves represent 50, 100, 150, and 200 lb (23, 45, 68, and 91 kg). Then slide the small upper rider until the beam balances. Add the upper and lower rider figures *to determine the weight.* (The upper rider is calibrated to eighths of a pound.)
• If you're using a multiple-weight scale, move the appropriate ratio weights onto the weight holder to balance the scale; ratio weights are labeled 50, 100, and 200 lb. Add ratio weights until the next weight causes the main beam to fall. Then adjust the main beam poise until the scale balances. Next, add the sum of the ratio weights to the figure on the main beam *to obtain the patient's weight.*
• Return ratio weights to their rack and the weight holder to its proper place.
• If you use a scale with a digital display, make sure the display reads 0 before use. Read the display with the patient on the scale and standing as still as possible.
• If you're measuring height, tell the patient to stand erect on the platform of the scale. Raise the measuring bar beyond the top of the patient's head, extend the horizontal arm, and lower the bar until it touches the top of the patient's head. Then read the patient's height.
• Help the patient off the scale, and give him his robe and slippers or shoes. Then return the measuring bar to its initial position.

### Using a chair scale

• Transport the patient to the weighing area or the scale to the patient's bedside.
• Lock the scale in place *to prevent it from moving accidentally.*
• If you're using a scale with a swing-away chair arm, unlock the arm. When unlocked, the arm swings back 180 degrees to permit easy patient access.
• Position the scale beside the patient's bed or wheelchair with the chair arm open. Transfer the patient onto the scale, swing the chair arm to the front of the scale, and lock it in place.
• Weigh the patient by adding ratio weights and adjusting the main beam poise. Then unlock the swing-away chair arm as before, and transfer the patient back to his bed or wheelchair.
• Lock the main beam *to avoid damaging the scale during transport.* Unlock the wheels and remove the scale from the patient's room.

### Using a multiple-weight bed scale

• Provide privacy, and tell the patient that you're going to weigh him on a special bed scale.
• Position the scale next to the patient's bed and lock the scale's wheels. Then turn the patient on his side, facing away from the scale.
• Release the stretcher frame to the horizontal position, and pump the hand lever until the stretcher is positioned over the mattress. Lower the stretcher onto the mattress, and roll the patient onto the stretcher.
• Raise the stretcher 2″ (5 cm) above the mattress. Then add ratio weights, and adjust the main beam poise as for the standing and chair scales.
• After weighing the patient, lower the stretcher onto the mattress, turn the patient on his side, and remove the stretcher. Be sure to leave the patient in a comfortable position.

### Using a digital bed scale

• Provide privacy, and tell the patient that you're going to weigh him on a special bed scale. If the patient is being weighed for the first time, demonstrate the scale's operation.
• Release the stretcher to the horizontal position, then lock it in place.
• Turn the patient on his side, facing away from the scale.
• Roll the base of the scale under the patient's bed. Adjust the lever *to widen the base of the scale, providing stability.* After doing so, lock the scale's wheels.
• Center the stretcher above the bed, lower it onto the mattress, and roll the patient onto the stretcher. Then position the circular weighing arms of the scale over the patient, and attach them securely to the stretcher bars.
• Pump the handle with long, slow strokes *to raise the patient a few inches off the bed.* Ensure that the patient doesn't lean on or touch the headboard, side rails, or other bed equipment *because this will affect weight measurement.*
• Depress the operate button, and read the patient's weight on the digital display panel. Then press in the scale's handle *to lower the patient slowly onto the bed.*
• Detach the circular weighing arms from the stretcher bars, roll the patient off the stretcher and remove it, and position him comfortably in bed.
• Release the wheel lock and withdraw the scale. Return the stretcher to its vertical position for storage.

### Special considerations

Reassure and steady patients who might lose their balance on a scale.

Weigh the patient at the same time each day (usually before breakfast), in similar clothing, and using the same scale. If the patient uses crutches, weigh him with the crutches. Then weigh the crutches and any heavy clothing and subtract their weight from the total to determine the patient's weight. If the patient is markedly obese, check scale capacity. (Although some newer scales can measure up to 600 lb [272 kg], most scales can measure a maximum of 250 lb [113 kg].) You may have to weigh the patient on a large commercial scale (usually located on the loading dock or in the dietary department).

Before using a bed scale, cover its stretcher with a disposable cover sheet *to avoid stains from perspiration, drainage, or excretions.* Balance the scale before use with the cover sheet in place *to ensure accurate weighing.*

When rolling the patient onto the stretcher, have bedside rails up and be careful not to dislodge I.V. lines, indwelling catheters, and other supportive equipment.

### Documentation

Record the patient's height and weight on the nursing assessment form and other medical records, as required by your hospital.

# Monitoring anthropometric arm measurements

Measuring midarm circumference, triceps skin-fold thickness, and midarm muscle circumference provides information about skeletal muscle and adipose tissue. In turn, this helps indicate the patient's protein and calorie reserves. By obtaining serial measurements, it's possible to identify any change in the patient's nutritional status. Also, in an overweight patient, measuring triceps skin-fold thickness can help determine whether the patient's excess weight is the result of an excess amount of adipose tissue or an excess amount of muscle.

Although a nurse may perform skin-fold thickness measurements, some facilities prefer that a dietician obtain the measurement.

### Equipment

Nonstretchable tape measure ▪ skin-fold calipers ▪ felt-tip pen.

## Implementation
• Explain the procedure to the patient.

### Measuring the midarm circumference
• Extend the tape measure from the tip of the patient's shoulder (acromion process) to his elbow (olecranon process) on his nondominant arm.
• Identify the midpoint between those two landmarks. Mark that point on the patient's arm using a felt-tip pen.
• Now, wrap the tape measure gently but firmly around the patient's arm at the point marked. Pull the tape measure tight enough to avoid soft-tissue compression.
• Read the measurement to the nearest millimeter.

### Measuring triceps skin-fold thickness
• Grasp the patient's skin between thumb and forefinger about 1 cm above the midpoint.
• Place the calipers at the midpoint and squeeze the calipers for about 3 seconds.
• Record the measurement registered on the handle gauge to the nearest 0.5 mm.
• Take two more readings; then average all three to compensate for possible error.

### Calculating midarm muscle circumference
• Multiply the triceps skin-fold thickness (in centimeters) by 3.143. Then subtract the result from the midarm circumference.

## Special considerations
Compare the patient's actual measurement with the standard to determine the percentage measurement. (See *Evaluating anthropometric arm measurements*.)

A measurement under 90% of the standard indicates caloric deprivation; a measurement over 90% indicates adequate or more than adequate energy reserves.

Laboratory tests the doctor may order to evaluate a patient with a suspected nutritional prob-

## Evaluating anthropometric arm measurements

For all three measurements—triceps skin-fold thickness, midarm circumference, and midarm muscle circumference—determine the percentages of the standard measurements by using the following formula:

$$\frac{\text{Actual measurement}}{\text{Standard measurement}} \times 100$$

Then, compare the patient's percentage measurement with the standard. A measurement less than 90% of the standard indicates caloric deprivation; a measurement over 90% indicates adequate or more than adequate energy reserves.

| MEASUREMENT | STANDARD | 90% |
|---|---|---|
| Triceps skin-fold thickness | *Men:* 11.3 mm | *Men:* 12.5 mm |
| | *Women:* 14.9 mm | *Women:* 16.5 mm |
| Midarm circumference | *Men:* 26.4 cm | *Men:* 29.3 cm |
| | *Women:* 25.7 cm | *Women:* 28.5 cm |
| Midarm muscle circumference | *Men:* 22.8 cm | *Men:* 25.3 cm |
| | *Women:* 20.9 cm | *Women:* 23.2 cm |

lem include nitrogen balance testing (to determine the amount of protein being used by the body) and creatinine-height index (to identify protein and calorie deficiencies and to estimate lean body mass and muscle protein reserve).

When measuring skin-fold thickness, you may measure either the triceps or subscapular skin fold. Although the subscapular skin fold is less accessible, its results are more reliable. When measuring skin-fold thickness, keep in mind that adipose tissue, and therefore fat stores, may not be distributed evenly. Also, edema may distort results. In addition, note that normal skin-fold thickness varies greatly in older patients.

## Precautions for giving lipid emulsions

You may administer lipid emulsions as part of a total parenteral nutrition solution along with a peripheral parenteral nutrition solution, or separately through either a central venous line or a peripheral I.V. line. No matter which of these methods you use, be sure to observe these precautions.

**Before the infusion**
• Use a particulate filter according to the manufacturer's recommendations (usually a 1.2-micron filter). Standard 0.22-micron filters are insufficient because lipid particles clog the filter and disturb the emulsion.
• Always check the lipid emulsion for separation or an oily appearance. If either condition exists, the emulsion may have been disturbed and shouldn't be used. Never shake the lipid container excessively or use the emulsion if you see any inconsistency in texture or color.
• Never add anything to the lipid emulsion; doing so could cause instability. Also protect the emulsion from freezing.

**During the infusion**
• Monitor the patient's vital signs. The flow rate shouldn't exceed 1 ml/minute for the first 30 minutes.

• Check for signs and symptoms of an adverse reaction. Indications of an immediate adverse reaction, which can occur within 2½ hours, include increased temperature, flushing, sweating, pressure sensations over the eyes, nausea, vomiting, headache, chest and back pain, dyspnea, and cyanosis. Indications of a delayed reaction, which occurs up to 10 days after the infusion, include hepatomegaly, splenomegaly, thrombocytopenia, focal seizures, hyperlipidemia, hepatic damage, jaundice, hemorrhagic diathesis, and gastroduodenal ulcer.

**After the infusion**
• Be aware of the biochemical and clinical signs and symptoms of essential fatty acid disease that may be associated with impaired wound healing, adverse effects on red blood cells, and ineffective prostaglandin synthesis. Check for dry or scaly skin, thinning hair, liver function abnormalities, and thrombocytopenia.
• Discard any unused emulsion; if contaminated, it can support microbial growth. The Centers for Disease Control and Prevention guidelines recommend hanging lipid emulsions for no longer than 12 hours. Follow the manufacturer's recommendations.

## Documentation
Document the date and time of the evaluation; the measurements for midarm circumference, triceps skin-fold thickness, and midarm muscle circumference; and the percentages of the standard for each.

# Patient monitoring during TPN

TPN requires careful monitoring to assess the patient's response to the nutrient solution and to detect early signs of complications. Because the typical patient is in a protein-wasting state, TPN therapy causes marked changes in fluid and electrolyte status and in glucose, amino acid, mineral, and vitamin levels. If the patient displays an adverse reaction or signs of complications, the TPN regimen can be changed as needed.

Assessment of the patient's nutritional status includes physical examination, anthropometric measurements, biochemical determinations, and tests of cell-mediated immunity. Assessment of the patient's condition to detect complications requires recognition of the signs and symptoms of possible complications, understanding of laboratory test results, and careful record keeping.

Because the TPN solution is high in glucose, the infusion must start slowly to allow the patient's pancreatic beta cells to adapt to it by increasing insulin output. Usually, if the adult patient tolerates the TPN solution the first day, the doctor increases the intake to 1 liter every 12 hours for at least 2 days. Within the first 3 to 5 days of TPN, the typical adult patient can tolerate 3 liters of solution daily without adverse reactions. Lipid emulsions also require monitoring. (See *Precautions for giving lipid emulsions*.)

## Equipment

Test kits for blood and urine glucose and urine ketones ▪ stethoscope ▪ sphygmomanometer ▪ watch with second hand ▪ scale ▪ input and output chart ▪ time tape ▪ additional equipment for nutritional assessment, as ordered ▪ optional: 10% dextrose in water ($D_{10}W$).

If the patient is receiving cephalosporins, methyldopa, aspirin, or large doses of ascorbic acid, Tes-Tape should be used in place of Clinitest reagent tablets *to avoid false-positive results in urine glucose and ketone determinations.*

## Preparation of equipment

Prepare the infusion pump and TPN solution in accordance with hospital policy. Attach a time tape to the TPN container to allow approximate measurement of fluid intake. Make sure each bag or bottle has a label listing the expiration date, glucose concentration, and total volume of solution. (If the bag or bottle is damaged and you don't have an immediate replacement, hang a bag of $D_{10}W$ until the new container is ready. For more information, see *Administering TPN solutions through a central venous line,* page 158.)

## Implementation

• Explain the procedure to the patient *to diminish his anxiety and encourage cooperation.* Instruct the patient to inform you if he experiences any unusual sensations during the infusion. Begin the infusion at a slow rate (usually 40 ml/hour), as ordered, *to reduce the risk of hyperglycemia.* Then, as ordered, increase the adult patient's infusion rate (usually in 25 ml/hour increments) *to allow the pancreatic beta cells to increase endogenous insulin production, and to establish carbohydrate and water tolerances.*
• Record vital signs every 4 hours, or more often if necessary, *because increased temperature is one of the earliest signs of catheter-related sepsis.*
• Watch for swelling at the catheter site, *which may indicate extravasation of the TPN solution, possibly leading to tissue necrosis.*

• Check blood or urine for glucose and notify the doctor as appropriate.
• Perform I.V. site care and dressing changes at least three times a week (once a week for transparent semipermeable dressings), or whenever the dressing becomes wet, soiled, or nonocclusive. Use strict sterile technique.
• Expect to change the tubing and filter every 24 to 48 hours, using strict sterile technique. Make sure all tubing junctions are secure.
• Maintain flow rates, as prescribed, even if the flow falls behind schedule.
• Record daily fluid intake and output accurately. Specify the volume and type of each fluid, and calculate the daily caloric intake. *This record is a diagnostic tool for prompt, precise replacement of fluid and electrolyte deficits.*
• Physically assess the patient daily. If ordered, measure midarm circumference and skin-fold thickness over the triceps. Weigh the patient at the same time each morning (after voiding), in similar clothing, and on the same scale. Suspect fluid imbalance if the patient gains more than 1.1 lb (0.5 kg) daily.
• Monitor the results of routine laboratory tests and report abnormal findings to the doctor *to allow appropriate changes in the TPN solution.* Laboratory tests usually include serum electrolyte studies and blood urea nitrogen and blood glucose levels at least three times weekly; and liver function studies, complete blood count and differential, and levels of serum albumin, phosphorus, calcium, magnesium, and creatinine once weekly. Studies ordered less frequently include serum transferrin level, prothrombin time, creatinine-height index, nitrogen balance, total lymphocyte count, and skin tests.
• Monitor the patient for signs and symptoms of glucose metabolism disturbance, fluid and electrolyte imbalances, and nutritional aberrations. Remember that some patients may require supplementary insulin for the duration of TPN; the pharmacy usually adds insulin directly to the TPN solution.

## Administering TPN solutions through a central venous line

This illustration depicts the infusion of total parenteral nutrition (TPN) solution through a central vein. Because of its gentle arch, the left subclavian vein serves as a common site for central venous infusion.

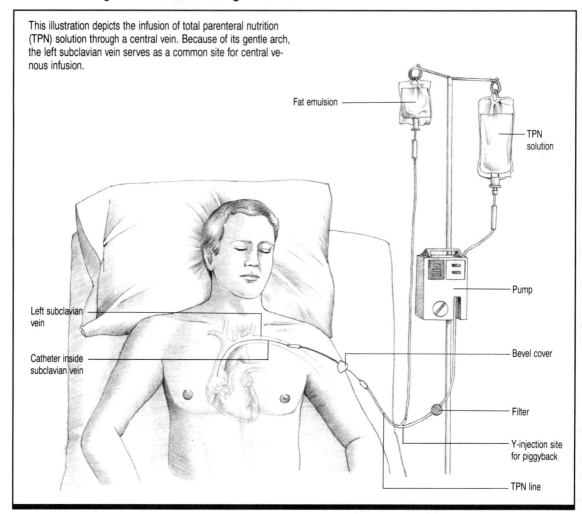

- Fat emulsion
- TPN solution
- Pump
- Bevel cover
- Filter
- Y-injection site for piggyback
- TPN line
- Left subclavian vein
- Catheter inside subclavian vein

• Provide emotional support. Keep in mind that patients often associate eating with positive feelings and become disturbed when eating is prohibited.
• Provide frequent mouth care.
• Keep the patient active *to enable him to utilize nutrients more fully.*
• When discontinuing TPN, decrease the infusion rate slowly, depending on the patient's current glucose intake, *to minimize the risk of hyperin-sulinemia and resulting hypoglycemia.* Weaning usually takes place over 24 to 48 hours but can be completed in 4 to 6 hours if the patient receives sufficient oral or I.V. carbohydrates. You may use a cyclic administration schedule, as ordered, to wean the patient from TPN to enteral feedings.

## Dealing with hazards of TPN

Potentially severe complications of total parenteral nutrition (TPN) include equipment-related problems and metabolic and nutritional problems caused by prolonged or overly rapid feedings.

### Equipment-related complications
Air embolism and infection are perhaps the most serious complications caused by the TPN equipment. Suspect *air embolism* if the patient reports chest pain and you detect cyanosis, dyspnea, and coughing. Treat this problem by clamping the catheter, placing the patient in the left Trendelenburg position, and having him perform Valsalva's maneuver. Then notify the doctor.

Suspect *infection* if the patient develops a fever or if redness, swelling, or drainage appears at the catheter insertion site. If he is lethargic, sweating profusely, or shivering, stop the TPN solution and replace it with dextrose 10% in water ($D_{10}W$). Change the I.V. tubing and dressing, and notify the doctor, who'll order cultures of the tubing, solution, and the patient's blood. If fever subsides within 6 hours of stopping TPN, suspect contamination of the solution or the delivery apparatus. If it persists, suspect catheter-related sepsis and again notify the doctor, who will then order blood and urine cultures. If necessary, he'll remove the catheter.

Be alert for other complications, such as pneumothorax, hydrothorax, extravasation, and injury to the brachial plexus.

### Metabolic and nutritional complications
A whole array of disturbances in nutrient metabolism, fluid and electrolyte balance, and nutrition can result from TPN. *Hyperglycemia*, for instance, can develop from overly rapid delivery of the solution, decreased glucose tolerance, or excessive total glucose load. If it develops, you'll need to add insulin to the solution.

*Hypoglycemia*, in contrast, can develop from excessive endogenous production of insulin after abrupt termination of feeding. It can also result from excessive addition of insulin to the TPN solution. To correct hypoglycemia, give carbohydrates orally if possible. Or you can infuse $D_{10}W$ or give a bolus of dextrose 50% in water. *Essential fatty acid deficiency*, which can result from absent or inadequate fat intake for a prolonged period, requires infusion of two or three bottles of 10% to 20% fat emulsion weekly. Deficiency of trace elements, such as *copper* and *zinc*, requires addition of these elements to the solution. *Fluid deficit or excess* can stem from inadequate or excessive replacement, electrolyte imbalance, or other problems. To correct fluid imbalance, adjust the patient's fluid intake as ordered. Electrolyte imbalances, such as *hypokalemia* and *hypocalcemia*, require addition of the deficient electrolyte to TPN the solution.

## Special considerations
Always maintain strict sterile technique when handling the equipment used to administer therapy. *Because the TPN solution serves as a medium for bacterial growth and the central venous (CV) line provides systemic access*, the patient risks infection and sepsis.

When using a filter, position it as close to the access site as possible. Check the filter's porosity and pressure capacity to make sure it exceeds the pounds per square inch exerted by the infusion pump.

Don't allow TPN solutions to hang for more than 24 hours.

Be careful when using the TPN line for other functions. If you're using a single-lumen CV catheter, don't use the line to infuse blood or blood products, to give a bolus injection, to administer simultaneous I.V. solutions, to measure CV pressure, or to draw blood for laboratory tests. Never add medication to a TPN solution container. Also, don't use a three-way stopcock, if possible, *because add-on devices increase the risk of infection.*

## Complications
Catheter-related, metabolic, and mechanical complications can occur during TPN administration. (See *Dealing with hazards of TPN*.)

## Documentation
Record serial monitoring indices on the appropriate flowchart to determine the patient's progress and response. Note any abnormal, adverse, or altered responses.

# 7

# MONITORING FETAL AND NEONATAL STATUS

## Introduction

More than 4 million infants were born in the United States in 1993. Many of them were born with considerably less medical intervention than was customary in previous decades, although many of them were conceived with considerably more intervention. Nurses today must be prepared to implement or assist with a wide range of procedures for monitoring fetal and neonatal status.

Neonatal care has changed over the past several years, thanks to advanced knowledge and techniques for improving fetal monitoring and promoting neonatal survival. Until recently, for example, admission to a neonatal care unit depended solely on birth weight. A neonate weighing less than 5.5 lb (2.5 kg) was considered premature. A neonate exceeding this weight was considered full-term. Today, it's possible to identify the 8-lb (3.5 kg), 35-week neonate of a diabetic mother as premature and large for gestational age.

New clinical evaluation methods, combined with advanced electronic and biochemical monitoring techniques, allow improved neonatal care. To apply these advances, you must be familiar with neonatal physiology, procedures, and equipment.

# Physiology review

To more fully understand the need for monitoring certain aspects of fetal and neonatal status, you should first review the stages of fetal development.

## Fertilization and early development

At ovulation, the mature ovarian follicle discharges its ovum, which promptly moves into the fallopian tube. When fertilization occurs, the egg nucleus fuses with a sperm. This fusion creates the full complement of 46 chromosomes and forms a zygote.

Shortly thereafter, the zygote begins moving down the fallopian tube toward the endome-trium. Along the way, it undergoes a series of mitotic divisions (known as *cleavage*). These divisions convert the zygote into a little ball of cells called a *morula*. The morula reaches the endometrial cavity about 3 days after fertilization and completes implantation about one week after fertilization. The amniotic sac then surrounds the embryo and grows with it. Eventually, the sac completely fills the chorionic cavity and fuses with the chorion.

Formative blood vessels within the growing villi attach to other rudimentary vessels in the chorion's connective tissue lining and in the *body stalk*, which later becomes the umbilical cord. When the embryo's heart starts to beat, blood begins to flow through this network of vessels — from the embryo through the body stalk, to the chorion, into the villi, and back to the embryo. This marks the beginning of *fetoplacental circulation* and occurs about 22 days after fertilization.

## Placenta formation and structure

Placenta formation begins during the third week of embryonic development, at the site of implantation. During pregnancy, the endometrium of the pregnant uterus, called the *decidua*, thickens to about ⅜″ (1 cm). This is the maternal portion of the placenta. The placental layer closest to the fetus is called the *amnion*. The developing placenta is divided into compartments, called *cotyledons*, in which the vascular systems formed by the villi become the junction of the maternal and fetal layers. This junction becomes the site of maternal-fetal transfer of gases and nutrients.

The umbilical cord develops from the body stalk. It extends from the fetal umbilicus to the placenta's fetal surface.

## Blood circulation in the placenta

The placenta has two kinds of blood circulation: fetoplacental and uteroplacental. *Fetoplacental circulation* delivers deoxygenated blood from the fetus through the umbilical arteries into the chorionic villi. It also carries oxygenated blood rich in nutrients to the fetus through the umbilical vein. *Uteroplacental circulation* delivers oxygenated maternal blood into the large vascular network called the *intervillous spaces.*

The maternal and fetal circulations don't normally mix within the placenta, but they do remain in close contact. This allows the transfer of oxygen and nutrients from maternal blood in the intervillous spaces to fetal blood in the villi. What's more, it permits the transport of fetal waste products to the maternal blood for elimination.

# Fetal heart rate monitoring

A major clue to fetal well-being during gestation and labor, fetal heart rate (FHR) may be assessed by auscultating with a fetoscope or a Doppler ultrasound stethoscope placed on the maternal abdomen. This ultrasound device emits low-energy, high-frequency sound waves that rebound from the fetal heart to a transducer, which transmits the impulses to a monitor strip for recording.

Because FHR normally ranges from 120 to 160 beats/minute, auscultation yields only an average rate at best. However, because auscultation can only detect gross fetal distress signs (tachycardia or bradycardia), the technique remains most useful in an uncomplicated, low-risk pregnancy. In a high-risk pregnancy, indirect external or direct internal electronic fetal monitoring gives more accurate information on fetal status.

## Equipment

Fetoscope or Doppler ultrasound stethoscope (see *Instruments for hearing fetal heart tones*) ▪ water-soluble lubricant (for ultrasound instrument) ▪ watch with second hand.

## Implementation

• Explain the procedure to the patient, wash your hands, don gloves, and provide privacy. Reassure the patient that you may reposition the listening instrument frequently *to hear the loudest fetal heart tones.*
• Assist the patient to a supine position, and drape her appropriately *to minimize exposure.* If you're using the Doppler ultrasound stethoscope, apply the water-soluble lubricant to the patient's abdomen. *This gel or paste creates an airtight seal between the skin and the instrument and promotes optimal ultrasound wave conduction and reception.*

### Calculating FHR during gestation

• *To assess FHR in a fetus age 20 weeks or less,* place the earpieces in your ears and position the bell of the fetoscope or Doppler ultrasound stethoscope on the abdominal midline above the pubic hairline. After 20 weeks, when you can palpate fetal position, use Leopold's maneuvers *to locate the back of the fetal thorax.* Then position the listening instrument over the fetal back. (See *Performing Leopold's maneuvers,* pages 164 and 165.)
• Using a Doppler ultrasound stethoscope, place the earpieces in your ears, and press the bell gently on the patient's abdomen. Start listening at the midline, midway between the umbilicus and the symphysis pubis. Or, using a fetoscope, place the earpieces in your ears with the fetoscope positioned centrally on your forehead. Gently press the bell about ½" (1.3 cm) into the patient's abdomen. Remove your hands from the fetoscope *to avoid extraneous noise.*
• Move the bell of either instrument slightly from side to side, as necessary, *to locate the loudest heart tones.* After locating these tones, palpate the maternal pulse.
• While monitoring the maternal pulse rate *(to avoid confusing maternal heart tones with fetal heart tones),* count the fetal heartbeats for at least 15 seconds. If the maternal radial pulse and the FHR are the same, try to locate the fetal thorax by using Leopold's maneuvers; then reassess FHR. Usually, the fetal heart beats faster than the maternal heart. Record the FHR.

## Instruments for hearing fetal heart tones

The fetoscope and the Doppler ultrasound stethoscope are basic instruments for auscultating fetal heart tones and assessing fetal heart rates.

### Fetoscope
This instrument can detect fetal heartbeats as early as the 18th gestational week. As an assessment tool during labor, it's helpful for hearing fetal heart tones when contractions are mild and infrequent.

### Doppler ultrasound stethoscope
This instrument can detect fetal heartbeats as early as the 10th gestational week. Useful throughout labor, the Doppler stethoscope has greater sensitivity than the fetoscope.

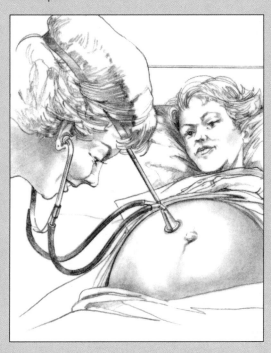

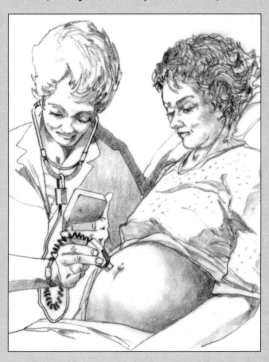

### Counting FHR during labor
• Allow the mother and her support person to listen to the fetal heart if they wish. *This helps to make the fetus a greater reality for them.* Record their participation.

• Position the fetoscope or Doppler ultrasound stethoscope on the abdomen — midway between the umbilicus and symphysis pubis *for cephalic presentation,* or at the umbilicus or above *for breech presentation.* Locate the loudest heartbeats, and simultaneously palpate the maternal pulse *to*

ensure that you're monitoring fetal rather than maternal pulse.

• Monitor maternal pulse rate and count fetal heartbeats for 60 seconds during the relaxation period between contractions *to determine baseline FHR.* In a low-risk labor, assess FHR every 60 minutes during the latent phase, every 30 minutes during the active phase, and every 15 minutes during the second stage of labor. In a high-risk labor, assess FHR every 30 minutes during the latent phase, every 15 minutes during

## Performing Leopold's maneuvers

You can determine fetal position by performing Leopold's maneuvers. Ask the patient to empty her bladder, assist her to a supine position, and expose her abdomen. Then perform the following four maneuvers in order.

### First maneuver
Face the patient and warm your hands. Place them on her abdomen to determine fetal position in the uterine fundus. Curl your fingers around the fundus. With the fetus in vertex position, you'll feel the buttocks—irregularly shaped and firm. With the fetus in breech position, you'll feel the head—hard, round, and movable.

### Second maneuver
Move your hands down the sides of the abdomen and apply gentle pressure. If the fetus lies in vertex position, you'll feel a smooth, hard surface on one side—the fetal back. On the other side, you'll feel lumps and knobs—the knees, hands, feet, and elbows. If the fetus lies in breech position, you may not feel the back at all.

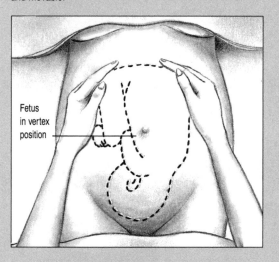

Fetus in vertex position

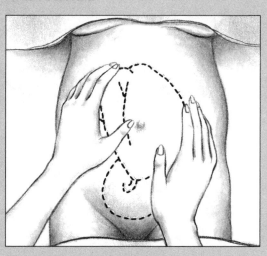

the active phase, and every 5 minutes during the second stage of labor. Preferably, perform this assessment immediately following a contraction.

• Notify the doctor or nurse-midwife immediately if you observe marked changes in FHR from baseline values (especially during or immediately after a contraction when signs of fetal distress typically occur). If fetal distress develops, begin indirect or direct electronic fetal monitoring.

• Repeat the procedure, as ordered.

### Special considerations
If you're auscultating FHR with a Doppler ultrasound stethoscope, be aware that obesity and hydramnios can interfere with sound-wave transmission, making accurate results more difficult to obtain. If the doctor orders continuous FHR monitoring, strap the ultrasound transducer to the patient's abdomen. The monitor will provide a printed record of the FHR.

### Documentation
Record both the FHR and the maternal pulse rate on the flowchart. Also note the patient's blood pressure and temperature, her membrane status, her cervical status (if known), any ox-

### Third maneuver

Spread apart the thumb and fingers of one hand. Place them just above the patient's symphysis pubis. Bring your fingers together. If the fetus lies in vertex position (and hasn't descended), you'll feel the head. If the fetus lies in vertex position (and has descended), you'll feel a less distinct mass.

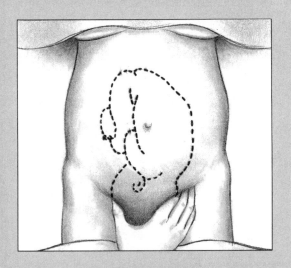

### Fourth maneuver

Use this maneuver in late pregnancy. Place your hands on both sides of the lower abdomen. Apply gentle pressure with your fingers as you slide your hands downward, toward the symphysis pubis. If the head presents, one hand's descent will be stopped by the cephalic prominence. The other hand will be unobstructed.

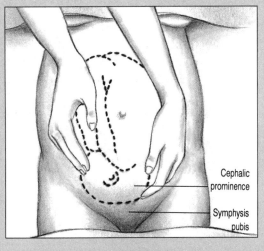

Cephalic prominence

Symphysis pubis

ygen or drug administration, and her position in bed.

## External fetal monitoring

An indirect, noninvasive procedure, external fetal monitoring has major advantages over auscultation with the fetoscope. Through the use of two devices strapped to the mother's abdomen, electronic monitoring evaluates fetal well-being during labor. By continuously monitoring the FHR throughout a contraction, external fetal monitoring can detect signs of fetal distress at an early stage.

One device, an ultrasound transducer, transmits high-frequency sound waves through soft body tissues to the fetal heart. The waves rebound from the heart through the abdominal wall, where the transducer relays them to a monitor. The other, a pressure-sensitive tocotransducer, responds to the pressure exerted by uterine contractions and simultaneously records their duration and frequency. (See *Applying external fetal monitoring devices,* page 166.) The monitoring apparatus traces FHR and uterine contraction data onto the same printout paper. The disadvantage of this method of monitoring is that it cannot assess the intensity of contractions.

## Applying external fetal monitoring devices

To ensure clear tracings that define fetal status and labor progress, be sure you precisely position external monitoring devices, such as an ultrasound transducer and a tocotransducer.

### Fetal heart rate monitor
Palpate the uterus to locate the fetus's back. If possible, place the ultrasound transducer over this site where the fetal heartbeat sounds the loudest. Then tighten the belt. Use the fetal heart tracing on the monitor strip to validate the transducer's position.

### Labor monitor
A tocotransducer records uterine motion during contractions. Place the tocotransducer over the uterine fundus where it contracts, either midline or slightly to one side. Place your hand on the fundus and palpate a contraction to verify proper placement. Secure the tocotransducer's belt; then adjust the pen set so that the baseline values read between 5 and 15 mm Hg on the monitor strip.

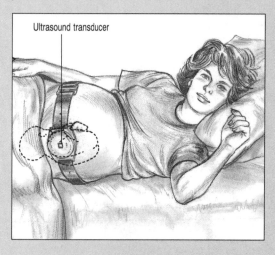

Ultrasound transducer

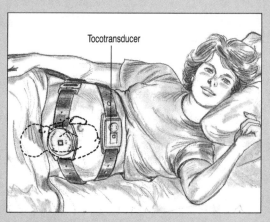

Tocotransducer

Indications for external fetal monitoring include high-risk pregnancy, oxytocin-induced labor, and antepartal nonstress and contraction stress tests. Many labor and delivery units use external fetal monitoring for all patients. The procedure has no contraindications, but may be difficult to perform on patients with hydramnios, on obese patients, or on hyperactive or premature fetuses.

### Equipment
Electronic fetal monitor ▪ ultrasound transducer ▪ tocotransducer ▪ conduction gel ▪ transducer straps ▪ damp cloth ▪ printout paper.

Monitoring devices, such as phonotransducers and abdominal electrocardiogram (ECG) trans-

ducers, are commercially available. However, hospitals use these devices less frequently than the ultrasound transducer.

### Preparation of equipment
Because fetal monitor features and complexity vary, review the operator's manual before proceeding. If the monitor has two paper speeds, select the slower speed (typically 3 cm/minute) *to ensure an easy-to-read tracing.* At higher speeds (for example, 1 cm/minute), the printed tracings are condensed, making results difficult to decipher and interpret accurately.

Next, plug the tocotransducer cable into the uterine activity jack and the ultrasound transducer cable into the phono-ultrasound jack. Attach the straps to the tocotransducer and the ultrasound transducer.

Label the printout paper with the patient's hospital number or birthdate and name, the date, maternal vital signs and position, cervical and membrane status, the presence of oxygen or drug administration, the paper speed, and the number of the strip paper *to maintain accurate, consecutive monitoring records.*

## Implementation

• Explain the procedure to the patient and provide emotional support. Inform her that the monitor may make noise if the pen set tracer moves above or below the grids on the printout paper. Reassure her that this doesn't indicate fetal distress. As appropriate, explain other aspects of the monitor *to help reduce maternal anxiety about fetal well-being.*
• Make sure the patient has signed a consent form, if required.
• Wash your hands and provide privacy.

### Beginning the procedure

• Assist the patient to a semi-Fowler or a left-lateral position with her abdomen exposed. Don't let her lie supine *because pressure from the gravid uterus on the maternal inferior vena cava may cause maternal hypotension,* decrease uterine perfusion, and induce fetal hypoxia.
• Palpate the patient's abdomen to locate the fundus—the area of greatest muscle density in the uterus. Then, using transducer straps, secure the tocotransducer over the fundus.
• Adjust the pen set tracer controls so that the baseline values read between 5 and 15 mm Hg on the monitor strip. *This prevents triggering the alarm that indicates the tracer has dropped below the paper's margins.* The proper setting varies among tocotransducers.
• Apply conduction gel to the ultrasound transducer crystals *to promote an airtight seal and optimal sound-wave transmission.*

• Use Leopold's maneuvers to palpate the fetal back, through which fetal heart tones resound most audibly.
• Start the monitor. Then apply the ultrasound transducer directly over the site having the strongest heart tones.
• Activate the control that begins the printout. On the printout paper, note any coughing, position changes, drug administration, vaginal examinations, and blood pressure readings that may affect interpretation of the tracings.
• Explain to the patient and her support person how to time and control contractions with the monitor. To time contractions, inform them that the distance from one dark vertical line to the next on the printout grid represents 1 minute. The support person can use this information to prepare the patient for the onset of a contraction and to guide and slow her breathing as the contraction subsides.

### Monitoring the patient

• Observe the tracings *to identify frequency and duration of uterine contractions,* but palpate the uterus *to determine intensity of contractions.*
• Mentally note the baseline FHR—the "resting" heart rate between contractions when fetal movement diminishes—*to compare with suspicious-looking deviations.* FHR normally ranges from 120 to 160 beats/minute.
• Assess periodic accelerations or decelerations from the baseline FHR. Compare the FHR patterns with those of the uterine contractions. Note the time relationship between the onset of an FHR deceleration and the onset of a uterine contraction, the time relationship of the lowest level of an FHR deceleration to the peak of a uterine contraction, and the range of FHR deceleration. *These data help distinguish fetal distress from benign head compression.*
• Move the tocotransducer and the ultrasound transducer *to accommodate changes in maternal or fetal position.* Readjust both transducers every hour and assess the patient's skin for reddened

areas caused by the strap pressure. Document skin condition.

• Clean the ultrasound transducer periodically with a damp cloth *to remove dried conduction gel that can interfere with ultrasound transmission.* Apply fresh gel, as necessary. After use, place the cover over the ultrasound transducer.

### Special considerations

If the monitor fails to record uterine activity, palpate for contractions. Check for equipment problems as the manufacturer directs, and readjust the tocotransducer.

If the patient reports discomfort in the position that provides the clearest signal, try to obtain a satisfactory 5- or 10-minute tracing with the patient in this position before assisting her to a more comfortable position. As the patient progresses through labor and abdominal pressure increases, the pen set tracer may exceed the alarm boundaries.

### Documentation

Check to make sure you numbered each monitor strip in sequence and labeled each printout sheet with the patient's hospital number or birthdate and name, the date, the time, and the paper speed. Record the time of any vaginal examinations, membrane rupture, drug administration, and maternal or fetal movements. Record maternal vital signs and the intensity of uterine contractions. Document each time that you moved or readjusted the tocotransducer and ultrasound transducer, and summarize this information in your notes.

# Internal electronic fetal monitoring

Also known as direct fetal monitoring, internal electronic fetal monitoring utilizes a spiral electrode and an intrauterine catheter to evaluate fetal status during labor. A doctor or a nurse with special skills performs this invasive procedure only after the amniotic sac ruptures and the cervix dilates at least 2 cm. Typically used when external (indirect) fetal monitoring provides insufficient or unusual information about fetal well-being, internal monitoring furnishes information on beat-to-beat variability and precisely measures intrauterine pressure and labor progress. This helps the health care team determine the need for intervention.

Contraindications to direct fetal monitoring include maternal blood dyscrasias, suspected fetal immune deficiency, placenta previa, face presentation or uncertainty regarding the presenting part, and cervical or vaginal herpetic lesions.

### Equipment

Electronic fetal monitor ▪ printout paper ▪ strain gauge and mounting bracket ▪ 20-ml syringe ▪ intrauterine catheter and guide ▪ three-way stopcock ▪ sterile water for injection ▪ conduction gel ▪ spiral electrode with drive tube and guide tube ▪ leg plate ▪ Velcro straps or 2″ tape ▪ hypoallergenic tape ▪ two pairs of sterile gloves ▪ sterile drape.

Commercially available kits for direct fetal monitoring contain the intrauterine catheter and guide, syringe, and three-way stopcock.

### Preparation of equipment

Because fetal monitor models vary in features and complexity, review the operator's manual before proceeding.

If the monitor has two paper speeds, set the monitor to 3 cm/minute *to ensure a readable tracing.* You may interpret a 1 cm/minute tracing less accurately because it's more condensed.

On the printout paper, record the number of the strip, the date, the patient's name and hospital number or birthdate, the printing speed, the type of procedure, and the reason for the procedure.

Place the strain gauge on the appropriate mounting bracket. Then attach this bracket to the side of the monitor. Connect the strain-gauge cable to the uterine activity outlet on the monitor.

Wash your hands and open the sterile equipment, maintaining sterile technique. Fill the 20-ml syringe with sterile water.

## Implementation

• Explain the procedure to the patient and provide emotional support.
• Confirm that the patient has signed a consent form, if required.

### *Monitoring uterine contractions*

• Assist the patient to the lithotomy position as the doctor or specially skilled nurse puts on sterile gloves. Inform the patient that she'll have a vaginal examination *to identify the position of the fetus.* During the examination, the intrauterine catheter will be inserted.
• Cover the perineum with a sterile drape. Then clean the perineum according to hospital policy. Using sterile technique, the doctor or nurse will insert the uterine end of the catheter into a catheter guide *to advance the catheter.*
• Attach the syringe holding 20 ml of sterile water to the three-way stopcock at the monitor end of the catheter. Avoid touching the inside of the catheter *to prevent contamination.*
• Flush the catheter with about 5 ml of sterile water and leave the syringe in place.
• Secure the three-way stopcock to the angle fitting of the strain gauge. Avoid touching the stopcock ports *to prevent contamination.*
• Position the strain gauge level with the patient's xiphoid process *to ensure accurate measurements.*
• Prepare the patient for catheter insertion. Explain that the guide will be placed about ¾" (2 cm) into the cervical opening. The catheter will be advanced into the uterus alongside the fetus for about 18" (45.7 cm) until a premarked level (on the tubing) reaches the introitus. Then the catheter guide will be removed and the catheter attached to the side fitting on the three-way stopcock.

• Refill the syringe with 20 ml of sterile water and secure the syringe to the upright fitting of the stopcock.
• Tape the catheter to the patient's inner thigh with the hypoallergenic tape.
• Turn the stopcock lever to the right *to open the connection between the syringe and the catheter.* Inject 5 ml of sterile water *to clear air bubbles or vernix that could invalidate pressure measurements.*
• Turn the stopcock lever to the left *to close off the catheter.* Then lift the pressure-release cap, and inject water *to flush air bubbles from the strain gauge's dome.*
• Test the monitoring system. First, disconnect the syringe from the stopcock fitting *to open the strain gauge to atmospheric pressure.* Next, turn on the monitor. Observe the lower grid on the printout paper. (This shows uterine activity and contraction pressures.) Look for a zero level reading, which indicates a properly operating system. Reconnect the syringe to the stopcock fitting.
• Turn the stopcock lever to the upright position *to open the connection between the strain gauge and the catheter.* Begin monitoring.
• Inform the patient that the monitor may make noise if the tracer arm swings off the printout paper. Reassure her that this doesn't indicate fetal distress.

### *Monitoring FHR*

• Apply conduction gel to the leg plate. Then secure the leg plate to the patient's inner thigh with Velcro straps or 2" tape. Next, connect the leg plate to the ECG outlet on the monitor.
• Tell the patient that she will have a vaginal examination *to identify the fetal presenting part and determine its level of descent and to apply the electrode.* Explain that this examination ensures against attaching the electrode to fetal suture lines or fontanels, the face, or the genitalia. The spiral electrode will be engaged in a drive tube and advanced through the vagina to the fetal presenting part. *To secure the electrode,* mild pressure will be applied and the drive tube turned clockwise 360 degrees.

## Reading a fetal monitor strip

Presented in two parallel recordings, the fetal monitor strip records the fetal heart rate (FHR) in beats per minute in the top recording and uterine activity (UA) in mm Hg in the bottom recording. You can obtain information on fetal status and labor progress by reading the strips horizontally and vertically.

Each small block (when you're reading horizontally on the FHR or UA strip) represents 10 seconds. Six consecutive small blocks, separated by a dark vertical line, represent 1 minute. When you read vertically, each block on the FHR

strip represents an amplitude of 10 beats/minute. On the UA strip, each block read vertically represents 5 mm Hg of pressure.

Assess the baseline FHR – the "resting" heart rate between uterine contractions when fetal movement diminishes. This baseline FHR (normal range: 120 to 160 beats/minute) pattern serves as a reference for subsequent FHR tracings produced during contractions.

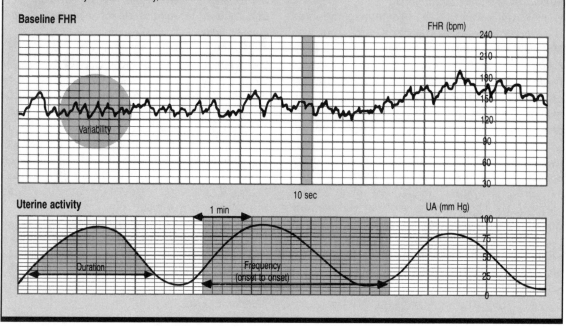

**Baseline FHR**

FHR (bpm)

Variability

10 sec

**Uterine activity**

1 min

Duration

Frequency
(onset to onset)

UA (mm Hg)

• After the electrode is in place and the drive tube is removed, connect the color-coded electrode wires to the corresponding color-coded leg plate posts.
• Turn on the recorder. Note the time on the printout paper.
• Assist the patient to a comfortable position, and read the strip.

### Monitoring the patient
• Note the frequency, duration, and intensity of uterine contractions. (See *Reading a fetal monitor strip*.) Normal intrauterine pressure ranges from 8 to 12 mm Hg.
• Check the baseline FHR, which normally ranges from 120 to 160 beats/minute.
• Assess periodic accelerations or decelerations from the baseline FHR. Compare the FHR pattern with the uterine contraction pattern. Note the time between the onset of an FHR deceleration and the onset of a uterine contraction, the time between the lowest level of an FHR decel-

eration and the peak of a uterine contraction, and the range of FHR deceleration.

• Check for FHR variability, a measure of fetal reserve and neurologic integrity and stability.

## Special considerations

Take care to ensure a level strain-gauge position when monitoring contractions. Positioning the strain gauge too low will yield false-high values; positioning the strain gauge too high will yield false-low values.

During labor, clean the leg plate and reapply conduction gel, as necessary. Periodically flush the intrauterine catheter *to remove air and vernix that prevent accurate pressure measurement.* Also flush the catheter if the monitor stops recording contractions. If the FHR tracing diminishes, tug gently on the electrode wire *to ensure electrode attachment.* Internal electronic fetal monitoring is often used without internal uterine monitoring. However, internal electronic uterine monitoring is seldom used without internal fetal monitoring.

## Complications

Possible maternal complications include uterine perforation and intrauterine infection. Possible fetal complications include abscess, hematoma, or infection.

## Documentation

Make sure you've numbered each printout sheet and labeled it with the patient's hospital number or birthdate and name, the date, the time, the printing speed, the type of procedure, and the reason for the procedure.

Record any information related to the insertion of the catheter or electrode or both, drug administration, vaginal examinations, or position changes on the printout.

Periodically summarize this information in your notes. Follow hospital policy for required documentation.

# Apgar score monitoring

Named after its developer, Virginia Apgar, the Apgar score quantifies the neonatal heart rate, respiratory effort, muscle tone, reflexes, and color. Each category is assessed 1 minute after birth and again 5 minutes later. Scores in each category range from 0 to 2. The highest Apgar score is 10 – the greatest possible sum of the five categories.

The evaluation at 1 minute indicates the neonate's initial adaptation to extrauterine life. The evaluation at 5 minutes gives a clearer picture of overall status. If the neonate doesn't breathe or his heart beats fewer than 100 times a minute, call for help and begin resuscitation at once. Don't wait for a 1-minute Apgar test score.

## Equipment

Apgar score sheet or neonatal assessment sheet (see *Recording the Apgar score,* page 172) ▪ stethoscope ▪ clock with second hand or Apgar timer ▪ gloves.

## Preparation of equipment

If you use Apgar timers, make sure both timers are on at the instant of birth.

## Implementation

• Note the exact time of delivery. Wear gloves *for protection from blood and body fluids.* Place the neonate on a heated radiant warmer and then dry the neonate *to prevent heat loss.*

• Place the neonate in a 15-degree Trendelenburg's position to promote mucus drainage. Then position his head with the nose slightly tilted upward *to straighten the airway.*

• Assess the neonate's respiratory efforts. If necessary, supply stimulation by rubbing his back or gently flicking his foot.

• With abnormal respiratory responses, begin neonatal resuscitation according to the guidelines of the American Heart Association and the American Academy of Pediatrics. Then, use the Apgar score to judge the progress and success of resuscitation efforts. Should resuscitation ef-

## Recording the Apgar score

Use this chart to record the neonatal Apgar score at 1 minute and at 5 minutes after birth. A score of 7 to 10 indicates good condition; 4 to 6, fair condition – the infant may have moderate central nervous system depression, muscle flaccidity, cyanosis, and poor respirations; 0 to 3, danger – the infant needs immediate resuscitation, as ordered.

| SIGN | APGAR SCORE | | |
| | 0 | 1 | 2 |
| --- | --- | --- | --- |
| Heart rate | Absent | Less than 100 beats/ minute (slow) | More than 100 beats/ minute |
| Respiratory effort | Absent | Slow, irregular | Good crying |
| Muscle tone | Flaccid | Some flexion and resistance to extension of extremities | Active motion |
| Reflex irritability | No response | Grimace or weak cry | Vigorous cry |
| Color | Pallor, cyanosis | Pink body, blue extremities | Completely pink |

forts prove futile, you'll need to implement measures for dealing with stillbirth.
• If the neonate exhibits normal responses, proceed to assign the Apgar score at 1 minute after birth.
• Repeat the evaluation and record the score at 5 minutes after birth.

### Assessing neonatal heart rate
• Using a stethoscope, listen to the heartbeat for 30 seconds, and record the rate. In order to obtain beats/minute, double the rate. Or palpate the umbilical cord where it joins the abdomen. Monitor pulsations for 6 seconds and multiply by 10 to obtain beats/minute. Assign a 0 for no heart rate, a 1 for a rate under 100 beats/minute, and a 2 for a rate over 100 beats/minute.

### Assessing respiratory effort
• Count unassisted respirations for 60 seconds, noting quality and regularity (a normal rate is 30 to 60 respirations/minute). Assign a 0 for no

respirations; a 1 for slow, irregular, shallow, or gasping respirations; and a 2 for regular respirations and vigorous crying.

### Assessing muscle tone
• Observe the extremities for flexion and resistance to extension. This can be done by extending the limbs and observing their rapid return to flexion—the neonate's normal state. Assign a 0 for flaccid muscle tone; a 1 for some flexion and resistance to extension; and a 2 for normal flexion of elbows, knees, and hips, with good resistance to extension.

### Assessing reflex irritability
• Observe the neonate's response to nasal suctioning or to flicking the sole of his foot. Assign a 0 for no response, a 1 for a grimace or weak cry, and a 2 for a vigorous cry.

### Assessing color

• Observe skin color, especially at the extremities. Assign a 0 for complete pallor and cyanosis, a 1 for a pink body with blue extremities (acrocyanosis), and a 2 for a completely pink body. To assess color in a dark-skinned neonate, inspect the oral mucous membranes and conjunctiva, the lips, the palms, and the soles.

### Special considerations

If the patient and her support person don't know about the Apgar score, discuss it with them during early labor, when they will be more receptive to new knowledge. *To prevent confusion or misunderstanding at delivery,* explain to them what will occur and why. Add that this is a routine procedure.

If the neonate requires emergency care, make sure that a member of the delivery team offers appropriate support.

Closely observe the neonate whose mother receives heavy sedation just before delivery. Despite a high Apgar score at birth, he may show secondary effects of sedation in the nursery. Be alert for depression or unresponsiveness.

### Documentation

Record the Apgar score on the Apgar score sheet or the neonatal assessment sheet required by your hospital. Be sure to indicate the total score and the signs for which points were deducted *to guide postnatal care.*

# Neonatal vital sign monitoring

Measuring vital signs establishes the baseline of any neonatal assessment. Typically, you'll visually assess the respiratory rate by watching and counting the neonate's breaths, although you may auscultate the lungs with a pediatric stethoscope and watch for labored or abnormal breathing. You'll measure the heart rate apically — also with a pediatric stethoscope. To assess blood pressure you'll either use a sphygmomanometer or perform palpation or auscultation. An elec-

tronic vital signs monitor may also be used. (See "Temperature monitoring," "Pulse monitoring," "Respiration monitoring," and "Blood pressure monitoring" in Chapter 1.)

When the neonate arrives in the nursery, additional procedures may be required. Depending on hospital policy, some procedures to ensure the neonate's safety and progress in the nursery include an identification and weight check; placement in radiant warming equipment; rectal temperature measurement; a vitamin $K_1$ injection to stimulate neonatal clotting mechanisms; and eye treatments with an antibiotic or silver nitrate to guard against infections.

### Equipment

Pediatric stethoscope ▪ watch with second hand ▪ thermometer (mercury or electronic with rectal probe and cover) ▪ water-soluble lubricant ▪ gloves ▪ sphygmomanometer with 1″ (2.5-cm) cuff ▪ optional: Doppler ultrasound stethoscope with conduction gel or an electronic vital signs monitor.

### Preparation of equipment

Assemble the equipment beside the patient. If you're using a mercury thermometer, shake it until the mercury drops under 96° F (35.5° C). If you have an electronic thermometer, apply the cover to the rectal probe. Using water-soluble lubricant, coat the thermometer or probe cover before taking a rectal temperature.

### Implementation

• Wash your hands.

### Determining respiratory rate

• Observe respirations first, before the neonate becomes too active or agitated. Watch and count respiratory movements for 1 minute. Then record the result.

• Expect to see mostly diaphragmatic respirations. Also expect an irregular respiratory rate and pattern, varying from slow and shallow to rapid and deep. (See *Normal vital signs in full-term neonates,* page 174.) Abnormally fast breath-

## Normal vital signs in full-term neonates

Use these ranges (or those established by your hospital) to guide assessment of neonatal status.

**Respiratory rate**
30 to 60 breaths/minute

**Heart rate (apical)**
110 to 160 beats/minute

**Temperature**
Axillary: 97.5° to 99° F (36.4° to 37.2° C)
Rectal: one degree higher

**Blood pressure**
Systolic: 60 to 80 mm Hg
Diastolic: 40 to 50 mm Hg

ing (tachypnea) may signal a perinatal problem. A lapse of 15 seconds or more after a complete respiratory cycle (one expiration and one inspiration) indicates apnea.
• Check for labored breathing (sometimes resulting from blocked nasal passages). Observe for uneven chest expansion, nasal flaring, visible chest retractions, expiratory grunts, and inspiratory stridor (a high-pitched sound audible without a stethoscope).
• *To evaluate breath sounds,* auscultate the anterior and posterior lung fields, placing the stethoscope over each lung lobe for at least 5 seconds for a total time of 1 minute. Normal breath sounds are clear and the same bilaterally. However, immediately after birth, you may hear a few crackles *resulting from retained fetal lung fluid.*
• Observe the chest as it rises and falls; normal movement should be symmetrical. Also, determine any difference between the anterior and posterior diameters of the chest, which normally should be equal. *Unequal diameters suggest hyperinflated lungs or respiratory distress.*

### Assessing heart rate
• Place the stethoscope over the apical pulse on the fourth or fifth intercostal space at the left midclavicular line over the cardiac apex. Listen to and count the heartbeats for 1 minute *to learn the heart rate and to detect any abnormalities in quality or rhythm.*
• If you hear an unorthodox rhythm, assess whether the irregularity follows a definite or random pattern. *This evaluation helps to identify the type of abnormality.* For example, atrial fibrillation is an irregular rhythm with an irregular pattern.
• Auscultate for variations from the normal "lub-dub" systole-diastole sounds. Determine whether the first and second heart sounds are separate and distinct or split into two sounds. Assess for extra heartbeats and sounds that stretch into the next sound. *Such abnormal sounds may indicate a heart murmur—from patent ductus arteriosus,* for example, as blood rushes through the ductus opening.

### Taking temperature rectally
• Wash your hands and put on gloves.
• With the neonate lying supine, firmly grasp his ankles with your index finger between them *to prevent skin trauma.* Place a diaper over the penis of a male neonate *to absorb urine if he urinates.*
• Still holding the neonate's ankles, insert the lubricated thermometer no more than ½" (1.3 cm)—*any farther could cause rectal injury.* Place the palm of your hand on his buttocks and hold the thermometer between your index and middle fingers. *This stabilizes the thermometer and prevents breakage* if the neonate moves suddenly. To inhibit the defecation response induced by inserting a rectal thermometer, press the buttocks together. If you meet resistance during insertion, withdraw the thermometer, and notify the doctor.
• Hold a mercury thermometer in place for 3 minutes and an electronic thermometer until the temperature registers (see "Temperature monitoring," Chapter 1). Remove the thermom-

eter and read the number on the scale where the mercury stops or on the digital display panel. Record the result.

### Taking an axillary temperature

• Dry the axillary skin. Then place the thermometer in the axilla and hold it along the outer aspect of the neonate's chest between the axillary line and the arm for at least 3 minutes *because axillary temperature takes this long to register.* Hold an electronic thermometer in place until the temperature registers.

• Reassess axillary temperature in 15 to 30 minutes if it registers outside the normal range. If the temperature remains abnormal, notify the doctor or nurse practitioner. *A subnormal temperature may result from infection, and an elevated temperature may result from dehydration or reflect the environment,* such as a malfunctioning overhead warmer.

• Document the temperature.

### Determining blood pressure

• Measure blood pressure in a quiet neonate.

• Be sure that the blood pressure cuff is small enough for the patient (cuff width: about half the circumference of the neonate's arm) because *the cuff size affects accurate readings.*

• Wrap the cuff one or two fingerbreadths above the antecubital or popliteal area. With the stethoscope held directly over the chosen artery, hold the cuffed extremity firmly with the same hand *to keep it extended* and then inflate the cuff no faster than 5 mm Hg/second.

• *To determine whether subsequent blood pressures measure within the neonate's normal range,* compare the readings to baseline values. Report any significant deviation.

### Special considerations

If desired, count respirations while auscultating the heart rate.

When listening to neonatal heart tones immediately after birth, you may hear murmurs. These may result from a delayed closing of fetal blood shunts.

Excessive neonatal activity—restlessness and crying during a vital signs assessment, for example—may elevate the heart rate above normal. For this reason, describe the neonate's activity along with measured findings.

### Documentation

Record vital signs and related measurements in your notes, on a special neonatal appraisal form, or on a flowchart. Include any observations about the neonate's condition, such as abnormal breath sounds.

## Neonatal size and weight monitoring

A beginning point for many neonatal assessments, measuring anthropometric dimensions and weight establishes the baseline for accurately monitoring normal growth. Size and weight measurements help detect such disorders as intrauterine growth retardation, small for gestational age, and hydrocephalus. You'll take these measurements in the nursery during routine checkups and sometimes at the neonate's home. You'll then compare the results with previous measurements and with normal values.

Normally the neonate's head circumference measures the same as or more than his chest circumference. The exception: the first 24 hours after birth when head molding leaves the head circumference slightly smaller than chest circumference. The head's contour usually returns to normal in 2 to 3 days.

The neonate's weight varies with sex, gestational age, heredity, and other factors. A first-born usually weighs less at birth than his siblings. The neonate with a diabetic mother tends to be large. Because of an erratic feeding pattern and passage of urine and meconium, the normal neonate loses between 5% and 10% of his birth weight during the first few days. However, he usually regains this weight in 10 days.

Normal weight gain for the neonate is 5 to 7 oz (140 to 200 g) weekly.

### Equipment
Crib or examination table with a firm surface ▪ scale with tray ▪ scale paper, if necessary ▪ tape measure ▪ length board ▪ gloves.

Disposable paper tape measures are available. Cloth tapes aren't recommended *because they can stretch, leading to inaccurate measurements.*

### Preparation of equipment
Put clean paper on the scale to promote warmth and prevent cold stress. Balance the scale at zero as directed by the manufacturer.

### Implementation
• Explain the procedure to the parents, if present. Wash your hands, and put on gloves.
• To begin, position the neonate supine in the crib or on the examination table. Remove all clothing but his diaper (if he has one). Be sure to record all measurements. (See *Average neonatal size and weight.*)

#### *Measuring head circumference*
• Slide the tape measure under the neonate's head at the occiput. *To arrive at the greatest circumference,* draw the tape snugly around, just above the eyebrows.

#### *Measuring chest circumference*
• Place the tape under the back and wrap it snugly around the chest at the nipple line. *To ensure accuracy,* keep the back and front of the tape level.
• Take the measurement after the neonate inspires and before he begins to exhale.

#### *Measuring head-to-heel length*
• Fully extend the neonate's legs with the toes pointing up. Measure the distance from the heel to the top of the head. If possible, have someone extend the legs by pressing down gently on the knees. Or use a length board, if available.

#### *Measuring crown-to-rump length*
• Place the neonate on his side and measure from the crown of his head to his buttocks. This measurement should approximate the head circumference.

#### *Weighing the neonate*
• Take this measurement before, not after, a feeding. Remove the neonate's diaper before placing him in the middle of the scale tray.
• Note the neonate's weight. Keep one hand poised over him at all times *to prevent accidents.* Work quickly *to avoid having the scale become soiled or wet and to prevent neonatal heat loss.*
• Return the neonate to the crib or examination table.
• If the neonate has clothing or equipment on him (such as an I.V. armband), be sure to record this information.
• Clean the scale tray *to prevent cross-contamination between neonates.*

#### *Measuring abdominal girth*
• Place the neonate supine, and measure his girth just above the umbilicus. Though not an anthropometric measurement, *the size of this expanse may suggest abnormalities—an obstruction, for example.*
• When you finish, dress and diaper the neonate. Return him to his crib, if necessary, or give him to a parent who can hold and comfort him.

### Special considerations
Keep in mind that head swelling or molding after delivery may skew initial head circumference measurements.

Another way to measure length is to place the neonate on paper, such as that used on examination tables. Mark the paper at the heel, with the toes pointing straight up, and at the head; measure the distance between the marks.

Various scale models are available. Be sure to learn how to read and operate the one available to you. If you use a model that measures met-

# Average neonatal size and weight

Besides weight, anthropometric measurements include head and chest circumferences, crown-to-rump length, and head-to-heel length (as shown below). These measurements serve as a baseline and show whether neonatal size is within normal ranges or whether there may be a significant problem or anomaly—especially if values stray far from the mean.

Initial average anthropometric ranges for a neonate follow:
• Head circumference: 13″ to 14″ (33 to 35 cm)
• Chest circumference: 12″ to 13″ (30 to 33 cm)
• Head-to-heel length: 18″ to 21″ (45 to 53 cm)
• Crown-to-rump length: about the same as head circumference
• Weight: 5 lb 8 oz to 8 lb 13 oz (2,500 to 4,000 g)

**Head circumference**

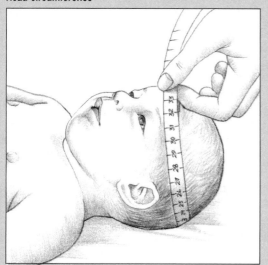

**Chest circumference**

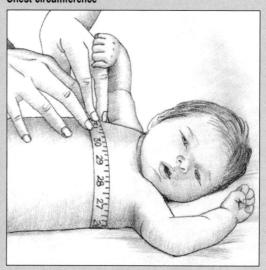

**Head-to-heel length**

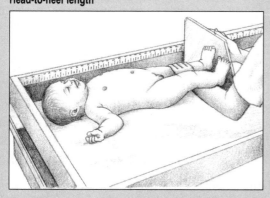

**Crown-to-rump length**

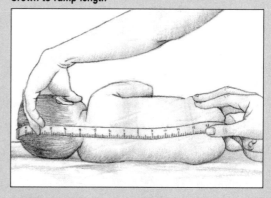

## Using a home apnea monitor

If a neonate in your care will require home apnea monitoring equipment, you'll need to prepare his parents to operate it safely, correctly, and confidently.

First, review the neonate's breathing problem with his parents. Explain that the monitor will warn them of breathing or heart rate changes. Then, offer the following guidelines:

• Advise parents to prepare their home and family for the equipment, for instance by providing a sturdy, flat surface for the monitor and by posting emergency telephone numbers (for the doctor, nurse, equipment supplier, ambulance) accessibly.

• Teach other responsible family members how to use the monitor safely. Also suggest that older siblings, grandparents, babysitters, and other caregivers learn cardiopulmonary resuscitation (CPR).

• Instruct parents to notify local service authorities—the police and ambulance, telephone, and electric companies—if their neonate uses an apnea monitor so that alternative power can be supplied if a failure occurs.

• Explain how a monitor with electrodes works. Teach parents to make sure the respirator indicator goes on each time the neonate breathes. If it doesn't, describe troubleshooting techniques, such as moving the electrodes slightly. Tell them to try this technique several times.

• Show parents how to respond to either the apnea or bradycardia alarm. Direct them to check the color of the neonate's oral tissues. If they appear bluish and the neonate isn't breathing, tell them to call loudly and touch him—gently at first, then more urgently as needed. Tell them to stop short of shaking him. If he doesn't respond, urge them to begin CPR.

• Also advise the parents to keep the operator's manual attached to or beside the monitor and to consult it as needed. Explain that an activated loose-lead alarm, for example, may indicate a dirty electrode, a loose electrode patch, a loose belt, or a disconnected or malfunctioning wire or monitor.

rically, supply the parents with a table of metric equivalents for use at home.

### Documentation

Record each weight and dimension measurement in your notes or on a neonatal assessment sheet.

During routine checkups, remember to share information with the parents, who may carry a booklet in which they also document weight and dimensions.

# Apnea monitoring in infants

If detected and treated at onset, apneic episodes may be reversed. Using an apnea monitor that signals when the breathing rate falls dangerously low may save the neonate who's vulnerable to apnea.

Apnea monitors may be used for vulnerable neonates, such as those born prematurely or those with neurologic disorders, neonatal respiratory distress syndrome, seizure disorders, congenital heart disease with congestive heart failure, a tracheostomy, a personal history of sleep-induced apnea, a family history of sudden infant death syndrome, or acute drug withdrawal.

In most common use are two types of monitors. The *thoracic impedance monitor* uses chest electrodes to detect conduction changes caused by respirations. Some monitors of this type also detect bradycardia. The *apnea mattress, or underpad monitor,* relies on a transducer connected to a pressure-sensitive pad, which detects pressure changes resulting from altered chest movements.

To guard against potentially life-threatening apneic episodes in vulnerable neonates, monitoring begins in the hospital and continues at home. Parents need to learn how to operate the monitor, what actions to take when the alarm sounds, and how to revive a neonate or an infant with cardiopulmonary resuscitation (CPR). Crucial steps for correctly using a monitor include testing the alarm system, positioning the sensor properly, and setting the controls correctly. (See *Using a home apnea monitor.*)

### Equipment

Monitor unit ▪ electrodes ▪ leadwires ▪ electrode belt ▪ electrode gel, if needed ▪ pressure transducer pad, if using apnea mattress ▪ stable surface for monitor placement.

Prepackaged and pretreated disposable electrodes are available.

## Implementation

• Explain the procedure to the parents, as appropriate, and wash your hands.

• Plug the monitor's power cord into a grounded wall outlet. Attach the leadwires to the electrodes, and attach the electrodes to the belt.

• To hold the electrodes securely in position, wrap the belt snugly but not restrictively around the neonate's chest at the point of greatest movement — optimally at the right and left midaxillary line about ⅘″ (2 cm) below the axilla. Be sure to position the leadwires according to the manufacturer's instructions.

• Follow the color code to connect the leadwires to the patient cable. Then connect the cable to the proper jack at the rear of the monitoring unit.

• Turn the sensitivity controls to maximum *to facilitate tuning when adjusting the system.*

• Set the alarms according to recommendations *so that an apneic period lasting for a specified time activates the signal.*

• Turn on the monitor. If the monitor has two alarms — one to signal apnea, one to signal bradycardia — both will sound until you adjust the monitor and reset the alarms according to the manufacturer's instructions.

• Adjust the sensitivity controls until the indicator lights blink with each breath and heartbeat.

• If you use an apnea mattress, assemble the monitor and pressure transducer pad according to the manufacturer's directions.

• Plug the monitor into a grounded wall outlet. Then plug the cable of the transducer pad into the monitor.

• Touch the pad to make sure it works. Watch for the monitor's respiration light to blink.

• Follow the manufacturer's instructions for pad placement.

• If you have difficulty obtaining a signal, place a foam rubber pad under the mattress, and sandwich the transducer pad between the foam pad and the mattress.

• If you hear the apnea or bradycardia alarm during monitoring, immediately check the neonate's respirations and color, but don't touch or disturb him *until you confirm apnea.*

• If he's still breathing and his color is good, readjust the sensitivity controls or reposition the electrodes, if necessary.

• If he isn't breathing, but his color looks normal, wait 10 seconds *to see if he starts breathing spontaneously.* If he isn't breathing and he appears pale, dusky, or blue, immediately try to stimulate breathing in these ways: Sequentially, place your hand on the neonate's back, rub him gently, or flick his soles gently. If he doesn't begin to breathe at once, start CPR and have someone call the doctor.

## Special considerations

*To ensure accurate operation,* don't put the monitor on top of any other electrical device. Make sure it's on a level surface and can't be bumped easily.

Avoid applying lotions, oils, or powders to the neonate's chest, *where they could cause the electrode belt to slip.* Periodically check the alarm by disconnecting the sensor plug. Then listen for the alarm to sound after the preset time delay.

## Complications

An apneic episode resulting from upper airway obstruction may not trigger the alarm if the neonate continues to make respiratory efforts without gas exchange. However, the monitor's bradycardia alarm may be triggered by the decreased heart rate resulting from vagal stimulation (which accompanies obstruction).

If you're using a thoracic impedance monitor without a bradycardia alarm, you may interpret bradycardia during apnea as shallow breathing. *That's because this type of monitor fails to distinguish between respiratory movement and the large cardiac stroke volume associated with bradycardia.* In this case, the alarm won't sound until the heart rate drops below the apnea limit.

## Neonatal pulse oximetry

Another noninvasive technique for monitoring oxygenation is pulse oximetry. The sensor of the pulse oximeter, which is attached to the neonate's foot, measures beat-to-beat arterial oxygen saturation. Normally, oxygenation values should drop no lower than 90%.

Don't be guided only by oximetric findings, though. Every 3 to 4 hours, you'll need to correlate laboratory values (from arterial blood gas analyses) with oximetric values for a reliable overview of neonatal status.

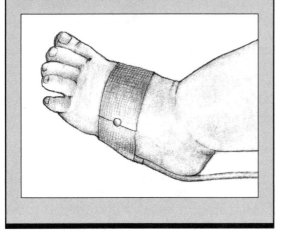

## Documentation
Record all alarm incidents. Document the time and duration of apnea. Describe the neonate's color, the stimulation measures implemented, and any other pertinent information.

# TcPO₂ monitoring in infants
A transcutaneous partial pressure of oxygen (TcPO$_2$) monitor measures the amount of oxygen diffusing through skin from capillaries directly beneath the surface. This measurement, which correlates closely with the neonate's partial pressure of oxygen in arterial blood (PaO$_2$), supplements traditional methods (observing skin color and taking periodic arterial blood gas [ABG] measurements) for detecting hypoxemia and hyperoxemia.

The monitor relies on a tiny electrode sensor applied to the skin. This sensor—a metallic, oxygen-sensitive device—warms to between 107.6° and 115° F (42° and 46° C). As the electrode's temperature increases (typically, to slightly higher than skin temperature), so does capillary blood flow. The increased vasodilation in cutaneous vessels enhances oxygen diffusion, which the electrode measures. The device may also be used to measure transcutaneous carbon dioxide.

This procedure is widely used in neonatal intensive care units by staff nurses trained to use the monitor. Because neonatal skin is thin with little subcutaneous fat, TcPO$_2$ monitoring produces accurate findings. However, in neonates with shock or hypoperfusion, the results seldom accurately reflect arterial oxygen levels. In these neonates, peripheral blood flow decreases as blood is shunted to the heart, brain, and lungs.

Another device for monitoring arterial oxygen levels is the pulse oximeter. (See *Neonatal pulse oximetry*.)

## Equipment
TcPO$_2$ monitor and electrode ■ cotton balls ■ soap and water ■ alcohol sponge ■ adhesive ring for electrode.

## Preparation of equipment
Set up the monitor, and calibrate it, if necessary, following manufacturer's instructions. Ensure that the strip chart recorder works properly.

## Implementation
• Wash your hands, don gloves, and decide where to place the electrode. Choose a flat site, with good capillary blood flow, few fatty deposits, and no bony prominences. Common sites include the neonate's upper chest, abdomen, and inner thigh.
• Clean the site first with a cotton ball and soap and water. Then wipe the site with an alcohol sponge *to remove dirt and oils and to ensure good electrode contact.*

• Dry the skin, attach the adhesive ring to the electrode, and moisten the skin site with a drop of water, according to the manufacturer's instructions, *to seal out all air.*
• Place the electrode on the site, and make sure that the adhesive ring is tight.
• Set the alarm switches and the electrode temperature according to the manufacturer's instructions or hospital policy.
• Expect the monitor reading to stabilize in 10 to 20 minutes. Normal oxygen pressures range from 50 to 80 mm Hg, but normal values also vary with the neonate and the equipment. TcPO₂ monitors usually have digital readouts and strip chart recorders to show trends.
• Rotate the electrode site every 4 hours *to prevent skin irritation, breakdown, or burns.*

### Special considerations

Expect TcPO₂ values to vary with neonatal movement and treatment. Also expect them to drop markedly whenever the neonate cries vigorously. But be prepared to start resuscitation if a sudden, significant drop in TcPO₂ occurs.

Remember that TcPO₂ monitoring doesn't replace ABG measurements, because it doesn't give information about partial pressure of arterial carbon dioxide and pH.

### Complications

Be alert for burns and blisters from the electrode and skin reactions to the adhesive ring.

### Documentation

Place graphic or printout results on the neonate's chart. Record the range of values observed during monitoring in your notes. Also record any skin disorders related to the electrode.

# APPENDICES

# Appendix 1: MANAGING PAIN

A common and always serious complaint, pain affects all areas of your patient's life. By learning more about pain and strategies to control it, you'll be better equipped to help relieve your patient's suffering.

## Understanding pain

Although pain originates in a physical stimulus, the mind shapes and defines its perception, making pain a highly subjective experience. Each person's pain is distinctive, shaped by his physiology, emotions, and life experiences.

As you provide care, accommodate your nursing assessment and interventions to your patient's type of pain—acute or chronic pain, for example. (See *Acute and chronic pain: How they differ,* page 184.)

### Acute pain

For the most part, you'll deal with acute pain more often in emergency rooms, surgical suites, and intensive care units. Sudden in onset, acute pain may trigger sympathetic nervous system responses, including sweating, tachycardia, and elevated blood pressure. If your patient has acute pain, you also may observe behavioral changes, such as grimacing, crying, restlessness, or other signs of distress.

### Chronic pain

Dealing with chronic pain can be overwhelming for the patient. In chronic pain, autonomic nervous system responses give way to depression and exhaustion. Without relief, chronic pain sufferers may undergo complete personality changes and isolate themselves from their family and friends.

## Compiling the pain history

To assess pain thoroughly, you'll need to consider the patient's description and your observations of his physical and behavioral responses. As you compile the pain history, keep your patient's assessment of his own pain paramount in your mind. Because pain is subjective, the person who can judge it most accurately is the patient.

Before you compile the history, consider any preconceptions you may have about pain that could interfere with your assessment. For instance, don't assume that a patient must appear to be in pain to be suffering intensely. Everyone responds to pain differently. Some patients bear their suffering stoically.

Consider also that the extent of the patient's disease or injury may not be a reliable indicator of his pain. How intensely your patient suffers depends, in part, on the meaning and context the pain has for him. Family, cultural, and spiritual values may increase or decrease his pain. What's more, physiologic factors make some patients more or less susceptible to pain.

As you continue the pain history, establish trust and rapport with your patient. The pain history may be his first opportunity to express his feelings about his pain. Another step toward helping the patient is believing him when he says he has pain. If he senses that you don't believe his responses, he may feel hopeless and be inclined to minimize or exaggerate his pain report.

When gathering information, use open-ended questions. Avoid asking questions that can be answered with a yes or a no—especially leading questions, such as "Would you describe your pain as throbbing?" Instead, use an open-ended statement such as "Tell me what your pain feels like."

## Acute and chronic pain: How they differ

Acute pain differs significantly from chronic pain in several ways. Technically, acute pain lasts less than 6 months; chronic pain lasts more than 6 months. This chart describes additional differences and related nursing considerations.

| TYPE | CHARACTERISTICS | NURSING CONSIDERATIONS |
|---|---|---|
| Acute | • Typically well localized<br>• Usually sharp; may radiate<br>• Generally arises from an acute injury or disease and subsides relatively quickly<br>• Associated with autonomic nervous system response | • Observe the patient for related signs and symptoms, including increased blood pressure, tachycardia, tachypnea, diaphoresis, pallor, mydriasis, restlessness, distractibility, apprehension, grimacing, and anxiety.<br>• Encourage the patient to express feelings about pain treatment. Typically, he expects pain to subside completely with therapy. |
| Chronic | • Commonly general; not well localized<br>• Typically described as dull, aching, diffuse, constant, nagging, intractable<br>• May be associated with an ongoing chronic disease or an aftereffect of previous disease or injury | • Expect the patient to exhibit such symptoms as extreme fatigue or exhaustion, listlessness, depression, and social withdrawal.<br>• Promote discussion of the patient's perception of pain and its treatment. Typically, he realizes that pain may continue, with treatment reducing (not necessarily eliminating) pain. |

Be sure you explore all aspects of the patient's pain, including onset and duration, location, quality and character, aggravating and mitigating factors, and related influences.

### Investigating onset and duration

Ask the patient when his pain began and how long he's had it. Find out if he recognizes any pattern to his pain. Does the pain occur suddenly? Is it episodic or long-term? Also inquire if your patient has more than one type of pain concurrently. For example, a cancer patient with shoulder pain may suddenly develop severe pain in the hip, which may represent metastasis or a fracture.

### Determining location

To help the patient accurately locate his pain, ask him to point to the painful areas of his body. Or provide him with a body diagram and ask him to mark the painful areas. If his pain radiates, ask him to indicate its most severe point and to trace its path.

### Describing quality and character

An accurate pain description may provide a clue to the condition causing the pain. For example, a patient with an ulcer may describe stomach pain as burning or gnawing.

Eliciting a good pain description, however, isn't always easy. Often, a patient can show you where he hurts but can't find the words to describe the pain. In such a case, try using a standard pain assessment tool. For example, ask the patient to scan a list of descriptive words and pick out terms that best describe his pain (see *Using pain assessment tools*).

### Identifying aggravating or mitigating factors

Explore the patient's history to find out what factors precipitate or hasten the occurrence of pain. For example, position changes, certain foods, and bodily functions, such as defecation and micturition, can aggravate some types of pain.

(Text continues on page 188.)

# Using pain assessment tools

Certain standardized formats offer ways to measure pain with more consistency and accuracy than do simple verbal reports. Used properly, the following assessment tools—the McGill-Melzack Pain Questionnaire, the Initial Pain Assessment Tool (developed by McCaffery and Beebe), a pain flow sheet, and visual and graphic rating scales—will provide a solid foundation for your nursing diagnoses and care planning.

### McGill-Melzack Pain Questionnaire
If your patient has chronic pain, the McGill-Melzack Pain Questionnaire may be the pain assessment tool for him. This form helps your patient describe the nature and intensity of his pain. Most patients can answer the self-explanatory questions and complete the form with little assistance from you.

## McGill-Melzack Pain Questionnaire

Patient's name _____ Age _____

File no. _____ Date _____

Clinical category (cardiac, neurologic, other) _____

Diagnosis _____

_____

_____

**Analgesic** (if already administered)

Type _____

Dosage _____

Time given in relation to this test _____

### Where is your pain?
Please mark on the drawings below the areas where you feel pain. Put *E* if external or *I* if internal near the areas you mark. Put *EI* if both external and internal.

### What does your pain feel like?
Some of the words below describe your *present* pain. Circle *ONLY* those words that best describe it. Leave out any category that is not suitable. Use only a single word in each appropriate category—the one that applies best.

| 1 | 5 | 9 | 14 | 18 |
|---|---|---|----|----|
| Flickering | Pinching | Dull | Punishing | Tight |
| Quivering | Pressing | Sore | Greuling | Numb |
| Pulsing | Gnawing | Hurting | Cruel | Drawing |
| Throbbing | Cramping | Aching | Vicious | Squeezing |
| Beating | Crushing | Heavy | Killing | Tearing |
| Pounding | | | | |
| | **6** | **10** | **15** | **19** |
| **2** | Tugging | Tender | Wretched | Cool |
| Jumping | Pulling | Taut | Blinding | Cold |
| Flashing | Wrenching | Rasping | | Freezing |
| Shooting | **7** | Splitting | **16** | |
| | Hot | | Annoying | **20** |
| **3** | Burning | **11** | Troublesome | Nagging |
| Pricking | Scalding | Tiring | Miserable | Nauseating |
| Boring | Searing | Exhausting | Intense | Agonizing |
| Drilling | | **12** | Unbearable | Dreadful |
| Stabbing | **8** | Sickening | | Torturing |
| Lancinating | Tingling | Suffocating | **17** | |
| | Itchy | | Spreading | |
| **4** | Smarting | **13** | Radiating | |
| Sharp | Stinging | Fearful | Penetrating | |
| Cutting | | Frightful | Piercing | |
| Lacerating | | Terrifying | | |

### How does your pain change with time?
Circle the word or words in each group that describe the *pattern* of your pain.

| Continuous | Constant | Periodic | Brief | Transient |
|---|---|---|---|---|
| Steady | Rhythmic | Intermittent | Momentary | |

What *relieves* your pain? _____

What *increases* your pain? _____

### How strong is your pain?
The following 5 words represent pain of increasing intensity. They are: 1 Mild  2 Discomforting  3 Distressing  4 Horrible  5 Excruciating

Write the number of the most appropriate word in the space beside the question.

- Which word describes your pain right now? _____
- Which word describes it at its worst? _____
- Which word describes it when it is lease severe? _____
- Which word describes the worst toothache you ever had? _____
- Which word describes the worst headache you ever had? _____
- Which word describes the worst stomachache you ever had? _____

Adapted from Melzack, R. *Pain*, vol.1. Amsterdam: Elsevier Science Publishing Co., 1975, with permission of the publisher.

*(continued)*

## Using pain assessment tools *(continued)*

### Initial Pain Assessment Tool

Another assessment tool that's useful for patients with chronic pain is the Initial Pain Assessment Tool, developed by Mc- Caffery and Beebe. This tool is well suited to clinical use. If you wish, use it as you interview the patient.

**Initial Pain Assessment Tool**

Date _____

Patient's name _____ Age _____ Room _____

Diagnosis _____ Doctor _____

Nurse _____

**Location** (Patient or nurse marks drawing.)

**Intensity scale** (Patient rates pain.): Present pain _____

Most severe pain _____ Least severe pain _____

Acceptable level of pain _____

**Quality** (Use patient's own words, for example, prick, ache, burn, throb, pull, sharp.) _____

**Onset, duration variations, rhythms** _____

**Manner of expressing pain** _____

**What relieves the pain?** _____

**What causes or increases the pain?** _____

**Effects of pain** (Note decreased function, decreased quality of life.)

Accompanying symptoms (for example, nausea) _____

Sleep _____

Appetite _____

Physical activity _____

Relationship with others (for example, irritability) _____

Emotions (such as anger, crying) _____

Concentration _____

**Treatment** _____

Adapted from McCaffery, M. and Beebe, A. *Pain: Clinical Manual for Nursing Practice.* Chicago: Mosby-Year Book, Inc., 1989, with permission of the publisher.

## Using pain assessment tools *(continued)*

### Pain flow sheet

The flow sheet may be the most convenient tool for pain assessment. Designed for ongoing assessment, this tool provides a standard for reevaluating the patient's pain at regular intervals. It's also beneficial for patients and families, who may feel too overwhelmed by the pain experience to answer a long, detailed questionnaire.

If possible, incorporate pain assessment into the flow sheet you're already using. Generally, the easier the flow sheet is to use, the more likely you and your patient will be to use it.

**PAIN FLOW SHEET**

| Date and time | Pain rating (0 to 10) | Patient behaviors | Vital signs | Pain rating after intervention | Comments |
|---|---|---|---|---|---|
| | | | | | |
| | | | | | |
| | | | | | |
| | | | | | |

### Visual analog pain scale

In a visual analog pain scale, the patient marks a linear scale with words or numbers that correspond to his perceived degree of pain. You can easily draw a scale to represent a continuum of pain intensity. Verbal anchors describe the pain's intensity; for example, "no pain" begins the scale and "pain as bad as it could possibly be" ends it.

To use this scale, simply ask the patient to mark the point on the continuum that best describes his pain. These scales are especially useful for assessing acute postoperative pain.

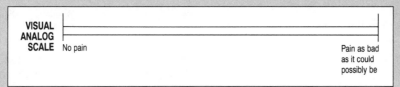

### Graphic rating scales

Other types of rating scales that are useful for acute pain have words that represent pain intensity. Use these graphic rating scales as you would the visual analog scale. Have the patient mark the spot on the continuum that best describes his pain.

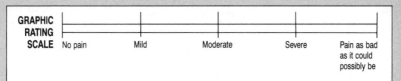

Perform a psychosocial assessment to evaluate how personal, emotional, and social conditions may contribute to the pain experience. If the patient feels depressed, socially isolated, or under stress, his perception of pain may be intensified. Likewise, explore measures the patient uses to cope with pain, such as relaxation or distraction. By knowing what's likely to worsen or relieve your patient's pain, you can devise a more effective plan of care.

### Examining attitudes

Find out how the patient's background shapes his responses to pain. Ask such questions as:
• How do you think your pain affects your family? (Is it bringing them closer together, causing problems, or having no effect?)
• How do you think your pain affects your daily life? (Does it interfere with your work? Does it affect your social activities?)
• What activities or remedies have you and your family tried to relieve your pain? For example, do you ever try to distract yourself by listening to music, by reading, or by watching television?
• How do you view your illness in general? How do you feel about your control over it?
• What do you think causes your pain?

### Assessing associated physical effects

Finally, assess your patient for signs and symptoms related to pain, such as:
• blood pressure changes
• tachycardia
• skin color changes
• diminished pulses
• diaphoresis
• hyperventilation.

Observe closely for facial expressions and body postures that reflect pain and anxiety. Be sure to record your findings.

## Reviewing the physiology of pain

The more you know about pain physiology, the better you'll understand pain-relief strategies. Over the years, several theories have evolved to explain how and why we feel pain.

### Pain theories

The oldest explanation of pain — *the specificity theory* — assumes the existence of specific pain receptors that respond only to painful stimuli. Pain travels from these receptors along specific neural pathways to the spinal cord and brain.

Though useful for explaining how pain travels along neural pathways, this theory has several flaws. A major flaw assumes that specific fibers carry only pain impulses. Scientists now know that some nerve fibers carry several types of sensory impulses, such as pain, thermal, and pressure sensations.

According to the *pattern theory*, receptors generate pain impulses that form a pattern. This pattern informs the central nervous system (CNS) of pain's presence. The pattern theory proposes that different patterns of activity in the same neuron can signal a painful or nonpainful stimulus. For example, a light tap on the skin might cause receptors to discharge impulses at a low frequency, signaling touch. But a sharp pinch might cause the same receptors to fire at a higher rate, signaling pain.

Known as the *gate theory*, the most recent and widely accepted explanation of pain borrows elements from the specificity and pattern theories. This theory proposes that pain is modulated by a gating mechanism located in the spinal cord and by activity in higher CNS structures. According to this theory, pain impulses travel to the dorsal horn of the spinal cord, where they encounter a gate, thought to be substantia gelatinosa cells.

If the gate is open, pain impulses ascend the spinal cord to the brain, resulting in pain perception. If the gate is closed, pain impulses can't proceed. According to this theory, various factors control the gate, thereby influencing pain perception. (See *Gate theory of pain*.)

## Structures of pain perception

Pain receptors, also called nociceptors, are free nerve endings sensitive to painful mechanical, thermal, electrical, or chemical stimuli. Located in many areas of the body, these nerve endings, when stimulated, generate afferent (sensory) impulses. These impulses transmit the pain message to the spinal cord, then to the brain, which interprets the message and perceives pain.

Pain impulses travel to the spinal cord along two types of small-diameter nerve fibers: A-delta and C fibers. A-delta fibers, which are myelinated, transmit fast pain. Fast pain is a brief, well-localized sensation — for example, a pinprick or a sharp pinch. Pain receptors attached to A-delta fibers are mostly found in the skin and muscle and respond primarily to mechanical stimuli.

C fibers are unmyelinated or poorly myelinated. These fibers transmit slow pain: dull, aching, or burning sensations that are poorly localized. Stimulation of the pain receptors attached to these fibers produces more continuous and constant pain, primarily in response to thermal, chemical, and mechanical stimuli. Pain receptors that convey slow pain are typically found in deep tissues, such as internal organs, joints, and muscles.

Pain impulses from both types of fibers enter the spinal cord at the dorsal nerve root. There they form a synapse at the substantia gelatinosa, cross over to the lateral spinothalamic tract, ascend to the thalamus, and eventually reach the higher cortical centers responsible for pain perception.

Large-diameter fibers, called A-beta fibers, from the body's periphery, mainly the skin, transmit impulses to the same area as the small-diameter nerve fibers. Stimulation of these large fibers may override the nociceptive impulses from the small fibers, blocking transmission of the pain impulse at the dorsal horn of the brain.

## Pain centers in the brain

Various areas within the brain work together to raise awareness of pain, to interpret painful stimuli, and to produce motor and affective responses to pain. Among the most important brain centers for pain perception are:
- the thalamus, which receives sensory input from the spinothalamic tract and relays it to other parts of the brain
- the midbrain, which signals the cerebral cortex to increase awareness of noxious stimuli
- the cerebral cortex, which discerns well-localized pain and the cognitive aspects of pain perception.

Certain brain structures may also modulate pain perception. For example, under some circumstances, the cerebral cortex may actually suppress pain. The brain relays its responses along descending pathways of efferent fibers that extend from the cerebral cortex and brain stem down the spinal cord. In theory, these pathways act to close the gate in the substantia gelatinosa, inhibiting the transmission of pain impulses.

## Role of neuromodulators

In addition, several neuromodulators play an important role in pain transmission. Neuromodulators are polypeptides that act on postsynaptic membranes to inhibit or amplify the effects of neurotransmitters.

Among the most significant neuromodulators are the endogenous opioid peptides: alpha- and beta-endorphins and enkephalins. These natural opiate-like substances produce analgesic effects. By binding with opiate receptors throughout the nervous system, they inhibit the release of certain neurotransmitters involved in pain transmission.

The larger peptides, the endorphins, are produced by the anterior pituitary gland and the hypothalamus. They exert more prolonged analgesic effects than enkephalin. Enkephalin, a small polypeptide, is found in the dorsal horn of the spinal cord and various parts of the brain. Certain palliative therapies, such as acupuncture and transcutaneous electrical nerve stimulation, may work because they stimulate release of endogenous opioids.

Endorphin and enkephalin activity may also be enhanced by vigorous exercise and antidepressant therapy. Pain and stress also activate the endogenous opiates, triggering an internal feedback loop that promotes analgesia in response to pain and stress.

# Appendix 2: LABORATORY TEST VALUES

## A

**AChR antibodies, serum**
negative or ≤ 0.03 nmol/liter

**Acid mucopolysaccharides, urine**
age 2: 8 to 30 mg glucuronic acid/
g of creatinine
age 4: 7 to 27
age 6: 6 to 24
age 8: 4 to 22
age 10: 2 to 18
age 12: 0 to 15
age 14: 0 to 12

**Acid phosphatase, serum**
0.5 to 1.9 U/liter

**ACTH, plasma**
< 60 pg/ml

**ACTH, rapid test, plasma**
Cortisol rises 7 to 18 μg/dl above
baseline, 60 minutes after injection

**Activated partial thromboplastin time**
25 to 36 seconds

**Alanine aminotransferase**
*Men:* 10 to 32 U/liter
*Women:* 9 to 24 U/liter

**Albumin, peritoneal fluid**
50% to 70% of total protein

**Albumin, serum**
3.3 to 4.5 g/dl

**Aldosterone, serum**
1 to 16 ng/dl
4 to 31 ng/dl (standing for 2 hours)

**Aldosterone, urine**
2 to 16 μg/24 hours

**Alkaline phosphatase, peritoneal fluid**
*Men:* > age 18, 90 to 239 U/liter
*Women:* < age 45, 76 to 196 U/liter;
> age 45, 87 to 250 U/liter

**Alkaline phosphatase, serum**
1.5 to 4 Bodansky units/dl
4 to 13.5 King-Armstrong units/dl
*Chemical inhibition method:*
Men, 90 to 239 U/liter
Women < age 45, 76 to 196 U/liter
Women > age 45, 87 to 250 U/liter

**Alpha-fetoprotein, amniotic fluid**
≤ 18.5 μg/ml at 13 or 14 weeks

**Alpha-fetoprotein, serum**
*Nonpregnant women:* 0 to 6.4 IU/ml

**Amino acids, urine**
50 to 200 mg/24 hours

**Ammonia, peritoneal fluid**
< 50 μg/dl

**Ammonia, plasma**
< 50 μg/dl

**Amniotic fluid**
*Lecithin/sphingomyelin ratio:* > 2
*Meconium:* Absent
*Phosphatidiglycerol:* Present

**Amylase, peritoneal fluid**
138 to 404 amylase units/liter

**Amylase, serum**
30 to 220 U/liter

**Amylase, urine**
10 to 80 amylase units/hour

**Androstenedione**
*Men:* 0.9 to 1.7 ng/ml
*Menstruating women:* 0.6 to 3 ng/ml
*Postmenopausal women:* 0.3 to 8 ng/ml

**Angiotensin-converting enzyme**
> age 20: 18 to 67 U/liter

**Anion gap**
8 to 14 mEq/liter

**Antibodies to extractable nuclear antigens**
Negative

**Antibody screening, serum**
Negative

**Anti-deoxyribonucleic acid antibodies, serum**
< 7.0 IU/ml

**Antidiuretic hormone, serum**
1 to 5 pg/ml

**Antiglobulin test, direct**
Negative

**Antimitochondrial antibodies, serum**
Negative at titer < 20

**Antinuclear antibodies, serum**
Negative at ≤ 1:40 using Hep-2 cell

**Anti-Smith antibodies**
Negative

**Anti-smooth-muscle antibodies, serum**
Normal titer < 1:20

**Antistreptolysin-O, serum**
< 120 Todd units/ml

**Antithrombin III**
> 50% of normal control values

**Antithyroid antibodies, serum**
Normal titer < 1:100

**Arginine test**
*Men:* hgH increases to > 10 ng/ml
*Women:* hgH increases to > 15 ng/ml

**Arterial blood gases**
*pH:* 7.35 to 7.42
*Pa$O_2$:* 75 to 100 mm Hg
*Pa$CO_2$:* 35 to 45 mm Hg
*$O_2$CT:* 15% to 23%
*Sa$O_2$:* 94% to 100%
*$HCO_3^-$:* 22 to 26 mEq/liter

**Arylsulfatase A, urine**
*Men:* 1.4 to 19.3 U/liter
*Women:* 1.4 to 11 U/liter

**Aspartate aminotransferase**
8 to 20 U/liter

**Aspergillosis antibody, serum**
Normal titer < 1:8

**Atrial natriuretic factor, plasma**
20 to 77 pg/ml

**B**

**B-hydroxybutyrate**
< 0.4 mmol/liter

**B-lymphocyte count**
270 to 640/mm$^3$

**Bacterial meningitis antigen**
Negative

**Bence Jones protein, urine**
Negative

**Bilirubin, amniotic fluid**
Absent at term

**Bilirubin, serum**
*Adult:* Direct, < 0.5 mg/dl;
indirect, ≤ 1.1 mg/dl
*Neonate:* Total, 1.0 to 12.0 mg/dl

**Bilirubin, urine**
Negative

**Blastomycosis antibody, serum**
Normal titer < 1:8

**Bleeding time**
*Modified template:* 2 to 10 minutes
*Template:* 2 to 8 minutes
*Ivy:* 1 to 7 minutes
*Duke:* 1 to 3 minutes

**Blood urea nitrogen**
8 to 20 mg/dl

**C**

**C-reactive protein, serum**
Negative

**Calcitonin, plasma**
*Baseline:* Males, ≤ 0.155 ng/ml;
females, ≤ 0.105 ng/ml
*Calcium infusion:* Males, 0.265 ng/ml;
females, 0.120 ng/ml
*Pentagastrin infusion:* Males, 0.210 ng/ml;
females, 0.105 ng/ml

**Calcium, serum**
4.5 to 5.5 mEq/liter
*Atomic absorption:* 8.9 to 10.1 mg/dl

**Calcium, urine**
*Men:* < 275 mg/24 hours
*Women:* < 250 mg/24 hours
***Candida* antibody, serum**
Negative
**Capillary fragility**

| *Petechiae per 5 cm:* | *Score:* |
|---|---|
| 0 to 10 | 1 + |
| 10 to 20 | 2 + |
| 20 to 50 | 3 + |
| 50 | 4 + |

**Carbon dioxide, total, blood**
22 to 34 mEq/liter
**Carcinoembryonic antigen, serum**
< 5 ng/ml
**Cardiolipin antibodies**
1:2 titer: negative
1:8 titer: positive
**Carotene, serum**
48 to 200 µg/dl
**Catecholamines, plasma**
*Supine:* Epinephrine, 0 to 110 pg/ml;
norepinephrine, 70 to 750 pg/ml;
dopamine, 0 to 30 pg/ml
*Standing:* Epinephrine, 0 to 140 pg/ml;
norepinephrine, 200 to 1,700 pg/ml;
dopamine, 0 to 30 pg/ml
**Catecholamines, urine**
*24-hour specimen:* 0 to 135 µg
*Random specimen:* 0 to 18 µg/dl
**Cerebrospinal fluid**
*Pressure:* 50 to 180 mm $H_2O$
*Appearance:* Clear, colorless
*Gram stain:* No organisms
**Ceruloplasmin, serum**
25 to 43 mg/dl
**Chloride, cerebrospinal fluid**
118 to 130 mEq/liter
**Chloride, serum**
100 to 108 mEq/liter

**Chloride, sweat**
10 to 35 mEq/liter
**Chloride, urine**
110 to 250 mEq/24 hours
**Cholesterol, total, serum**
0 to 240 mg/dl
**Cholinesterase (pseudocholinesterase)**
8 to 18 U/ml
**Chorionic gonadotropin, serum**
< 3 mIU/ml
**Chorionic gonadotropin, urine**
*Pregnant women:* First trimester,
≤ 500,000 IU/24 hours; second
trimester, 10,000 to 25,000 IU/
24 hours; third trimester, 5,000 to
15,000 IU/24 hours
**Clot retraction**
50%
**Coccidioidomycosis antibody, serum**
Normal titer < 1:2
**Cold agglutinins, serum**
Normal titer < 1:32
**Complement, serum**
*Total:* 330 to 730 $CH_{50}$ units
*C1 esterase inhibitor:* 7.8 to 23.4 mg/dl
*C3:* 57 to 125 mg/dl
*C4:* 10 to 54 mg/dl
**Complement, synovial fluid**
*10 mg protein/dl:* 3.7 to 33.7 units/ml
*20 mg protein/dl:* 7.7 to 37.7 units/ml
**Copper, urine**
15 to 60 µg/24 hours
**Copper reduction test, urine**
Negative
**Coproporphyrin, urine**
*Men:* 0 to 96 µg/24 hours
*Women:* 1 to 57 µg/24 hours
**Cortisol, free, urine**
24 to 108 µg/24 hours

**Cortisol, plasma**
    *Morning:* 7 to 28 µg/dl
    *Afternoon:* 2 to 18 µg/dl
**Creatine kinase**
    *Total:* Men, 25 to 130 U/liter;
       women, 10 to 150 U/liter
    *CK-BB:* None
    *CK-MB:* 0 to 7 U/liter
    *CK-MM:* 5 to 70 U/liter
    *CK-MB$_2$:* < 1 U/liter
    *CK-MB$_2$/CK-MB$_1$:* < 5 U/liter
**Creatine, serum**
    *Men:* 0.2 to 0.6 mg/dl
    *Women:* 0.6 to 1 mg/dl
**Creatinine, amniotic fluid**
    > 2 mg/dl in mature fetus
**Creatinine clearance**
    *Men:* 107 to 139 ml/minute
    *Women:* 87 to 107 ml/minute
**Creatinine, serum**
    *Men:* 0.8 to 1.2 mg/dl
    *Women:* 0.6 to 0.9 mg/dl
**Creatinine, urine**
    *Men:* 1 to 1.9 g/24 hours
    *Women:* 0.8 to 1.7 g/24 hours
**Cryoglobulins, serum**
    Negative
**Cryptococcosis antigen, serum**
    Negative
**Cyclic adenosine monophosphate, urine**
    *Parathyroid hormone infusion:* 3.6- to
       4-µmol increase
**Cytomegalovirus antibody, serum**
    Negative

**D**
**Delta-aminolevulinic acid, urine**
    1.5 to 7.5 mg/dl/24 hours

**D-xylose absorption**
    *Blood:* Children, > 30 mg/dl in 1 hour;
       adults, 25 to 40 mg/dl in 2 hours
    *Urine:* Children, 16% to 33% excreted in
       5 hours; adults, > 3.5 g excreted in
       5 hours

**E**
**Epstein-Barr virus antibodies**
    Negative
**Erythrocyte distribution, fetal-maternal**
    No fetal RBCs
**Erythrocyte sedimentation rate**
    *Men:* 0 to 10 mm/hour
    *Women:* 0 to 20 mm/hour
**Esophageal acidity**
    pH > 5.0
**Estriol, amniotic fluid**
    *16 to 20 weeks:* 25.7 ng/ml
    *Term:* < 1,000 ng/ml
**Estrogens, serum**
    *Menstruating women:*
       day 1 to 10, 24 to 68 pg/ml;
       day 11 to 20, 50 to 186 pg/ml;
       day 21 to 30, 73 to 149 pg/ml
    *Men:* 12 to 34 pg/ml
**Estrogens, total urine**
    *Menstruating women:* follicular phase, 5 to
       25 µg/24 hours; ovulatory phase, 24
       to 100 µg/24 hours; luteal phase, 12 to
       80 µg/24 hours
    *Postmenopausal women:* < 10 µg/24 hours
    *Men:* 4 to 25 µg/24 hours
**Euglobulin lysis time**
    ≥ 2 hours

**F**
**Factor assay**
    50% to 150% of normal activity

**Febrile agglutination, serum**
 Salmonella *antibody:* < 1:80
 *Brucellosis antibody:* < 1:80
 *Tularemia antibody:* < 1:40
 *Rickettsial antibody:* < 1:40
**Ferritin, serum**
 *Men:* 20 to 300 ng/ml
 *Women:* 20 to 120 ng/ml
**Fibrin split products**
 *Screening assay:* < 10 μg/ml
 *Quantitative assay:* < 3 μg/ml
**Fibrinogen, peritoneal fluid**
 0.3% to 4.5% of total protein
**Fibrinogen, plasma**
 195 to 365 mg/dl
**Fibrinogen, pleural fluid**
 *Transudate:* Absent
 *Exudate:* Present
**Fluorescent treponemal absorption, serum**
 Negative
**Folic acid, serum**
 3 to 16 ng/ml
**Follicle-stimulating hormone, serum**
 *Menstruating women:* Follicular phase, 5
 to 20 mIU/ml; ovulatory phase, 15 to
 30 mIU/ml; luteal phase, 5 to 15 mIU/
 ml
 *Menopausal women:* 5 to 100 mIU/ml
 *Men:* 5 to 20 mIU/ml
**Free thyroxine, serum**
 0.8 to 3.3 ng/dl
**Free triiodothyronine**
 0.2 to 0.6 ng/dl

**G**
**Galactose-1-phosphate uridyltransferase**
 *Qualitative:* negative
 *Quantitative:* 18.5 to 28.5 mU/g of
 hemoglobin

**Gamma-glutamyltransferase**
 *Men:* 8 to 37 U/liter
 *Women:* < age 45, 5 to 27 U/liter;
 > age 45, 6 to 37 U/liter
**Gastric acid stimulation**
 *Men:* 18 to 28 mEq/hour
 *Women:* 11 to 21 mEq/hour
**Gastric secretion, basal**
 *Men:* 1 to 5 mEq/hour
 *Women:* 0.2 to 3.8 mEq/hour
**Gastrin, serum**
 < 300 pg/ml
**Globulin, peritoneal fluid**
 30% to 45% of total protein
**Globulin, serum**
 *Alpha$_2$:* 0.1 to 0.4 g/dl
 *Alpha$_2$:* 0.5 to 1.0 g/dl
 *Beta:* 0.7 to 1.2 g/dl
 *Gamma:* 0.5 to 1.6 g/dl
**Glucagon, serum, fasting**
 < 250 pg/ml
**Glucose, amniotic fluid**
 < 45 mg/dl
**Glucose, cerebrospinal fluid**
 50 to 80 mg/dl
**Glucose, peritoneal fluid**
 70 to 100 mg/dl
**Glucose, plasma, fasting**
 70 to 100 mg/dl
**Glucose, plasma, oral tolerance**
 Peak at 160 to 180 mg/dl, 30 to
 60 minutes after challenge dose
**Glucose, plasma, 2-hour postprandial**
 < 145 mg/dl
**Glucose-6-phosphate dehydrogenase**
 8.6 to 18.6 U/g of hemoglobin
**Glucose, synovial fluid**
 70 to 100 mg/dl
**Glucose, urine**
 Negative

**Glutathione reductase activity index**
0.9 to 1.3
**Growth hormone, serum**
*Men:* 0 to 5 ng/ml
*Women:* 0 to 10 ng/ml
**Growth hormone suppression**
0 to 3 ng/ml after 30 minutes to 2 hours

**H**
**HAM (acidified serum lysis test)**
Negative RBC hemolysis
**Haptoglobin, serum**
38 to 270 mg/dl
**Heinz bodies**
Negative
**Hematocrit**
*Men:* 42% to 54%
*Women:* 38% to 46%
**Hemoglobin electrophoresis**
*Hb A:* 95%
*Hb A₂:* 2% to 3%
*Hb F:* < 1%
**Hemoglobin, glycosylated**
*Hb $A_{1a}$:* 1.6% of total RBC Hb
*Hb $A_{1b}$:* 0.8% of total RBC Hb
*Hb $A_{1c}$:* 5% of total RBC Hb
*Total glycosylated Hb:* 5.5% to 9%
**Hemoglobin, total**
*Men:* 14 to 18 g/dl
*Women:* 12 to 16 g/dl
**Hemoglobin, urine**
Negative
**Hemoglobins, unstable**
*Heat stability:* Negative
*Isopropanol:* Stable
**Hemosiderin, urine**
Negative
**Hepatitis-B surface antigen, serum**
Negative

**Herpes simplex antibodies, serum**
Negative
**Heterophil agglutination, serum**
Normal titer < 1:56
**Hexosaminidase A and B, serum**
*Total:* 5 to 12.9 U/liter
(Hex A is 55% to 76% of total)
**Histoplasmosis antibody, serum**
*Normal titer:* < 1:8
**Homovanillic acid, urine**
< 8 mg/24 hours
**Human immunodeficiency virus antibody, serum**
Negative
**Hydroxybutyric dehydrogenase**
*Serum HBD:* 114 to 290 U/ml
*LD/HBD ratio:* 1.2 to 1.6:1
**17-Hydroxycorticosteroids, urine**
*Men:* 4.5 to 12 mg/24 hours
*Women:* 2.5 to 10 mg/24 hours
**5-Hydroxyindoleacetic acid, urine**
< 6 mg/24 hours

**I**
**Immune complex assays, serum**
Negative
**Immunoglobulins, serum**
*IgG:* 700 to 1,800 ng/dl
*IgA:* 70 to 440 ng/dl
*IgM:* 60 to 290 ng/dl
**Insulin, serum**
0 to 25 μU/ml
**Insulin tolerance test**
10 to 20 ng/dl increase over baseline
human growth hormone and ACTH
**Inulin clearance, urine**
≥ *Age 21:* 90 to 130 ml/minute
**Iron, serum**
*Men:* 70 to 150 μg/dl
*Women:* 80 to 150 μg/dl

**Iron, total binding capacity, serum**
*Men:* 300 to 400 µg/dl
*Women:* 300 to 450 µg/dl
**Isocitrate dehydrogenase**
1.2 to 7 units/liter

**JK**
**17-Ketogenic steroids, urine**
*Men:* 4 to 14 mg/24 hours
*Women:* 2 to 12 mg/24 hours
**Ketones, urine**
Negative
**17-Ketosteroids, urine**
*Men:* 6 to 21 mg/24 hours
*Women:* 4 to 17 mg/24 hours

**L**
**Lactate dehydrogenase**
*Total:* 48 to 115 IU/liter
*LD$_1$:* 14% to 26%
*LD$_2$:* 29% to 39%
*LD$_3$:* 20% to 26%
*LD$_4$:* 8% to 16%
*LD$_5$:* 6% to 16%
**Lactic acid, blood**
0.93 to 1.65 mEq/liter
**Leucine aminopeptidase**
< 50 units/liter
**Leukoagglutinins**
Negative
**Lipase**
< 300 U/liter
**Lipids, amniotic fluid**
> 20% of lipid-coated cells stain orange
**Lipids, fecal**
< 20% of excreted solids;
< 7 g/24 hours
**Lipoproteins, serum**
*High-density lipoproteins:* 29 to 77 mg/dl
*Low-density lipoproteins:* 62 to 185 mg/dl

**Long-acting thyroid stimulator, serum**
Negative
**Lupus erythematosus cell preparation**
Negative
**Luteinizing hormone, plasma**
*Menstruating women:* Follicular phase,
5 to 15 mIU/ml; ovulatory phase,
30 to 60 mIU/ml; luteal phase, 5 to
15 mIU/ml
*Postmenopausal women:* 50 to 100 mIU/ml
*Men:* 5 to 20 mIU/ml
**Lyme disease antibody**
Normal titer < 90
**Lymphocyte transformation**
60% to 90% of lymphocytes respond
**Lysozyme, urine**
< 3 mg/24 hours

**M**
**Magnesium, serum**
1.5 to 2.5 mEq/liter
*Atomic absorption:* 1.7 to 2.1 mg/dl
**Magnesium, urine**
< 150 mg/24 hours
**Manganese, serum**
0.04 to 1.4 µg/dl
**Melanin, urine**
Negative
**Myoglobin, urine**
Negative

**N**
**Neonatal thyroid-stimulating hormone**
≤ Age 2 days: 25 to 30 µIU/ml
> Age 2 days: < 25 µIU/ml
**5'-Nucleotidase**
2 to 17 U/liter

## O

**Occult blood, fecal**
< 2.5 ml/24 hours
**Ornithine carbamoyltransferase, serum**
0 to 500 Sigma units/ml
**Oxalate, urine**
≤ 40 mg/24 hours

## PQ

**Para-aminohippuric acid excretion, urine**
*Age 20:* 400 to 700 ml/minute (decrease of 17 ml/minute each decade after age 20)
**Parathyroid hormone, serum**
*Intact PTH:* 210 to 310 pg/ml
*N-terminal fraction:* 230 to 630 pg/ml
*C-terminal fraction:* 410 to 1,760 pg/ml
**Pericardial fluid**
*Amount:* 10 to 50 ml
*Appearance:* Clear, straw-colored
*White blood cell count:* < 1,000/mm³
*Glucose:* approximately whole blood level
**Peritoneal fluid**
*Amount:* < 50 ml
*Appearance:* Clear, straw-colored
**Phenolsulfonphthalein excretion, urine**
*15 minutes:* 25% of dose excreted
*30 minutes:* 50% to 60% of dose excreted
*1 hour:* 60% to 70% of dose excreted
*2 hours:* 70% to 80% of dose excreted
**Phenylalanine, serum, screening**
*Negative:* < 2 mg/dl
**Phosphate, tubular reabsorption, urine and plasma**
80% reabsorption
**Phosphates, serum**
1.8 to 2.6 mEq/liter
*Atomic absorption:* 2.5 to 4.5 mg/dl
**Phosphates, urine**
< 1,000 mg/24 hours

**Phospholipids, plasma**
180 to 320 mg/dl
**Placental lactogen, serum**
*Pregnant women:* 5 to 27 weeks, < 4.6 µg/ml; 28 to 31 weeks, 2.4 to 6.1 µg/ml; 32 to 35 weeks, 3.7 to 7.7 µg/ml; 36 weeks to term, 5 to 8.6 µg/ml
*Nonpregnant women:* < 0.5 µg/ml
*Men:* < 0.5 µg/ml
**Plasma plasminogen**
*Immunologic method:* 10 to 20 ng/ml
*Functional method:* 80 to 120 U/ml
**Plasma renin activity**
*Sodium-depleted, peripheral vein (upright position):* Ages 18 to 39, 2.9 to 24 ng/ml/hour; age 40 and over, 2.9 to 10.8 ng/ml/hour
*Sodium-replete, peripheral vein (upright position):* Ages 18 to 39, 0.6 to 4.3 ng/ml/hour; age 40 and over, 0.6 to 3.0 ng/ml/hour
**Platelet aggregation**
3 to 5 minutes
**Platelet count**
130,000 to 370,000/mm³
**Platelet survival**
50% tagged platelets disappear within 84 to 116 hours; 100% disappear within 8 to 10 days
**Pleural fluid**
*Appearance:* Clear (transudate); cloudy, turbulent (exudate)
*Specific gravity:* < 1.016 (transudate); > 1.016 (exudate)
**Porphobilinogen, urine**
≤ 1.5 mg/24 hours
**Porphyrins, total**
16 to 60 mg/dl of packed RBCs
**Potassium, serum**
3.8 to 5.5 mEq/liter

**Potassium, urine**
25 to 125 mEq/24 hours
**Pregnanediol, urine**
*Men:* 1.5 mg/24 hours
*Women:* 0.5 to 1.5 mg/24 hours
*Postmenopausal women:* 0.2 to 1 mg/
24 hours
**Pregnanetriol, urine**
< 3.5 mg/24 hours
**Progesterone, plasma**
*Menstrual cycle:*
Follicular phase, < 150 ng/dl
Luteal phase, 300 ng/dl
Midluteal phase, 2,000 ng/dl
*Pregnancy:* First trimester, 1,500 to 5,000
ng/dl; second and third trimesters,
8,000 to 20,000 ng/dl
**Prolactin, serum**
0 to 23 ng/dl
**Protein, cerebrospinal fluid**
15 to 45 mg/dl
**Protein, pleural fluid**
*Transudate:* < 3 g/dl
*Exudate:* > 3 g/dl
**Protein, total, peritoneal fluid**
0.3 to 4.1 g/dl
**Protein, total, serum**
6.6 to 7.9 g/dl
*Albumin fraction:* 3.3 to 4.5 g/dl
*Globulin levels:*
alpha$_1$-globulin, 0.1 to 0.4 g/dl
alpha$_2$-globulin, 0.5 to 1 g/dl
beta globulin, 0.7 to 1.2 g/dl
gamma globulin, 0.5 to 1.6 g/dl
**Protein, total, synovial fluid**
10.7 to 21.3 mg/dl
**Protein, urine**
≤ 150 mg/24 hours
**Protein C, plasma**
70% to 140%

**Prothrombin consumption time**
20 seconds
**Prothrombin time**
10 to 14 seconds
**Protoporphyrins**
16 to 60 mg/dl
**Pulmonary artery pressure**
*Right atrial pressure:* 1 to 6 mm Hg
*Right ventricular systolic:* 20 to 30 mm Hg
*Right ventricular end-diastolic:* < 5 mm Hg
*Pulmonary artery systolic pressure:* 20 to
30 mm Hg
*Pulmonary artery diastolic pressure:*
approximately 10 mm Hg
*Mean PAP:* < 20 mm Hg
*PAWP:* 6 to 12 mm Hg
*Left atrial pressure:* approximately
10 mm Hg
**Pyruvate kinase**
*Ultraviolet:* 9 to 22 units/g hemoglobin
*Low substrate assay:* 1.7 to 6.8 units/g
hemoglobin
**Pyruvic acid, blood**
0.08 to 0.16 mEq/liter

**R**
**Radioallergosorbent test**
*Negative:* < 150% of control
**Red blood cell count**
*Men:* 4.5 to 6.2 million/μL venous blood
*Women:* 4.2 to 5.4 million/μL venous
blood
**Red blood cell survival time**
25 to 35 days
**Red blood cells, pleural fluid**
*Transudate:* Few
*Exudate:* Variable
**Red blood cells, urine**
0 to 3 per high-power field

**Red cell indices**
  *MCV:* 84 to 99 fL
  *MCH:* 26 to 32 fL
  *MCHC:* 30 to 36 g/dl
**Respiratory syncytial virus antibodies, serum**
  Negative
**Reticulocyte count**
  0.5% to 2% of total RBC count
**Rheumatoid factor, serum**
  Negative
**Ribonucleoprotein antibodies**
  Negative
**Rubella antibodies, serum**
  Titer of 1:8 or less indicates little or no
  immunity

**S**
**Semen**
  *Volume:* 0.7 to 6.5 ml
  *pH:* 7.3 to 7.9
  *Liquefaction:* 20 minutes
  *Sperm:* 20 million to 150 million/ml
  *Cervical mucus:* ≥ 10 motile sperm per
  high-power field
**Sickle cell test**
  Negative
**Sjögren's antibodies**
  Negative
**Sodium, serum**
  135 to 145 mEq/liter
**Sodium, sweat**
  10 to 30 mEq/liter
**Sodium, urine**
  30 to 280 mEq/24 hours
**Sodium chloride, urine**
  5 to 20 g/24 hours
**Sporotrichosis antibody, serum**
  Normal titers < 1:40

**Synovial fluid**
  *Color:* Colorless to pale yellow
  *Clarity:* Clear
  *Quantity* (in knee): 0.3 to 3.5 ml
  *Viscosity:* 5.7 to 1,160
  *pH:* 7.2 to 7.4
  *Mucin clot:* Good
  *Pa$O_2$:* 40 to 80 mm Hg
  *Pac$O_2$:* 40 to 60 mm Hg

**T**
**T-lymphocyte count**
  1,400 to 2,700/mm$^3$
**$T_3$ resin uptake**
  25% to 35% of radioactive $T_3$ ($T_3$*) binds
  resin
**Terminal deoxynucleotidyl transferase, serum**
  < 2% in bone marrow; undetectable in
  blood
**Testosterone, plasma or serum**
  *Men:* 300 to 1,200 ng/dl
  *Women:* 30 to 95 ng/dl
**Thrombin time, plasma**
  10 to 15 seconds
**Thyroid-stimulating hormone, serum**
  0 to 15 μIU/ml
**Thyroid-stimulating immunoglobulin, serum**
  Negative
**Thyroxine, total, serum**
  5 to 13.5 μg/dl
**Thyroxine-binding globulin, serum**
  *Electrophoresis:* 10 to 26 μg $T_4$ (binding
  capacity)/dl
  *Radioimmunoassay:* 1.3 to 2 ng/dl
**Tolbutamide tolerance**
  Plasma glucose drops to one-half fasting
  level for 30 minutes, recovers in 1½ to
  3 hours
**Transferrin, serum**
  220 to 400 mg/dl

**Triglycerides, serum**
*Males:* 40 to 160 mg/dl
*Females:* 35 to 135 mg/dl
**Triiodothyronine, serum**
90 to 230 ng/dl

# U
**Urea, urine**
*Maximal clearance:* 64 to 99 ml/minute
**Uric acid, serum**
*Men:* 4.3 to 8 mg/dl
*Women:* 2.3 to 6 mg/dl
**Uric acid, synovial fluid**
*Men:* 2 to 8 mg/dl
*Women:* 2 to 6 mg/dl
**Uric acid, urine**
250 to 750 mg/24 hours
**Urinalysis, routine**
*Color:* Straw
*Appearance:* Clear
*Specific gravity:* 1.005 to 1.035
*pH:* 4.5 to 8
*Epithelial cells:* Few
*Casts:* Occasional hyaline casts
*Crystals:* Present
**Urine concentration**
*Specific gravity:* 1.025 to 1.032
*Osmolality:* > 800 mOsm/kg water
**Urine dilution**
*Specific gravity:* < 1.003
*Osmolality:* < 100 mOsm/kg
80% of water excreted in 4 hours
**Urine hydroxyproline, total**
*Adult:* 14 to 45 mg/24 hours
**Urobilinogen, fecal**
50 to 300 mg/24 hours
**Urobilinogen, urine**
*Men:* 0.3 to 2.1 Ehrlich units/2 hours
*Women:* 0.1 to 1.1 Ehrlich units/2 hours

**Uroporphyrin, urine**
*Men:* 0 to 42 µg/24 hours
*Women:* 1 to 22 µg/24 hours
**Uroporphyrinogen I synthase**
≥ 7 nmol/sec/liter

# V
**Vanillylmandelic acid, urine**
0.7 to 6.8 mg/24 hours
**VDRL, cerebrospinal fluid**
Negative
**VDRL, serum**
Negative
**Vitamin A, serum**
30 to 65 µg/dl
**Vitamin $B_1$, urine**
100 to 200 µg/24 hours
**Vitamin $B_2$, urine**
0.9 to 1.3 activity index
**Vitamin $B_6$ (tryptophan), urine**
< 50 µg/24 hours
**Vitamin $B_{12}$, serum**
100 to 700 pg/ml
**Vitamin C, plasma**
≥ 0.3 mg/dl
**Vitamin C, urine**
30 mg/24 hours
**Vitamin $D_3$, serum**
10 to 55 ng/ml

# W
**White blood cell count, blood**
4,100 to 10,900 $10^9$/liter
**White blood cell count, cerebrospinal fluid**
0 to 5/mm³
**White blood cell count, peritoneal fluid**
< 300/µl
**White blood cell count, pleural fluid**
*Transudate:* Few
*Exudate:* Many (may be purulent)

**White blood cell count, synovial fluid**
   0 to 200/μl
**White blood cell count, urine**
   0 to 4 per high-power field
**White blood cell differential, blood**
   *Neutrophils:* 47.6% to 76.8%
   *Lymphocytes:* 16.2% to 43%
   *Monocytes:* 0.6% to 9.6%
   *Eosinophils:* 0.3% to 7%
   *Basophils:* 0.3% to 2%
**White blood cell differential, synovial fluid**
   *Lymphocytes:* 0 to 78/μl
   *Monocytes:* 0 to 71/μl
   *Clasmatocytes:* 0 to 26/μl
   *Polymorphonuclears:* 0 to 25/μl
   *Other phagocytes:* 0 to 21/μl
   *Synovial lining cells:* 0 to 12/μl
**Whole blood clotting time**
   5 to 15 minutes

**Z**
**Zinc, serum**
   70 to 150 μg/dl

# APPENDIX 3: RECOGNIZING COMMON ARRHYTHMIAS

## Sinus arrhythmia

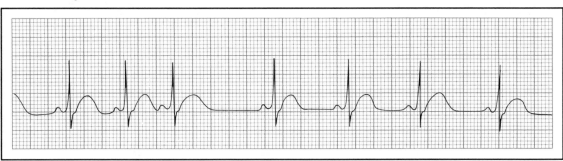

This arrhythmia is a normal variation in sinus rhythm related to the respiratory cycle. Unlike sinus bradycardia or tachycardia, the heart rate remains within normal limits.

A sinus arrhythmia results from vagal tone inhibition and may occur normally in athletes and young adults. Usually, it isn't significant. A marked variation in P-P intervals in an elderly patient may indicate sick sinus syndrome.

### ECG characteristics

• *Rhythm.* *Atrial* rhythm is irregular, corresponding to the respiratory cycle. P-P interval is shorter during inspiration, longer during expiration. The difference between the longest and shortest P-P intervals exceeds 0.12 second.

*Ventricular* rhythm is also irregular, corresponding to the respiratory cycle. R-R interval is shorter during inspiration, longer during expiration. The difference between the longest and shortest R-R intervals exceeds 0.12 second.

• *Rate.* Atrial and ventricular rates are within normal limits (60 to 100 beats/minute). They vary with respiration—faster with inspiration, slower with expiration.

• *P wave.* Normal size and configuration. P wave precedes each QRS complex.

• *PR interval.* May vary slightly within normal limits.

• *QRS complex.* Normal duration and configuration.

• *T wave.* Normal size and configuration.

• *QT interval.* May vary slightly, but usually within normal limits.

### Possible causes

• Reflex vagal tone inhibition related to the normal respiratory cycle

• Underlying conditions that increase vagal tone, such as digitalis glycoside toxicity, increased intracranial pressure, or inferior wall myocardial infarction

## Sinus bradycardia

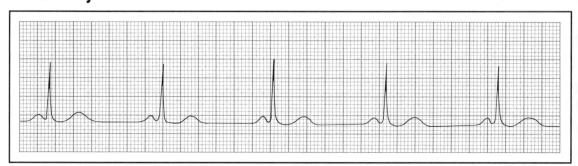

In this arrhythmia, the sinus rate is below 60 beats/minute, and all impulses come from the sinoatrial (SA) node. Its significance depends on the symptoms and the underlying cause. For example, many athletes develop sinus bradycardia because their hearts are well-conditioned and thus can maintain stroke volume with reduced effort. It may also occur during sleep. Sinus bradycardia is the most common arrhythmia seen in patients who have suffered a myocardial infarction (MI), regardless of its location.

### ECG characteristics

• *Rhythm.* Atrial and ventricular rhythms are regular.
• *Rate.* Atrial and ventricular rates are less than 60 beats/minute.
• *P wave.* Normal size and configuration. P wave precedes each QRS complex.
• *PR interval.* Within normal limits and constant.

• *QRS complex.* Normal duration and configuration.
• *T wave.* Normal size and configuration.
• *QT interval.* Within normal limits, but may be prolonged.

### Possible causes

• Hyperkalemia
• Increased intracranial pressure
• Increased vagal tone that accompanies straining at stool, vomiting, intubation, mechanical ventilation, sick sinus syndrome, hypothyroidism, or hard physical exertion
• Possible result of inferior wall MI involving the right coronary artery, which supplies blood to the SA node
• Treatment with beta blockers, sympatholytic drugs, digitalis, morphine, or meperidine (normal sinus rates return when drugs are stopped)

# Sinus tachycardia

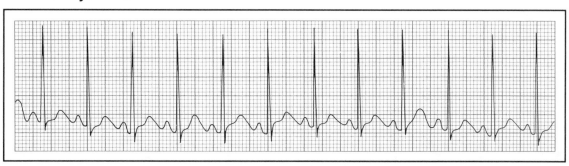

This arrhythmia is an acceleration of the firing of the sinoatrial (SA) node beyond its normal discharge rate, resulting in a heart rate between 100 and 160 beats/minute. Rates greater than 160 beats/minute may indicate an ectopic focus.

Sinus tachycardia commonly occurs in normal, healthy patients with no serious adverse effects. However, persistent sinus tachycardia, especially with acute myocardial infarction (MI), can be serious. It may lead to ischemia and myocardial damage by raising the oxygen requirements.

## ECG characteristics
• **Rhythm.** Atrial and ventricular rhythms are regular.
• **Rate.** Atrial and ventricular rates are greater than 100 beats/minute (usually between 100 and 160).
• **P wave.** Normal size and configuration. P wave precedes each QRS complex.
• **PR interval.** Within normal limits and constant.
• **QRS complex.** Normal duration and configuration.
• **T wave.** Normal size and configuration.
• **QT interval.** Within normal limits, but commonly shortened.

## Possible causes
• Caffeine, nicotine, or alcohol ingestion
• Digitalis glycoside toxicity
• Hypothyroidism or hyperthyroidism
• Normal cardiac response to demand for increased oxygen during fever, stress, pain, dehydration
• Any other occurrence that decreases vagal tone and increases sympathetic tone
• May develop as a normal part of inflammatory response after an MI. In acute MI, may be one of the first signs of congestive heart failure, cardiogenic shock, pulmonary embolism, or infarct extension.
• Treatment with adrenergics, anticholinergics, and some antiarrhythmics

## Sinus arrest

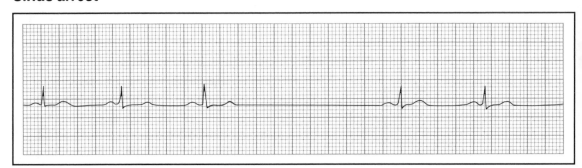

In sinus arrest, the normal sinus rhythm is interrupted by an occasional, prolonged failure of the sinoatrial (SA) node to initiate an impulse. The atria are not stimulated to contract, and an entire P-QRS-T complex will be missing from the ECG strip. Except for this missing complex (or pause), the ECG usually remains normal.

Sinus arrest is not usually significant unless symptoms of decreased cardiac output occur. However, extremely slow rates can give rise to other arrhythmias.

### ECG characteristics
• *Rhythm.* Atrial and ventricular rhythms are regular, except for the missing complex.
• *Rate.* Atrial and ventricular rates are usually within normal limits (60 to 100 beats/minute) but vary because of the pauses.
• *P wave.* Normal size and configuration. P wave precedes each QRS complex but is absent during a pause.
• *PR interval.* Within normal limits and constant when the P wave is present; not measurable when the P wave is absent.
• *QRS complex.* Normal duration and configuration; absent during a pause.

• *T wave.* Normal size and configuration; absent during a pause.
• *QT interval.* Within normal limits; not measurable during a pause.
• *Other.* With sinus arrest, the pause usually isn't equal to a multiple of the previous sinus rhythm. Junctional escape beats may occur with sinus arrest.

### Possible causes
• Acute infection
• Acute inferior wall myocardial infarction
• Cardiac glycoside, quinidine, or salicylate toxicity
• Carotid sinus massage or carotid sinus sensitivity
• Contrast dye
• Coronary artery disease
• Degenerative heart disease
• Pesticide poisoning
• Pharyngeal irritation, such as that caused by endotracheal intubation
• Sick sinus syndrome
• Vagal stimulation (overeating, caffeine, tobacco, or conditions that increase vagal tone)
• Valsalva's maneuver

# Premature atrial contraction

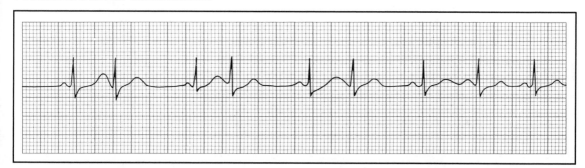

Originating outside the sinoatrial (SA) node, premature atrial contractions (PACs) usually arise from an irritable focus in the atria that supersedes the SA node as pacemaker for one or more beats. PACs can occur in groups of two (bigeminy) and are often followed by a pause as the SA node is reset.

PACs are rarely dangerous in patients free of heart disease. However, they may precipitate a more serious arrhythmia (such as atrial flutter or atrial fibrillation) in patients with heart disease. If PACs occur with an acute myocardial infarction (MI), they may signal congestive heart failure (CHF) or an electrolyte imbalance.

## ECG characteristics

• *Rhythm.* Atrial and ventricular rhythms are irregular as a result of PACs, but the underlying rhythm may be regular.
• *Rate.* Atrial and ventricular rates vary with the underlying rhythm.
• *P wave.* Premature and abnormally shaped; possibly lost in the previous T wave. Often results from increased automaticity caused by a longer refractory period in the SA node.
• *PR interval.* Usually within normal limits, but

may be shortened or slightly prolonged, depending on the origin of the ectopic focus.
• *QRS complex.* Duration and configuration are usually normal because ventricular depolarization and conduction are normal.
• *T wave.* Usually has a normal configuration. However, if the P wave is hidden in the T wave, the T wave may be distorted.
• *QT interval.* Usually within normal limits.
• *Other.* As previously mentioned, PACs can occur in bigeminy. A PAC is usually followed by a pause, which may be noncompensatory, compensatory, or longer than a compensatory pause.

## Possible causes

• Acute respiratory failure, chronic obstructive pulmonary disease, or hypoxia
• CHF
• Coronary and valvular heart disease
• Drugs that prolong the SA node's absolute refractory period such as digitalis, quinidine, and procainamide
• Excessive use of caffeine, tobacco, or alcohol
• Ischemic heart disease
• Stress, fatigue, or overeating

# Atrial tachycardia

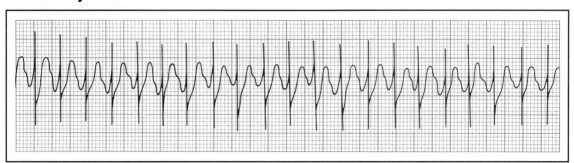

In atrial tachycardia, the atrial rhythm is ectopic, and the atrial rate ranges between 160 and 250 beats/minute. This arrhythmia is benign when it occurs in a healthy person. However, it can be dangerous when it occurs in a patient with an existing cardiac disorder.

### ECG characteristics
• *Rhythm.* Both atrial and ventricular rhythms are regular.
• *Rate.* The atrial rate is characterized by three or more consecutive ectopic atrial beats occurring at a rate between 160 and 250 beats/minute; the rate rarely exceeds 250 beats/minute. The ventricular rate depends on the atrioventricular (AV) conduction ratio.
• *P wave.* Usually positive, the P wave may be aberrant, invisible, or hidden in the previous T wave. If visible, it precedes each QRS complex.
• *PR interval.* May be unmeasurable if the P wave can't be distinguished from the preceding T wave.

• *QRS complex.* Duration and configuration are usually normal.
• *T wave.* Usually can't be distinguished.
• *QT interval.* Usually within normal limits, but may be shorter because of the rapid rate.

### Possible causes
• Digitalis glycoside toxicity (the most common cause)
• Primary cardiac disorders, such as myocardial infarction, congenital heart disease, cardiomyopathy, pericarditis, valvular heart disease, or Wolff-Parkinson-White syndrome
• Secondary cardiac problems, such as hyperthyroidism, cor pulmonale, or systemic hypertension
• Chronic obstructive pulmonary disease
• In healthy persons: physical or psychological stress, hypoxia, hypokalemia, excessive use of caffeine or other stimulants, or use of marijuana

# Paroxysmal atrial tachycardia

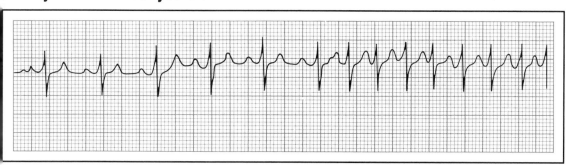

Also called paroxysmal supraventricular tachycardia (PSVT), paroxysmal atrial tachycardia (PAT) arises suddenly. It typically follows frequent premature atrial contractions (PACs), one of which precipitates the tachycardia. This arrhythmia is benign when it occurs in a healthy person, unless the PAT is sustained.

## ECG characteristics

• *Rhythm.* Both atrial and ventricular rhythms may be regular or irregular and start and stop abruptly.

• *Rate.* Atrial and ventricular rates range from 160 to 250 beats/minute.

• *P wave.* Upright, regular, but can be inverted or retrograde. It may not be visible or may be difficult to distinguish from the preceding T wave.

• *PR interval.* May be unmeasurable if the P wave can't be distinguished from the preceding T wave.

• *QRS complex.* Duration and configuration, usually normal, may become aberrant if the arrhythmia persists.

• *T wave.* Usually indistinguishable.

• *QT interval.* Usually shorter because of the rapid rate.

• *Other.* Sudden onset, typically initiated by a PAC.

## Possible causes

• Digitalis glycoside toxicity, commonly indicated by an atrial rate that's exactly twice the ventricular rate

• Primary cardiac disorders, such as myocardial infarction, congenital heart disease, cardiomyopathy, or Wolff-Parkinson-White syndrome

• Secondary cardiac problems, such as hyperthyroidism, cor pulmonale, systemic hypertension, or hypoxemia

• Chronic obstructive pulmonary disease

• In healthy persons: physical or psychological stress, hypoxia, hypokalemia or other electrolyte disturbances, excessive use of caffeine or other stimulants, or use of marijuana

# Atrial flutter

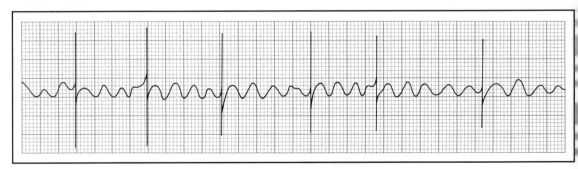

Atrial flutter is characterized by a rapid atrial rate. The rhythm, which originates in one atrial focus, results from circus reentry and possibly from increased automaticity.

The significance of atrial flutter depends on the extent to which the ventricular rate is accelerated. The faster this rate, the more dangerous the arrhythmia. Even a small rise in rate can cause angina, syncope, hypotension, congestive heart failure, or pulmonary edema.

## ECG characteristics
• *Rhythm.* Atrial rhythm is regular. Ventricular rhythm depends on the atrioventricular (AV) conduction pattern; it's often regular, although cycles may alternate. An irregular pattern may herald atrial fibrillation or indicate a block.
• *Rate.* Atrial rate is 250 to 400 beats/minute. Ventricular rate depends on the degree of AV block; usually, it's 60 to 100 beats/minute, but it may accelerate to 125 to 150.
• *P wave.* Saw-toothed, referred to as flutter or F waves.

• *PR interval.* Not measurable.
• *QRS complex.* Duration is usually within normal limits, but the complex may be widened if flutter waves are buried within.
• *T wave.* Not identifiable.
• *QT interval.* Not measurable because T wave can't be identified.
• *Other.* The patient may develop an atrial rhythm that frequently varies between a fibrillatory line and flutter waves. This is called *atrial fib-flutter*; the ventricular response is irregular.

## Possible causes
• Acute or chronic cardiac disorder, mitral or tricuspid valve disorder, cor pulmonale, and intracardiac infection, such as pericarditis
• Transient complication of inferior wall myocardial infarction
• Digoxin toxicity
• Hyperthyroidism
• Alcoholism

# Atrial fibrillation

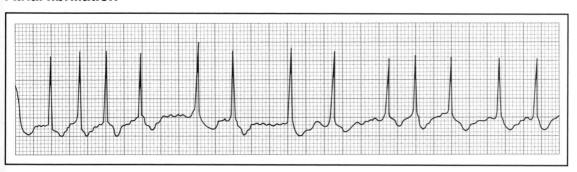

This arrhythmia results from impulses in multiple circus reentry pathways in the atria. These impulses usually fire at a rate of 400 to 600 per minute, causing the atria to quiver instead of contract regularly. The ventricles respond only to impulses that pass through the atrioventricular (AV) node.

Atrial fibrillation eliminates the atrial kick, which accounts for 10% to 20% of normal end-diastolic volume. If the ventricular rate is fast and diastolic filling time is diminished, cardiac output will decline.

If atrial fibrillation goes untreated, the ventricular rate is usually rapid, causing further decline in cardiac output. Congestive heart failure (CHF) and hypotension, as well as cardiogenic shock and myocardial ischemia, may follow.

## ECG characteristics

• *Rhythm.* Both atrial and ventricular rhythms are grossly irregular.
• *Rate.* The atrial rate, almost indiscernible, usually exceeds 400 beats/minute. The ventricular rate usually varies from 100 to 150 beats/minute but can be less than 100.

• *P wave.* Absent. Erratic baseline f (fibrillatory) waves appear instead. These chaotic f waves represent atrial tetanization from rapid atrial depolarizations.
• *PR interval.* Indiscernible.
• *QRS complex.* Duration and configuration are usually normal. If ventricular conduction is aberrant, the QRS complex may be wide and abnormally shaped.
• *T wave.* Indiscernible.
• *QT interval.* Not measurable.
• *Other.* Atrial fib-flutter, a rhythm that frequently varies between a fibrillatory line and flutter waves, may appear.

## Possible causes

• Rheumatic heart disease, valvular disorders (especially mitral stenosis), hypertension, myocardial infarction, coronary artery disease, CHF, cardiomyopathy, and pericarditis
• Thyrotoxicosis
• Chronic obstructive pulmonary disease
• Certain drugs, such as digitalis glycosides
• Occasionally increased sympathetic activity from exercise

## Junctional rhythm

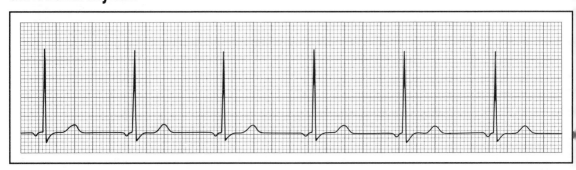

This arrhythmia originates in the atrioventricular (AV) junctional tissue at the rate of the inherent pacemaker—between 40 and 60 beats/minute. Its significance hinges on whether the patient can tolerate a reduced heart rate and lowered cardiac output.

In an accelerated junctional rhythm, the ectopic rhythm originates in the junctional tissue or bundle of His. The impulses control the ventricular rate at 60 to 100 beats/minute, which exceeds the rate of the junctional pacemaker.

### ECG characteristics
•*Rhythm.* Atrial and ventricular rhythms are regular.
•*Rate.* The atrial rate is 40 to 60 beats/minute. The ventricular rate is 40 to 60 beats/minute; however, with an accelerated junctional rhythm, the rate ranges from 60 to 100 beats/minute.
•*P wave.* Usually inverted. It may occur before or after the QRS complex, be hidden in it, or be missing.
•*PR interval.* If the P wave precedes the QRS complex, the PR interval is shortened (less than 0.12 second); otherwise, it can't be measured.
•*QRS complex.* Duration is usually within normal limits, though occasionally it may be prolonged. Configuration usually normal.
•*T wave.* Usually normal configuration.
•*QT interval.* Usually within normal limits.

### Possible causes
Extremely long pauses in the cardiac cycle, resulting from sinoatrial node ischemia, sick sinus syndrome, digitalis glycoside toxicity, and increased vagal tone

# Premature junctional contraction

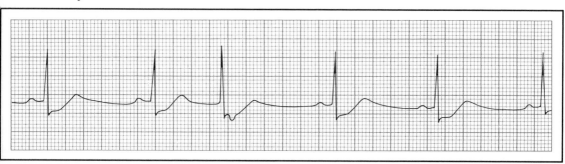

In a premature junctional contraction (PJC), a junctional beat occurs before the next normal sinus beat. Ectopic beats, PJCs commonly result from enhanced automaticity and are unusual in healthy people.

PJCs are generally considered harmless, unless they occur frequently (usually defined as more than six per minute). But frequent PJCs indicate junctional irritability and can precipitate a more dangerous arrhythmia, such as paroxysmal junctional tachycardia.

In patients taking digitalis glycosides, PJCs are a common early sign of toxicity.

## ECG characteristics
• *Rhythm.* Atrial and ventricular rhythms are irregular during PJCs; underlying rhythm may be regular.
• *Rate.* Atrial and ventricular rates follow the underlying rhythm.

• *P wave.* Usually inverted. May occur before or after the QRS complex or be hidden in the QRS complex; may also be absent.
• *PR interval.* If the P wave precedes the QRS complex, the PR interval is shortened (less than 0.12 second); otherwise, it can't be measured.
• *QRS complex.* Duration within normal limits; configuration usually normal.
• *T wave.* Usually normal configuration.
• *QT interval.* Usually within normal limits.
• *Other.* A noncompensatory pause reflectingretrograde atrial conduction commonly accompanies PJCs.

## Possible causes
• Digitalis glycoside toxicity is the most common cause (from enhanced automaticity).
• Excessive caffeine or amphetamine ingestion
• Myocardial infarction or ischemia

# Premature ventricular contractions

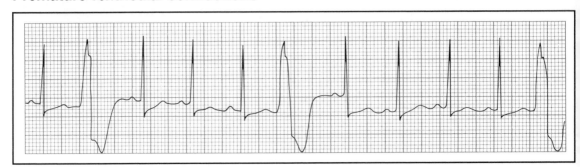

Among the most common arrhythmias, premature ventricular contractions (PVCs) are ectopic beats originating low in the ventricles (usually below the bundle of His) that occur earlier than you'd normally expect. PVCs may occur singly, in pairs, or in threes, and in many cases they are followed by a compensatory pause.

PVCs may be uniform, arising from the same ectopic focus; or they may be multiform, arising from two different ventricular sites or from one site with abnormal conduction.

Generally, PVCs are more serious if they occur in a patient with heart disease. They may be benign in a healthy asymptomatic patient. In an ischemic or damaged heart, PVCs will more likely develop into ventricular tachycardia, flutter, or fibrillation.

## ECG characteristics
• *Rhythm.* Atrial and ventricular rhythms are irregular during PVCs; the underlying rhythm may be regular.
• *Rate.* Atrial and ventricular rates follow the underlying rhythm.
• *P wave.* Absent.
• *PR interval.* Not measurable.

• *QRS complex.* Occurs earlier than expected. Duration exceeds 0.12 second. Bizarre configuration.
• *T wave.* Occurs in direction opposite QRS complex.
• *QT interval.* ot usually measured.
• *Other.* A horizontal baseline, called a compensatory pause, may follow the T wave. A compensatory pause exists if the P-P interval encompassing the PVC has twice the duration of a normal sinus beat's P-P interval. PVCs that don't have compensatory pauses are called interpolated PVCs and occur between two normal cardiac cycles.

## Possible causes
• Caffeine, tobacco, and alcohol ingestion
• Digitalis glycoside toxicity
• Exercise
• Hypocalcemia
• Hypokalemia
• Myocardial irritation by pacemaker electrodes
• Myocardial scarring secondary to myocardial infarction
• Sympathomimetic drugs (for example, epinephrine and isoproterenol)

# Ventricular tachycardia

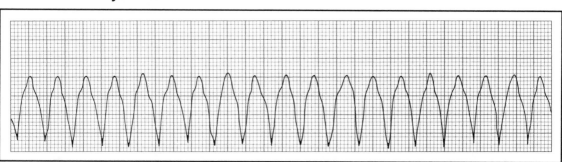

In this life-threatening arrhythmia, more than three premature ventricular contractions (PVCs) occur in succession, at a rate of more than 100 per minute. The arrhythmia may be paroxysmal or sustained. The rapid ventricular rate reduces effective ventricular filling time.

Because atrial and ventricular activity are dissociated, cardiac output may drop sharply. This puts the patient at risk for cardiovascular collapse. Continued ventricular tachycardia may lead to ventricular fibrillation.

## ECG characteristics
• ***Rhythm.*** Atrial rhythm not measurable. Ventricular rhythm usually regular.
• ***Rate.*** Atrial rate can't be measured. Ventricular rate is usually rapid (100 to 200 beats/minute).
• ***P wave.*** Usually absent. May be obscured by and is dissociated from the QRS complex. Retrograde P waves may be present.
• ***PR interval.*** Not measurable.
• ***QRS complex.*** Duration greater than 0.12 second; bizarre appearance, usually with increased amplitude.
• ***T wave.*** Occurs in opposite direction of QRS complex.

• ***QT interval.*** Not measurable.
• ***Other.*** Two other forms of ventricular tachycardia may occur. When the ventricular rate ranges from 150 to 300 beats/minute and the waveform shows a regular up-and-down pattern, the arrhythmia is called ventricular flutter. The other form, torsades de pointes, gets its name from the ECG configuration — the QRS complexes appear to spiral around the isoelectric line. The ventricular rate ranges from 150 to 250 beats/minute.

## Possible causes
• Usually caused by myocardial irritability, precipitated by a PVC in the vulnerable period of ventricular repolarization (R-on-T phenomenon).
• Acute myocardial infarction
• Cardiomyopathy
• Coronary artery disease
• Drug toxicity (digitalis glycoside, procainamide, quinidine, or epinephrine)
• Electrolyte imbalance (such as hypokalemia)
• Heart failure
• Mitral valve prolapse
• Pulmonary embolism
• Rheumatic heart disease

## Torsades de pointes

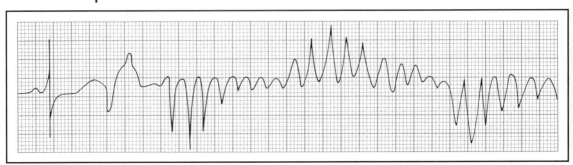

A life-threatening arrhythmia, torsades de pointes is marked by polymorphic ventricular tachycardia (the QRS polarity seems to spiral around the isoelectric line) and a prolonged QT interval. Any condition that causes a prolonged QT interval can also cause torsades de pointes.

Although the sinus rhythm sometimes resumes spontaneously, torsades de pointes usually degenerates to ventricular fibrillation.

### ECG characteristics
• *Rhythm.* Atrial rhythm can't be determined. Ventricular rhythm is regular or irregular.
• *Rate.* Atrial rate can't be determined. Ventricular rate is 150 to 250 beats/minute.
• *P wave.* Not identifiable because it's buried in the QRS complex.
• *PR interval.* Not applicable because P wave can't be identified.
• *QRS complex.* Usually wide with a phasic variation in its electrical polarity, shown by complexes that point downward for several beats and then turn upward for several beats, and vice versa.

• *ST segment.* Not discernible.
• *T wave.* Not discernible.
• *QT interval.* Prolonged (indicating delayed ventricular repolarization) while the patient is in sinus rhythm.
• *Other.* May be paroxysmal, starting and stopping suddenly.

### Possible causes
• Atrioventricular block
• Drug toxicity (particularly quinidine, procainamide, and related antiarrhythmics such as disopyramide)
• Electrolyte imbalance (hypokalemia, hypocalcemia, hypomagnesemia)
• Hereditary Q-T prolongation syndrome
• Myocardial ischemia
• Prinzmetal's angina
• Psychotropic drugs (phenothiazines and tricyclic antidepressants)
• Sinoatrial disease that results in profound bradycardia

# Ventricular fibrillation

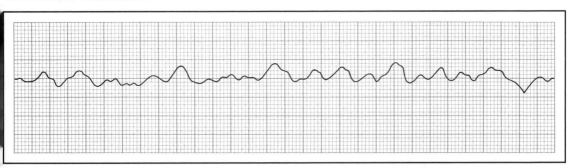

This life-threatening arrhythmia is marked by rapid, disorganized depolarizations of the ventricles and a disruption in the normal flow of electrical impulses through the cardiac conduction system. The ventricles quiver rather than contract. As a result, they fail to pump blood, and cardiac output falls to zero. If fibrillation continues, it eventually leads to ventricular asystole (or standstill), and death quickly follows.

## ECG characteristics
- *Rhythm.* Atrial rhythm is not measurable; ventricular rhythm has no pattern or regularity.
- *Rate.* Atrial and ventricular rates are not measurable.
- *P wave.* Not measurable.
- *PR interval.* Not measurable.
- *QRS complex.* Duration not measurable.
- *T wave.* Not measurable.
- *QT interval.* Not applicable.
- *Other.* Coarse fibrillation indicates more electrical activity in the ventricles than fine fibrillation, and it's easier to convert. The fibrillatory waves become finer as acidosis and hypoxemia develop.

## Possible causes
- Acute myocardial infarction
- Digitalis glycoside (rarely), epinephrine, or quinidine toxicity
- Electric shock
- Electrolyte imbalance (hypokalemia and alkalosis, hyperkalemia, and hypercalcemia)
- Hypothermia
- R-on-T phenomenon
- Untreated ventricular tachycardia

## Idioventricular rhythm

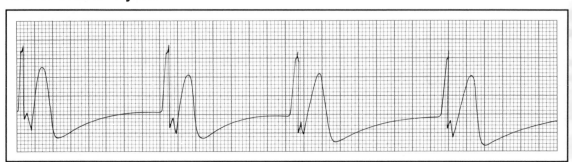

This extremely slow ventricular arrhythmia results when the cells of the His-Purkinje fibers take over as the heart's pacemaker. This occurs when all potential pacemakers above the ventricle fail to discharge or when a block prevents supraventricular impulses from reaching the ventricles. Because the ventricular rate is slow, atrial-ventricular synchrony is lost and no atrial kick occurs.

### ECG characteristics
• *Rhythm.* The atrial rhythm can't usually be determined. The ventricular rhythm is regular.
• *Rate.* The atrial rate can't usually be determined. The ventricular rate is 20 to 40 beats/minute.
• *P wave.* Absent.

• *PR interval.* Can't be measured because of the absent P wave.
• *QRS complex.* Wide and bizarre configuration; duration exceeds 0.12 second.
• *T wave.* Abnormal. Deflection usually occurs in the opposite direction from that of the QRS complex.
• *QT interval.* Usually prolonged.
• *Other.* Idioventricular rhythm commonly occurs with third-degree heart block.

### Possible causes
• Myocardial infarction
• Metabolic imbalances
• Digitalis glycoside toxicity, beta blockers, calcium antagonists, and tricyclic antidepressants

# First-degree AV block

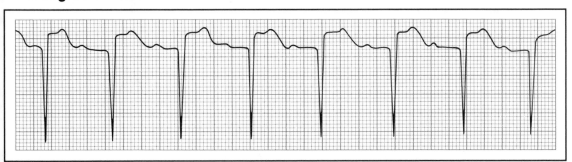

When conduction is normal through the sinoatrial node but delayed at the atrioventricular (AV) node or the His-Purkinje fibers, the AV block is classified as first degree. Depending on the duration of the PR interval, the block may be considered slight, moderate, or severe. The arrhythmia is usually considered clinically insignificant. In some cases, however, it may progress to complete AV block.

## ECG characteristics
• **Rhythm.** Both atrial and ventricular rhythms are regular.
• **Rate.** Both atrial and ventricular rates are the same and within normal limits.
• **P wave.** Normal size and configuration.
• **PR interval.** Prolonged (exceeding 0.2 second) but constant. A PR interval of 0.21 to 0.24 second indicates a slight first-degree AV block; a PR interval of 0.25 to 0.29 second, a moderate first-degree AV block; a PR interval of 0.3 second

or longer, a severe first-degree AV block. Usually, the PR interval doesn't last longer than 0.35 second. (If you see an exceptionally long PR interval, look for hidden P waves. These may indicate a second-degree AV block.)
• **QRS complex.** Duration usually remains within normal limits if the conduction delay occurs in the AV node. If the QRS duration exceeds 0.12 second, the conduction delay may be in the His-Purkinje fibers.
• **T wave.** Normal size and configuration.
• **QT interval.** Usually within normal limits.

## Possible causes
• Drug toxicity, especially digitalis glycoside, quinidine, procainamide, or propranolol
• Chronic degenerative disease of the conduction system or inferior wall myocardial infarction
• Hypokalemia or hyperkalemia
• Hypothermia
• Hypothyroidism

# Type I second-degree AV block

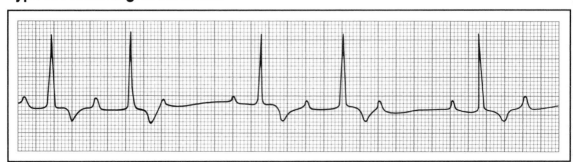

In Type I (Wenckebach or Mobitz I) second-degree atrioventricular (AV) block, diseased tissues in the AV node conduct successive impulses increasingly earlier in the refractory period. After several beats, an impulse arrives during the absolute refractory period, when the tissue can't conduct it. The next impulse arrives during the relative refractory period and is conducted normally. The cycle is then repeated.

Type I second-degree AV block is usually transient. An asymptomatic patient has a good prognosis. But the block may progress to a more serious type.

## ECG characteristics
• *Rhythm.* Atrial rhythm is regular, whereas the ventricular rhythm is irregular. The R-R interval shortens progressively until a P wave appears without a QRS complex. The cycle then repeats.
• *Rate.* The atrial rate exceeds the ventricular rate, but both usually remain within normal limits.
• *P wave.* Normal size and configuration.

• *PR interval.* Progressively, but typically only slightly, longer with each cycle until a P wave appears without a QRS complex. The PR interval after the nonconducted beat is shorter than the interval preceding it.
• *QRS complex.* Duration usually remains within normal limits because the block commonly lies above the bundle of His. The complex may be absent periodically.
• *T wave.* Has a normal size and configuration but its deflection may be opposite that of the QRS complex.
• *QT interval.* Usually within normal limits.
• *Other.* Usually distinguished by group beating, referred to as the footprints of Wenckebach.

## Possible causes
• Inferior wall myocardial infarction, cardiac surgery, electrolyte imbalance, vagal stimulation, and sinus tachycardia
• Digitalis glycoside toxicity and use of propranolol, quinidine, and procainamide

# Type II second-degree AV block

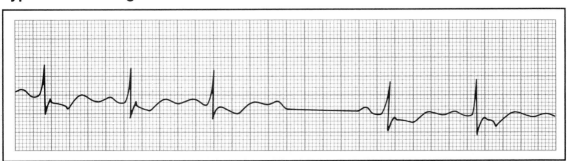

Produced by a conduction disturbance in the His-Purkinje fibers, a Type II (Mobitz II) second-degree atrioventricular (AV) block causes an intermittent conduction delay or block. On the ECG, you won't see any warning before a beat is dropped, as you do with Type I second-degree AV block. In Type II second-degree AV block, the PR and R-R intervals remain constant before the dropped beat. The arrhythmia frequently progresses to third-degree or complete heart block.

## ECG characteristics

• **Rhythm.** The atrial rhythm is regular, but the ventricular rhythm can be regular or irregular. Pauses correspond to the dropped beat. If the block is intermittent, the rhythm is often irregular. If the block stays constant (such as 2:1 or 3:1), the rhythm is regular.

• **Rate.** The atrial rate is usually within normal limits. The ventricular rate, slower than the atrial rate, may be within normal limits.

• **P wave.** Normal size and configuration, but some P waves aren't followed by a QRS complex. The P-P interval containing such a nonconducted P wave equals two normal P-P intervals.

• **PR interval.** Within normal limits or prolonged, but always constant for the conducted beats. The PR interval following a nonconducted beat may be shortened.

• **QRS complex.** Duration is within normal limits if the block occurs at the bundle of His; prolonged if it occurs below the bundle of His. The complex may be absent periodically.

• **T wave.** Usually normal size and configuration.

• **QT interval.** Usually within normal limits.

• **Other.** The PR and R-R intervals don't vary before a dropped beat, so no warning occurs.

## Possible causes

Organic heart disease, such as acute anterior wall myocardial infarction, severe coronary artery disease, acute myocarditis, or calcification of the cardiac conduction system

## Third-degree AV block

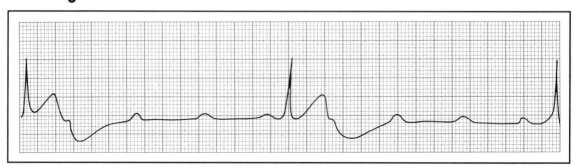

When all supraventricular impulses are prevented from reaching the ventricles, the patient has third-degree atrioventricular (AV) block, also known as complete heart block. Just how significant the block is depends on the patient's response to any decline in ventricular rate and on the stability of the escape rhythm. Junctional escape rhythms are typically stable and may resolve without intervention. Ventricular escape rhythms, however, are slower and less stable and pose the risk for intermittent or permanent ventricular standstill.

### ECG characteristics
• *Rhythm.* Both atrial and ventricular rhythms are regular.
• *Rate.* The atrial rate, which is usually within normal limits, exceeds the ventricular rate. The slow ventricular rate ranges from 25 to 40 beats/minute, but this rate is determined by the block's location and the origin of the subsidiary impulse.

• *P wave.* Normal size and configuration.
• *PR interval.* Not applicable or measurable because the atria and ventricles beat independently (AV dissociation).
• *QRS complex.* Configuration depends on where the ventricular beat originates. A high AV junctional pacemaker produces a narrow QRS complex; a pacemaker in the bundle of His produces a wide QRS complex; a ventricular pacemaker produces a wide, bizarre QRS complex.
• *T wave.* Normal size and configuration.
• *QT interval.* May or may not be within normal limits.

### Possible causes
• *Acute blocks.* Severe digitalis glycoside toxicity, beta blockers or calcium channel blockers, anterior or inferior wall myocardial infarction, cardiac catheterization, and myocarditis caused by Lyme disease

# Ventricular escape beat and rhythm

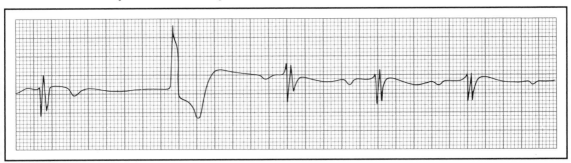

This arrhythmia is marked by a ventricular ectopic beat that occurs after an occasional, prolonged pause in which the supraventricular (SV) pacemakers fail to initiate an impulse. If a series of beats originate in this way, it's called a ventricular escape (idioventricular) rhythm.

Although this arrhythmia is a compensatory mechanism, it's considered serious because the slow rate can seriously reduce cardiac output. Ventricular escape beats indicate that a serious SV problem is present. For example, they're usually found in advanced heart disease.

## ECG characteristics
- **Rhythm.** Atrial and ventricular rhythms are irregular.
- **Rate.** Atrial and ventricular rates are usually between 20 to 40 beats/minute but vary depending on the rate of the underlying rhythm.
- **P wave.** May or may not be identifiable. If identifiable, the P wave may be normal in configuration if the sinoatrial (SA) node is firing, or abnormal in configuration if an alternate SV site is firing. In either case, the impulse generated is not conducted when the escape beat/rhythm occurs.
- **PR interval.** Not measurable.
- **QRS complex.** Altered contour and duration. Duration is wide, being greater than 0.12 second. Altered contour may also vary between escape beats if the ventricular pacemaker shifts its site of origin to other sites within the ventricles.
- **T wave.** T wave configuration and duration may differ from that of the underlying rhythm. In the escape beat/rhythm, T wave deflection is opposite that of the QRS complex.
- **QT interval.** Usually prolonged.
- **Other.** Atrioventricular (AV) block can be present if P waves are present but not conducted.

## Possible causes
- Presence of SA or AV block
- Suppression of SV pacemaker function from the effects of drugs (a digitalis glycoside or quinidine), ischemic process (such as coronary artery disease or myocardial infarction), an acute infection affecting cardiac tissue, or increased vagal tone

# Wandering pacemaker

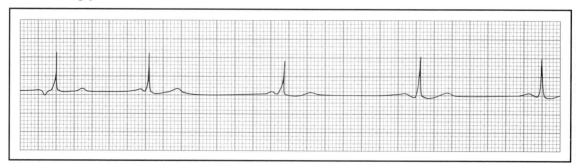

A wandering pacemaker is an atrial arrhythmia in which the site of the impulse shifts. Sometimes beats originate in the sinoatrial node; at other times, they originate in an irritable atrial focus or even in the atrioventricular node. Because of these shifts, the P wave may change shape, direction, or position in the cycle. If the pacemaker site moves to the junctional tissue, the P wave may be imperceptible.

A wandering pacemaker is rarely serious. However, if it's prolonged, it may indicate underlying heart disease. This arrhythmia is common in children, athletes, and elderly people.

## ECG characteristics
• *Rhythm.* Atrial rhythm varies slightly, with an irregular P-P interval. Ventricular rhythm varies slightly, with an irregular R-R interval.
• *Rate.* Atrial and ventricular rates vary but usually are within normal limits or less than 60 beats/minute.

• *P wave.* Changes size and configuration because of the changing pacemaker site. The P wave may also be absent or inverted or may follow the QRS complex. A combination of these variations may appear.
• *PR interval.* Varies. When the P wave is present, the PR interval may be normal or shortened.
• *QRS complex.* Duration usually within normal limits; normal configuration.
• *T wave.* Normal size and configuration.
• *QT interval.* Usually within normal limits, but may vary.

## Possible causes
• Accelerated atrial or junctional rhythm that results from digitalis glycoside toxicity
• Increased vagal tone
• Inflamed or irritated atrial tissue resulting from rheumatic carditis or other organic heart disease
• Pulmonary disease with hypoxemia

# Wolff-Parkinson-White syndrome

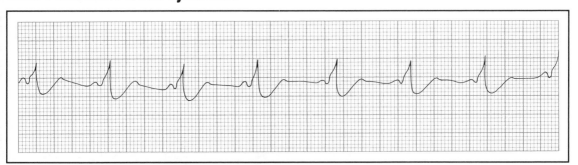

The most common preexcitation syndrome, Wolff-Parkinson-White (WPW) occurs when an anomalous atrial bypass develops outside the atrioventricular (AV) junction (probably in the bundle of Kent), connecting the atria and the ventricles. This pathway can conduct impulses either to the ventricles or to the atria. With retrograde conduction, circus reentry can arise, resulting in a reentrant tachycardia.

Usually, WPW syndrome is considered insignificant if tachycardia doesn't occur or if the patient has no associated cardiac disease. When tachycardia does occur in WPW, decreased cardiac output may develop.

The signs and symptoms of WPW first occur predominantly in young children and in adults ages 20 to 35.

## ECG characteristics

•*Rhythm.* Atrial and ventricular rhythms are regular.

•*Rate.* Atrial and ventricular rates are within normal limits, except when supraventricular tachycardia occurs.

•*P wave.* Normal in size and configuration.

•*PR interval.* Short (less than 0.12 second).

•*QRS complex.* Duration greater than 0.10 second. Beginning of the QRS may be slurred, from premature partial ventricular depolarization via the bypass tract. This slurring produces a delta wave.

•*ST segment.* Usually normal but may go in the direction opposite to the QRS complex.

•*QT interval.* Usually within normal limits.

•*T wave.* Usually normal but may be deflected in the direction opposite to the QRS complex.

•*Other.* The delta wave is the hallmark of WPW. The syndrome may develop abrupt episodes of premature supraventricular tachycardia, atrial fibrillation, and atrial flutter with rate as fast as 300 beats/minute.

## Possible causes

Most likely congenital in origin

# SELECTED REFERENCES

Andrus, C. "Intracranial Pressure: Dynamics and Nursing Management," *Journal of Neuroscience Nursing* 23(2):85-92, April 1991.

Bates, B. *A Guide to Physical Examination and History Taking,* 5th ed. Philadelphia: J.B. Lippincott Co., 1991.

Bavin, T.K. "Nursing Considerations for Patients Requiring Cardiopulmonary Support," *AACN Clinical Issues in Critical Care Nursing* 2(3):500-514, August 1991.

Bobak, I., et al. *Maternity and Gynecologic Care, the Nurse and the Family,* 4th ed. St. Louis: Mosby–Year Book, Inc., 1989.

Braunwald, E. "The Physical Examination," in *Heart Disease: A Textbook of Cardiovascular Medicine,* 4th ed. Edited by Braunwald, E. Philadelphia: W.B. Saunders Co., 1992.

Daily, E.K. "Hemodynamic Monitoring," in *Critical Care Nursing: Clinical Management through the Nursing Process.* Edited by Dolan, J. Philadelphia: F.A. Davis, 1991.

*Danger Signs and Symptoms.* Clinical Skillbuilders Series. Springhouse, Pa.: Springhouse Corp., 1990.

Dickman, C., et al. "Continuous Regional Cerebral Blood Flow Monitoring in Acute Craniocerebral Trauma," *Neurosurgery* 28(3):467-72, March 1991.

Dolan, J. *Critical Care Nursing: Clinical Management through the Nursing Process.* Philadelphia: F.A. Davis Co., 1991.

Gardner, P.E. "Cardiac Output: Theory, Technique, and Troubleshooting," *Critical Care Nursing Clinics of North America* 1(3):577-87, September 1989.

Guyton, A.C. *Textbook of Medical Physiology,* 8th ed. Philadelphia: W.B. Saunders Co., 1991.

Hickey, J. *Clinical Practice of Neurological and Neurosurgical Nursing,* 3rd ed. Philadelphia: J.B. Lippincott Co., 1992.

Holder, C., and Alexander, J. "A New and Improved Guide to I.V. Therapy," *AJN* 90(2):43-47, February 1990.

Ignatavicius, D., and Bayne, M. *Medical Surgical Nursing: A Nursing Process Approach.* Philadelphia: W.B. Saunders Co., 1991.

*Illustrated Manual of Nursing Practice,* 2nd ed. Springhouse, Pa.: Springhouse Corp., 1994.

Jansen, J.R.C., et al. "Reliability of Cardiac Output Measurements by the Thermodilution Method," in *Update in Intensive Care and Emergency Medicine.* Edited by Vincent, J.R. Berlin: Springer-Verlag, 408-441, 1989.

Kee, J.L. *Laboratory and Diagnostic Tests with Nursing Implications,* 3rd edition. East Norwalk, Conn: Appleton & Lange, 1991.

Kersten, L. *Comprehensive Respiratory Nursing: A Decision-Making Approach.* Philadelphia: W.B. Saunders Co., 1989.

Malasanos, L., et al. *Health Assessment,* 4th ed. St. Louis: Mosby–Year Book, Inc., 1990.

Marshall, S.B., et al. *Neuroscience Critical Care: Pathophysiology and Patient Management.* Philadelphia: W.B. Saunders Co., 1990.

*Mastering Advanced Assessment*, Advanced Skills Series. Springhouse, Pa.: Springhouse Corp., 1993.

Methany, N. *Fluid and Electrolyte Balance: Nursing Considerations,* 2nd ed. Philadelphia: J.B. Lippincott Co., 1992.

*Monitoring Critical Functions*, Advanced Skills Series. Springhouse, Pa.: Springhouse Corp., 1993.

*Nursing Procedures.* Springhouse, Pa.: Springhouse Corp., 1992.

Phillips, R., and Feeney, M. *The Cardiac Rhythms: A Systematic Approach to Interpretation,* 3rd ed. Philadelphia: W.B. Saunders Co., 1990.

Scott, J.R. *Danforth's Obstetrics and Gynecology,* 6th ed. Philadelphia: J.B. Lippincott Co., 1990.

Seidel, H., et al. *Mosby's Guide to Physical Examination,* 2nd ed. St. Louis: Mosby–Year Book, Inc., 1991.

Shapiro, B.A., et al. *Clinical Application of Respiratory Care,* 4th ed. St. Louis: Mosby–Year Book, Inc., 1991.

Smith, R.G., and Cleavinger, M. "Current Perspectives on the Use of Circulatory Assist Devices," *AACN Clinical Issues in Critical Care Nursing* 2(3):488-99, August 1991.

Sparks, S., and Taylor, C. *Nursing Diagnosis Reference Manual,* 2nd ed. Springhouse, Pa.: Springhouse Corp., 1993.

Traver, G.A., et al. *Respiratory Care: A Clinical Approach.* Rockville, Md.: Aspen Systems Corp., 1991.

Tucker, S. *Pocket Guide to Fetal Monitoring,* 2nd ed. St. Louis: Mosby–Year Book, Inc., 1992.

Tuman, K.J., et al. "Pitfalls in Interpretation of Pulmonary Artery Catheter Data," *Journal of Cardiothoracic Anesthesia* 3(5):625-41, October 1989.

Vonfrolio, L.G., and Bacon, K. "Abdominal Trauma," *RN* 54(6):30-34, June 1991.

Wardell, T. "Assessing and Managing a Gastric Ulcer," *Nursing91* 21(3):34-42, March 1991.

Wilson, J.D., et al. *Harrison's Principles of Internal Medicine,* 12th ed. New York: McGraw-Hill Book Co., 1991.

# INDEX

i refers to illustration; t refers to table

i refers to illustration; t refers to table

i refers to illustration; t refers to table

i refers to illustration; t refers to table

i refers to illustration; t refers to table

i refers to illustration; t refers to table

i refers to illustration; t refers to table

i refers to illustration; t refers to table